ANNUAL EDITIONS

Nutrition 10/11

Twenty-Second Edition

D1514743

EDITOR

Amy Strickland, MS, RD
University of North Carolina–Greensboro

Amy Strickland is an Academic Professional Instructor and the Director of the Didactic Program in Dietetics at the University of North Carolina at Greensboro. She currently teaches Nutrition Education, Management Practices in Dietetics, Nutrition Assessment, Medical Nutrition Therapy, and Clinical Dietetics. In past semesters she has taught sections of Introductory Nutrition and Food Safety/Sanitation and is a certified ServSafe Instructor/Proctor with the National Restaurant Association. Prior to teaching, she worked for six years as a clinical dietitian, one year as a consultant dietitian, and five years in a biomedical laboratory. In her free time, she takes business courses and by the time this book is published, will have earned her MBA. She is a member of The American Dietetic Association, American Society for Nutrition, American Society for Parenteral and Enteral Nutrition, North Carolina Dietetic Association, and the Greensboro District Dietetic Association.

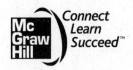

McGraw Hill

Connect
Learn
Succeed™

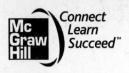

ANNUAL EDITIONS: NUTRITION, TWENTY-SECOND EDITION

Published by McGraw-Hill, a business unit of The McGraw-Hill Companies, Inc., 1221 Avenue
of the Americas, New York, NY 10020. Copyright © 2011 by The McGraw-Hill Companies,
Inc. All rights reserved. Previous edition(s) 2008, 2009, 2010. No part of this publication may be
reproduced or distributed in any form or by any means, or stored in a database or retrieval system,
without the prior written consent of The McGraw-Hill Companies, Inc., including, but not limited
to, in any network or other electronic storage or transmission, or broadcast for distance learning.

Some ancillaries, including electronic and print components, may not be available to customers
outside the United States.

Annual Editions® is a registered trademark of The McGraw-Hill Companies, Inc.

Annual Editions is published by the **Contemporary Learning Series** group within The McGraw-
Hill Higher Education division.

1 2 3 4 5 6 7 8 9 0 WDQ/WDQ 1 0 9 8 7 6 5 4 3 2 1 0

ISBN 978–0–07–351555–7
MHID 0–07–351555–8
ISSN 1055–6990

Managing Editor: *Larry Loeppke*
Developmental Editor: *Debra A. Henricks*
Editorial Coordinator: *Mary Foust*
Editorial Assistant: *Cindy Hedley*
Production Service Assistant: *Rita Hingtgen*
Permissions Coordinator: *DeAnna Dausner*
Senior Marketing Manager: *Julie Keck*
Senior Marketing Communications Specialist: *Mary Klein*
Marketing Coordinator: *Alice Link*
Director Specialized Production: *Faye Schilling*
Senior Project Manager: *Joyce Watters*
Design Specialist: *Margarite Reynolds*
Production Supervisor: *Sue Culbertson*

Compositor: Laserwords Private Limited
Cover Images: Getty Images/Blend Images (inset); Glow Images/Superstock (background)

Library in Congress Cataloging-in-Publication Data
Main entry under title: Annual Editions: Nutrition 2010/2011.
 1. Nutrition—Periodicals I. Strickland, Amy, *comp.* II. Title: Nutrition.
658'.05

Editors/Academic Advisory Board

Members of the Academic Advisory Board are instrumental in the final selection of articles for each edition of ANNUAL EDITIONS. Their review of articles for content, level, and appropriateness provides critical direction to the editors and staff. We think that you will find their careful consideration well reflected in this volume.

ANNUAL EDITIONS: Nutrition 10/11
22nd Edition

EDITOR

Amy Strickland, MS, RD
University of North Carolina–Greensboro

ACADEMIC ADVISORY BOARD MEMBERS

Editors/Academic Advisory Board continued

Preface

In publishing ANNUAL EDITIONS we recognize the enormous role played by the magazines, newspapers, and journals of the public press in providing current, first-rate educational information in a broad spectrum of interest areas. Many of these articles are appropriate for students, researchers, and professionals seeking accurate, current material to help bridge the gap between principles and theories and the real world. These articles, however, become more useful for study when those of lasting value are carefully collected, organized, indexed, and reproduced in a low-cost format, which provides easy and permanent access when the material is needed. That is the role played by ANNUAL EDITIONS.

Since nutrition is an evolving science, *Annual Editions: Nutrition* is updated annually with the latest topics and controversies in the field. Scientists around the world are discovering new substances, new pathways, and new explanations for the health benefits of certain components in healthy foods. In the last 100 years scientists have identified the macronutrients (protein, fat, carbs), the micronutrients (vitamins and minerals), and a new category of substances that improve health called bioactive food components and phytochemicals. Keeping up with all of the nutrition research is a challenging task, but thanks to books like the updated versions of *Annual Editions,* you can easily review the latest nutrition information taken from reputable sources.

The main goal of this anthology is to provide the reader with the most current information by presenting timely nutrition topics based on scientific evidence. *Annual Editions: Nutrition* also presents controversial topics in a balanced and unbiased manner and international perspectives where appropriate. We hope that the reader will develop critical thinking and be empowered to ask questions and to seek answers from credible sources.

Annual Editions: Nutrition 10/11 is composed of seven units that review current knowledge and controversies in the area of nutrition. The first unit describes current trends in the field of nutrition in the United States. Topics in this section cover a few of the initiatives that are contributing to a paradigm shift in how Americans view the food they eat. Also in this section are two articles that discuss the trend of municipalities regulating restaurants to ban trans fats or post nutrition information.

Unit 2 includes seven articles on the function and food sources of nutrients and antioxidants. These articles were chosen for their impressive content as well as the practical tips that can easily be incorporated into the lives of the readers.

Units 3 through 5 include topics that focus on the relationship between nutrition and chronic/degenerative diseases. Recent research findings on the role nutrients and diet play on diabetes, heart disease, cancer, Alzheimer's, and obesity are emphasized. An article on eating disorders is also included due to its increasing prevalence among children, teens, and college students.

Unit 6 covers food safety/technology including information on the growing incidence of bacteria and viruses in our food supply and what the reader can do to prevent contracting foodborne illness.

Finally, Unit 7 focuses on world hunger, nutrition, and sustainability of our food and water supply.

A topic guide will assist the reader in finding other articles on a given subject within this edition. A list of recommended Internet sites are presented to guide the student to the best sources of additional information on a topic.

Annual Editions: Nutrition 10/11 is to be used as a companion to a standard nutrition text so that it may update, expand, or emphasize certain topics that are covered in the text or present totally new topics not covered in a standard text.

Your input is most valuable to improve this anthology, which we update yearly. We would appreciate your comments.

Amy Strickland
Editor

Contents

Preface v

Correlation Guide xiv

Topic Guide xv

Internet References xvii

UNIT 1
Nutrition Trends

Unit Overview xx

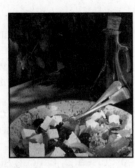

1. **Mission Organic 2010: Healthy People, Healthy Planet,** Carol M.
Bareuther, *Today's Dietitian,* April 2008
The Organic Center was founded in 2002 and has recently launched a campaign
titled Mission Organic 2010, with the goal to expand the sale of **organic foods** in
the American Market from its current 3 percent to 10 percent by 2010. This article
encourages people to buy organic and reminds them of the reasons why it is beneficial for their bodies as well as the earth's well-being. 2

2. **A Burger and Fries (Hold the Trans Fats),** Lindsey Getz, *Today's
Dietitian,* February 2009
Are you one of the average Americans who consumes 4.7 pounds of **trans fats** per
year? If you live in certain cities/states in the United States and avoid eating foods
rich in these fats, you may not be. This article will help you to determine if your
hometown has banned the use of trans fats by restaurants and how to avoid foods
high in trans fats at home. 6

3. **Fast Food: Would You Like 1000 Calories With That?,** Sean Gregory,
Time, June 29, 2009
The next time you go to your favorite restaurant, you may be in for a surprise.
Restaurants are encouraged (and in some areas, mandated) to **post calorie and
saturated fat information** on their menus. It may be cause to change your mind
about ordering your favorite appetizer that could contain close to the RDA for calories and exceed the RDA for saturated fat for three days. 9

4. **Smarter—and Healthier—Supermarket Shopping Made Simple,**
Tufts University Health & Nutrition Letter, September 2006
Beware when you enter your supermarket! Even though the **health claims on
packaged foods** have dramatically increased, consumers need to be educated
and vigilant as to the choices they make. Avoiding the center aisles, demanding
high nutrient density, reading and decoding food labels, and focusing on foods on
the perimeter of the supermarket will help the consumer make wise food choices. 11

5. **Eat Like a Greek,** *Consumer Reports on Health,* August 2009
The Mediterranean diet has been positively linked to lowering the risk of heart
disease, cancer, type 2 diabetes, and dementia. This diet isn't about foods you
should not eat, it's more of a style of eating that can easily be adopted with a little
planning. This easy-to-read article leads the reader through practical steps of how
to incorporate principles of the **Mediterranean lifestyle** into daily life. 14

The concepts in bold italics are developed in the article. For further expansion, please refer to the Topic Guide.

6. **The Slow Food Movement Picks up Speed,** Sharon Palmer, *Today's Dietitian,* November 2005

The slow food movement rose as a reaction to fast food, convenience cuisine, and a fast life pace. Buying **fresh local produce,** remembering the way grandparents cooked, slowing down and enjoying the taste of food, and preserving **traditional foods** and cooking methods is what the slow food movement is all about. A history of the origin of the movement and how it is starting to be introduced into the culinary arts and school wellness programs are discussed.   **16**

7. **Schools Can Taste Good,** Katherine Gigliotti, *State Legislatures,* December 2006

The **Edible Schoolyard Project** was founded by Alice Waters in order to address the hunger and nutrition problems of children in the Berkeley area by creating school gardens and farm-to-school programs. Building partnerships with the school system, state legislature, foundations, local nonprofits, the health community, and businesses helps reach at-risk children, prevents malnutrition, and teaches them healthy eating habits.   **20**

8. **The Potential of Farm-to-College Programs,** Kathleen A. Merrigan and Melissa Bailey, *Nutrition Today,* August 2008

Farm-to-college programs (FTC), in which colleges and universities purchase food directly from farms instead of large distributors, are becoming popular today with the increasing demand for locally grown food. More than 100 colleges and universities in the United States have begun or plan to implement an FTC program. This article uses Tufts University as a model to demonstrate the barriers to FTC's implementation and why it is especially difficult for schools in the Northeast region of the United States to have successful FTC programs.   **22**

9. **Produce to the People,** Constance Matthiessen and Anne Hamersky, *Sierra,* November/December 2006

Poor areas in the United States are being transformed with the creation of **community gardens** that grow fresh produce, offering benefits not only for health but also for food security and new skills for homeless teens. The advantages and benefits of community gardens and farmers' markets to the individual and society are presented.   **27**

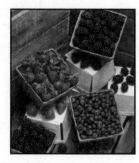

UNIT 2
Nutrients

Unit Overview   **30**

10. **Color Me Healthy: Eating for a Rainbow of Benefits,** Julian Schaeffer, *Today's Dietitian,* November 2008

What color is your diet? The mainstays of the Western diet are predominately beige (breads, crackers, snacks, potatoes, chicken, fries, baked goods, cookies, etc.). People who consume mostly beige foods are missing out on a **variety of nutrients and phytochemicals.** This article explains why it is important to eat a rainbow of natural colors.   **32**

11. **Antioxidants: Fruitful Research and Recommendations,** Pamela Brummit, *Today's Dietitian,* September 2008

Historically, the health benefits of foods has been explained by vitamins, minerals, fiber, protein, and healthy fats. Research on other bioactive food components, such as **phytochemicals** provides yet another aspect to the benefit of eating a variety of plant-based foods. This article reviews the functions of the antioxidants beta carotene, vitamin C, vitamin E, and selenium.   **36**

The concepts in bold italics are developed in the article. For further expansion, please refer to the Topic Guide.

12. **Confusion at the Vitamin Counter: Too Little or Too Much?,** Bonnie Liebman, *Nutrition Action HealthLetter,* November 2007

Forty percent of Americans are taking vitamins, but with the constantly changing scientific evidence on the **effects of vitamins on health and disease,** consumers are confused as to which vitamins and how much to take. Recent evidence on folic acid and selenium caution the use of high amounts of these nutrients especially when certain foods have been fortified with folic acid. On the other hand, scientists are concerned with the population taking too little vitamin D since this vitamin has been shown to be involved in diabetes, cancer, multiple sclerosis, arthritis, and periodontal disease.   **39**

13. **Minerals Matter: The Wrong Amounts Can Harm You,** *Consumer Reports on Health,* June 2006

Misconceptions abound about the **need and use of minerals.** Less than one-third of Americans consume the recommended amounts of calcium, magnesium, or potassium while sodium intakes are skyrocketing. Major food sources for these nutrients are presented.   **44**

14. **Fiber Free-for-All,** *Nutrition Action Health Letter,* July/August 2008

Most Americans are only consuming half of the **recommended levels of fiber** even though there is evidence that fiber is linked to a reduced risk of diabetes, colorectal cancer, and obesity. Now food companies have discovered how to put fiber into many foods that do not normally contain it. The only problem is that isolated fiber may not have the same benefits of intact, **naturally occurring fiber.** This article informs consumers on what they need to know about fiber and where they can find fiber in food in order to reap its benefits.   **47**

15. **The Fairest Fats of Them All (and Those to Avoid),** Sharon Palmer, *Today's Dietitian,* October 2008

If you think that all fats in your diet are bad, then this article is for you. Sharon Palmer walks the reader through the different types of fats, the good and the bad including MUFAs, PUFAs, omega-3s, saturated, trans, and cholesterol. Also included is a list of different oils, their fatty acid make up, and a description of each.   **51**

16. **Omega-3 Madness,** Bonnie Liebman, *Nutrition Action Health Letter,* October 2007

You have no doubt seen the numerous advertisements for **omega-3 fatty acids** on food labels throughout the grocery store. Most labels are misleading, however, and do not differentiate between the beneficial and the not-so-beneficial omega-3 fatty acids. This article provides advice on how to intelligently interpret the abundant claims about omega-3 fatty acids.   **54**

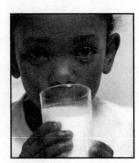

UNIT 3
Diet and Disease

Unit Overview   **56**

17. **Food for Thought: Exploring the Potential of Mindful Eating,** Sharon Palmer, *Environmental Nutrition,* June 1, 2009

Have you ever looked down at an empty plate, bag of chips, or cookies and asked, "Where did it go?" The busy lifestyle of Americans has changed our perception of food. We have desensitized ourselves of the normal homeostatic regulation of hunger cues. **Mindful eating** is a new concept that has proven beneficial in eating disorders treatment, cardiac disease risk, and overweight/obesity.   **58**

18. **Eating Disorders in Childhood: Prevention and Treatment Supports,** Catherine Cook-Cottone, *Childhood Education, Annual Theme,* 2009

The latest estimates of **eating disorders** among Americans is 36 million who suffer from anorexia, bulimia, or binge eating. Although the highest incidences are seen on college campuses, we are seeing increasing incidence of ED among children. This article addresses the types of ED, treatment recommendations, and school-based prevention practices.   **60**

The concepts in bold italics are developed in the article. For further expansion, please refer to the Topic Guide.

19. The Diet-Inflammation Connection, Sharon Palmer, *Today's Dietitian,* November 2007

The popular topic in nutrition these days seems to be the *"anti-inflammatory" diet.* Inflammation has been shown to be a risk factor in cardiovascular disease, obesity, diabetes, and a number of other chronic diseases. There are questions though, as to whether there is enough science to support dietary recommendation of an anti-inflammatory diet. The good news is that the diet makes sense even without the science to back it up—it's a traditionally healthy diet with little risk of harm.   66

20. The Best Diabetes Diet for Optimal Outcomes, Rita Carey, *Today's Dietitian,* August 2009

The American Diabetes Association recommends an individualized approach to meal planning for people with diabetes. This article addresses *several approaches to diets for people with diabetes.* Ms. Carey reviews three styles of diets, high fiber/vegetarian, Mediterranean, and low carbohydrate.   70

21. Diet Does Matter: Nutrition's Role in Cancer Prevention and Treatment, Marie Spano, *Today's Dietitian,* November 2006

Even though a large percentage of the population still views diet and nutrition as a tool for weight gain or loss, nutritionists have documentation on the *relationships between what we eat and cancer prevention and development.* Additionally, supporting the cancer patient nutritionally during cancer treatment leads to fewer side effects and improved outcomes.   73

22. Alzheimer's—The Case for Prevention, Oliver Tickell, *The Ecologist,* March 10, 2007

Alzheimer's disease is costly for both patients and the healthcare industry. It is time to put our wallets away however, because there are many cost-effective, scientifically proven ways to prevent this degenerative disease. A diet high in monounsaturated fats, long-chain omega-3 fatty acids, and antioxidants is just one of the few suggestions Oliver Tickell offers in this article.   77

23. Living Longer: Diet, Donna Jackson Nakazawa, *AARP The Magazine,* September/October 2006

Research has revealed that what we eat not only affects our health but is also a major factor of *longevity.* Researchers discuss the benefits of caloric restriction and the consumption of antioxidant-rich foods that can help add years to our lives.   79

UNIT 4
Obesity and Weight Control

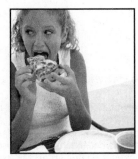

Unit Overview   82

24. Why We Overeat, David Kessler and Bonnie Liebman, *Nutrition Action Health Letter,* July/August 2009

Do you eat when you are not hungry? This article will help you understand why. David Kessler, the Commissioner of the FDA in the 1990s, has devoted his life to improving the health of Americans. This article, a manuscript of an interview, addresses his understanding of *why people overeat.*   84

25. Still Hungry?, Janet Raloff, *Science News,* April 2005

With the discovery of *ghrelin, the "hunger hormone,"* our understanding of individual differences in our ability to lose weight is better understood. This article documents from research the role of gut hormones, especially ghrelin, in obese humans and animals; the source of calories and their effect on gut hormones; and sleep deprivation and its effect on the "hunger" hormone.   88

The concepts in bold italics are developed in the article. For further expansion, please refer to the Topic Guide.

26. **The Health Diet Face-Off,** Christie Aschwanden, *Health Magazine,*
October 2005
This article compares four popular diets in real-life conditions and reports some of
the roadblocks dieters are faced with in order to lose and maintain weight.   **91**

27. **Will Your Child Be Fat?: How to Prevent Obesity—for Babies on Up,**
Jessica Snyder Sachs, *Parenting,* April 2006
The probability of being heavy as an adult depends, among other factors, on the weight
a baby gains before the age of 2. Also, eating and activity patterns learned in childhood
tend to persist over time. This article gives us practical advice on the *nutritional needs
and activity of infants, toddlers, preschoolers, and school kids to prevent obesity.*   **97**

28. **Are We Setting the Stage for Obesity and Poor Oral Health?,**
Terri Lisagor, *Today's Dietitian,* September 2007
This article discusses the many factors that have resulted in our country's *rising
childhood obesity rates and poor dental health.* Lisagor stresses the fact that
childhood is the time we must intervene in order to make positive changes and that
collaboration of parents, healthcare professionals, schools, government, the food
industry, and media is a must in order to deliver a consistent message to children.   **100**

29. **Cancer: How Extra Pounds Boost Your Risk,** Bonnie Liebman,
Nutrition Action Health Letter, September 2007
Researchers have recently observed a *strong association between different
types of cancer and excess weight.* The effects of insulin and estrogens on cancer of the liver, colon, pancreas, kidney, breast, and uterus are presented. Using
the BMI and waist circumference to assess your risk and suggestions to prevent
increase in central obesity are discussed.   **104**

30. **The World Is Fat,** Barry M. Popkin, *Scientific American,* September 2007
Globalization is causing third-world countries to mimic the unhealthy *Western
diet* that contributes to obesity. Sweetened beverages are just one example of
components of the Western diet that have crept into societies around the world.
It is not diet alone, but also the sedentary Western way of life also that has been
adopted by many developing countries. This article presents the need for intervention before it is too late.   **109**

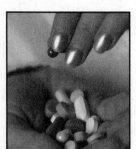

UNIT 5
Health Claims

Unit Overview   **114**

31. **Miscommunicating Science,** Sylvia Rowe and Nick Alexander, *Nutrition
Today,* May/June 2008
With the amount of technology we have in the twenty-first century, the speed of
communicating scientific results is greater than ever before and the possibility of miscommunication is equally as great. This article explains and makes us
aware that even if the scientific protocol, study design, data collection, and analysis
are impeccable, it is still possible to report the findings in a confusing and biased
manner.   **116**

32. **Shaping up the Dietary Supplement Industry,** Sharon Palmer, *Today's
Dietitian,* January 2007
With consumers spending more than 20 billion dollars on dietary supplements in
2004, a good look at the *safety and regulation of the dietary supplement industry*
needs to be taken. Consumer perceptions about supplements, the history of
dietary supplement regulation, and ways to protect the consumers are discussed.   **120**

The concepts in bold italics are developed in the article. For further expansion, please refer to the Topic Guide.

33. Why People Use Vitamin and Mineral Supplements, Elizabeth Sloan, *Nutrition Today,* March/April 2007

The supplement business is experiencing a huge transformation. Consumers are not buying the old single-nutrient supplements but opt for **combinations or condition-specific supplements.** This article reveals why the baby boomer generation is quickly embracing supplements for specific health conditions and why members of generation Y are going for nutrition and sports-performance type supplements.   **124**

34. "Fountain of Youth" Fact and Fantasy, *Tufts University Health & Nutrition Letter,* May 2008

Antioxidant supplements are extremely available in today's world. Most all Americans have a diet available to them that provides sufficient levels of the nutrients they need, but many choose to take supplements instead. This article describes what you really need to know about obtaining your antioxidants from diet alone versus getting them from supplements.   **129**

35. Brain Food, Linda Milo Ohr, *Food Technology,* September 2008

There has been a recent interest in brain health owing to the growing incidence of Alzheimer's and cognitive decline in old age. Because of this, there are several new products related to cognitive function in the market. This article provides information on foods, food components, and other products that are thought to **improve mental health.**   **134**

36. Phytosterols: Mother Nature's Cholesterol Fighters, Jill Weisenberger, *Today's Dietitian,* August 2006

Phytosterols are naturally occurring compounds of plants, which when added to foods are able to lower low-density lipoprotein cholesterol, decreasing the risk of heart disease. The **advantages and disadvantages of consuming phytosterol-fortified foods** are presented, along with practical suggestions on how to incorporate them into your diet.   **137**

37. The Benefits of Flax, *Consumer Reports on Health,* April 2009

Flax seeds are a natural source of fiber, protein, magnesium, and thiamin, but are marketed mostly for their omega-3 fatty acids. This article will address the benefits and possible negative consequences of consuming **flax seed oil supplements** and answer the question "Which is better, fish oil or flax seed oil supplements?"   **141**

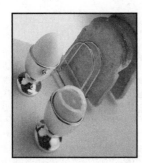

UNIT 6
Food Safety/Technology

Unit Overview   **142**

38. Is Your Food Contaminated?, Mark Fischetti, *Scientific American,* September 2007

New technologies are being developed in order to protect our food supply from bacterial contamination or even intentional contamination. Radio-frequency identification tags are one of the new technologies described in this article. However, widespread adoption of this new equipment will not happen until government regulations are enacted.   **144**

39. Dirty Birds: Even 'Premium' Chickens Harbor Dangerous Bacteria, *Consumer Reports,* January 2007

Controlling Salmonella and Campylobacter bacteria in chickens is of critical importance in preventing food-borne illness caused by chicken consumption independent of organic or conventionally grown practices. The role of the USDA's Food Safety and Inspection Service is explained, and what the consumer can do to prevent bacterial contamination is presented.   **148**

The concepts in bold italics are developed in the article. For further expansion, please refer to the Topic Guide.

40. Fear of Fresh: How to Avoid Food-Borne Illness from Fruits & Vegetables, Bonnie Liebman and Robert Tauxe, *Nutrition Action Health Letter,* December 2006

Dr. Robert Tauxe, at the Centers for Disease Control and Prevention, answers questions about **bacterial outbreaks in fruits and vegetables,** the reasons for food-borne illnesses to be on the rise, antibiotic resistance in humans, and others. Types of bacteria, major symptoms, foods causing outbreaks, and length of illness are tabulated.
152

41. Irradiation of Fresh Fruits and Vegetables, Xuetong Fan, Brendan A. Niemira, and Anuradha Prakash, *Food Technology,* March 2008

Meat products go through thermal treatment to kill bacteria and pathogens before consumption, but fresh fruits and vegetables are not treated and often consumed raw. **Irradiation** could offer a solution to this problem, inactivating the pathogens on fresh produce. This article describes different types of radiation and its positive and negative effects on different characteristics of produce.
157

42. The *E. Coli* Outbreak: Lettuce Learn a Lesson, Sharon Palmer, *Today's Dietitian,* January 2007

Food safety has focused primarily on the processing and handling of raw meat and poultry but after deaths occurred due to **spinach contamination by E.coli,** it necessitated the inclusion of produce farms. The reasons and interrelations among wandering livestock, worker hygiene, irrigation practices, animal husbandry, and feeding practices are explained. Steps taken by food processors and growers to eliminate new outbreaks are described.
163

43. Produce Safety: Back to Basics for Producers and Consumers, *Food Insight,* March/April 2007

Have you ever wondered what you can do to **protect yourself against food-borne illness?** This article informs consumers of steps they can take to reduce their chances and also summarizes what food producers and regulators are doing to protect their customers from harm.
168

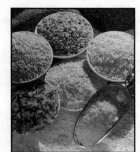

UNIT 7
World Hunger, Nutrition, and Sustainability

Unit Overview
170

44. In Search of Sustainability, Karen Nachay, *Food Technology,* July 2008

In response to consumer demands, food companies are finding ways to improve the **sustainability** of their processing and packaging operations and be more environmentally conscious. From green plants that save energy to reducing or modifying packaging material, this article will tell you how these companies are trying to deal with the problems facing our environment.
173

45. A Question of Sustenance, Gary Stix, *Scientific American,* September 2007

Thanks to globalization, the **Western diet** is now seen all over the world. This article points out that developing countries that are dealing with problems of starvation are simultaneously dealing with problems of obesity. With over-the-counter weight loss drugs and a questionable food guide pyramid, are we really solving the obesity epidemic or just masking the real problem?
178

46. Pushing Beyond the Earth's Limits, Lester R. Brown, *The Futurist,* May/June 2005

A global view of the increasing **demand for food and water** for irrigation and its effects on the shrinking water supplies is discussed by Lester Brown. The effects of **rapid industrialization,** rising incomes, and rising high temperatures signal the need for proactive measures to protect the environment and thus succeed in reaching the World's Food Summit goal of reducing the number of hungry people worldwide.
180

The concepts in bold italics are developed in the article. For further expansion, please refer to the Topic Guide.

47. Draining Our Future: The Growing Shortage of Freshwater,
Lester R. Brown, *The Futurist,* May/June 2008

Water tables all over the world are depleting at an alarming rate. What many people don't realize, though, is that with a shortage of water also comes a shortage of food; water is necessary to raise livestock and grow crops. This article raises awareness, reveals how serious the world's water crisis is, and puts forth ideas on how we can resolve the problem.   **186**

48. 10 Reasons Why Organic Can Feed the World, Ed Hamer and Mark Anslow, *The Ecologist,* January 3, 2008

Organic crops use 25 percent less energy than chemically produced crops, give higher yields, emit less greenhouse gases, and encourage biodiversity, which maintains soil fertility and supports natural pest control. These are just a few of the reasons for us to begin to implement organic farming practices if we are going to be able to feed the growing population.   **192**

Test-Your-Knowledge Form   **196**
Article Rating Form   **197**

The concepts in bold italics are developed in the article. For further expansion, please refer to the Topic Guide.

Correlation Guide

The *Annual Editions* series provides students with convenient, inexpensive access to current, carefully selected articles from the public press. **Annual Editions: Nutrition 10/11** is an easy-to-use reader that presents articles on important topics such as *nutrition trends, obesity and weight control, world hunger and malnutrition,* and many more. For more information on *Annual Editions* and other *McGraw-Hill Contemporary Learning Series* titles, visit www.mhhe.com/cls.

This convenient guide matches the units in **Annual Editions: Nutrition 10/11** with the corresponding chapters in two of our best-selling McGraw-Hill Nutrition textbooks by Schiff and Wardlaw/Smith.

Annual Editions: Nutrition 10/11	Nutrition for Healthy Living, 2/e by Schiff	Contemporary Nutrition, 8/e by Wardlaw/Smith
Unit 1: Nutrition Trends	**Chapter 1:** The Basics of Nutrition **Chapter 2:** Evaluating Nutrition Information **Chapter 3:** Planning Nutritious Diets **Chapter 13:** Nutrition for a Lifetime	**Chapter 1:** What You Eat and Why **Chapter 2:** Guidelines for Designing a Healthy Diet
Unit 2: Nutrients	**Chapter 5:** Carbohydrates **Chapter 6:** Fats and Other Lipids **Chapter 7:** Proteins **Chapter 8:** Vitamins **Chapter 9:** Water and Minerals	**Chapter 4:** Carbohydrates **Chapter 5:** Lipids **Chapter 8:** Vitamins **Chapter 9:** Water and Minerals
Unit 3: Diet and Disease	**Chapter 1:** The Basics of Nutrition **Chapter 5:** Carbohydrates **Chapter 10:** Energy Balance and Weight Control **Chapter 13:** Nutrition for a Lifetime	**Chapter 6:** Proteins **Chapter 7:** Energy Balance and Weight Control **Chapter 15:** Nutrition from Infancy through Adolescence **Chapter 16:** Nutrition during Adulthood
Unit 4: Obesity and Weight Control	**Chapter 10:** Energy Balance and Weight Control	**Chapter 7:** Energy Balance and Weight Control **Chapter 11:** Eating Disorders: Anorexia Nervosa, Bulimia Nervosa, and Other Conditions
Unit 5: Health Claims	**Chapter 1:** The Basics of Nutrition **Chapter 3:** Planning Nutritious Diets **Chapter 8:** Vitamins **Chapter 9:** Water and Minerals	**Chapter 3:** The Human Body: A Nutrition Perspective **Chapter 5:** Lipids **Chapter 8:** Vitamins **Chapter 9:** Water and Minerals
Unit 6: Food Safety/ Technology	**Chapter 12:** Food Safety Concerns	**Chapter 13:** Safety of Food and Water
Unit 7: World Hunger, Nutrition, and Sustainability	**Chapter 1:** The Basics of Nutrition **Chapter 13:** Nutrition for a Lifetime	**Chapter 12:** Undernutrition Throughout the World

Topic Guide

This topic guide suggests how the selections in this book relate to the subjects covered in your course. You may want to use the topics listed on these pages to search the Web more easily.

On the following pages a number of websites have been gathered specifically for this book. They are arranged to reflect the units of this Annual Editions reader. You can link to these sites by going to www.mhhe.com/cls.

All the articles that relate to each topic are listed below the bold-faced term.

Adolescents
- 9. Produce to the People
- 17. Food for Thought: Exploring the Potential of Mindful Eating

Agriculture
- 8. The Potential of Farm-to-College Programs
- 47. Draining Our Future: The Growing Shortage of Freshwater
- 48. 10 Reasons Why Organic Can Feed the World

Alzheimer's disease
- 19. The Diet-Inflammation Connection
- 22. Alzheimer's—The Case for Prevention
- 35. Brain Food

Attitudes/knowledge
- 4. Smarter—and Healthier—Supermarket Shopping Made Simple
- 5. Eat Like a Greek
- 6. The Slow Food Movement Picks up Speed
- 7. Schools Can Taste Good
- 15. The Fairest Fats of Them All (and Those to Avoid)
- 17. Food for Thought: Exploring the Potential of Mindful Eating

Cancer
- 11. Antioxidants: Fruitful Research and Recommendations
- 14. Fiber Free-for-All
- 19. The Diet-Inflammation Connection
- 21. Diet Does Matter: Nutrition's Role in Cancer Prevention and Treatment
- 29. Cancer: How Extra Pounds Boost Your Risk

Carbohydrates
- 20. The Best Diabetes Diet for Optimal Outcomes
- 28. Are We Setting the Stage for Obesity and Poor Oral Health?

Children
- 7. Schools Can Taste Good
- 18. Eating Disorders in Childhood: Prevention and Treatment Supports
- 27. Will Your Child Be Fat?: How to Prevent Obesity— for Babies on Up
- 28. Are We Setting the Stage for Obesity and Poor Oral Health?

Communication
- 3. Fast Food: Would You Like 1000 Calories With That?
- 31. Miscommunicating Science

Controversies
- 3. Fast Food: Would You Like 1000 Calories With That?
- 23. Living Longer: Diet
- 25. Still Hungry?
- 26. The Health Diet Face-Off
- 48. 10 Reasons Why Organic Can Feed the World

Coronary heart disease
- 2. A Burger and Fries (Hold the Trans Fats)
- 5. Eat Like a Greek
- 11. Antioxidants: Fruitful Research and Recommendations
- 15. The Fairest Fats of Them All (and Those to Avoid)

- 17. Food for Thought: Exploring the Potential of Mindful Eating
- 19. The Diet-Inflammation Connection
- 36. Phytosterols: Mother Nature's Cholesterol Fighters

Diet/disease
- 5. Eat Like a Greek
- 10. Color Me Healthy: Eating for a Rainbow of Benefits
- 12. Confusion at the Vitamin Counter: Too Little or Too Much?
- 17. Food for Thought: Exploring the Potential of Mindful Eating
- 19. The Diet-Inflammation Connection
- 20. The Best Diabetes Diet for Optimal Outcomes
- 21. Diet Does Matter: Nutrition's Role in Cancer Prevention and Treatment
- 22. Alzheimer's—The Case for Prevention
- 23. Living Longer: Diet
- 29. Cancer: How Extra Pounds Boost Your Risk

Diabetes
- 5. Eat Like a Greek
- 12. Confusion at the Vitamin Counter: Too Little or Too Much?
- 19. The Diet-Inflammation Connection

Food
- 4. Smarter—and Healthier—Supermarket Shopping Made Simple
- 5. Eat Like a Greek
- 6. The Slow Food Movement Picks up Speed
- 10. Color Me Healthy: Eating for a Rainbow of Benefits
- 15. The Fairest Fats of Them All (and Those to Avoid)

Food safety/technology
- 36. Phytosterols: Mother Nature's Cholesterol Fighters
- 38. Is Your Food Contaminated?
- 39. Dirty Birds: Even 'Premium' Chickens Harbor Dangerous Bacteria
- 40. Fear of Fresh: How to Avoid Food-Borne Illness from Fruits & Vegetables
- 41. Irradiation of Fresh Fruits and Vegetables
- 42. The *E. Coli* Outbreak: Lettuce Learn a Lesson
- 43. Produce Safety: Back to Basics for Producers and Consumers

Food security
- 7. Schools Can Taste Good
- 9. Produce to the People
- 45. A Question of Sustenance
- 47. Draining Our Future: The Growing Shortage of Freshwater

Food supply
- 8. The Potential of Farm-to-College Programs
- 9. Produce to the People
- 44. In Search of Sustainability
- 45. A Question of Sustenance
- 46. Pushing Beyond the Earth's Limits
- 47. Draining Our Future: The Growing Shortage of Freshwater
- 48. 10 Reasons Why Organic Can Feed the World

Functional foods
- 14. Fiber Free-for-All
- 16. Omega-3 Madness
- 35. Brain Food
- 36. Phytosterols: Mother Nature's Cholesterol Fighters

Guidelines

4. Smarter—and Healthier—Supermarket Shopping Made Simple
12. Confusion at the Vitamin Counter: Too Little or Too Much?
13. Minerals Matter: The Wrong Amounts Can Harm You

Hunger

45. A Question of Sustenance
46. Pushing Beyond the Earth's Limits

Minerals

13. Minerals Matter: The Wrong Amounts Can Harm You

Nutritional trends

1. Mission Organic 2010: Healthy People, Healthy Planet
2. A Burger and Fries (Hold the Trans Fats)
3. Fast Food: Would You Like 1000 Calories With That?
4. Smarter—and Healthier—Supermarket Shopping Made Simple
6. The Slow Food Movement Picks up Speed
7. Schools Can Taste Good
8. The Potential of Farm-to-College Programs
28. Are We Setting the Stage for Obesity and Poor Oral Health?

Nutrition claims

16. Omega-3 Madness
34. "Fountain of Youth" Fact and Fantasy
37. The Benefits of Flax

Obesity

3. Fast Food: Would You Like 1000 Calories With That?
14. Fiber Free-for-All
17. Food for Thought: Exploring the Potential of Mindful Eating
19. The Diet-Inflammation Connection
24. Why We Overeat
25. Still Hungry?
26. The Health Diet Face-Off
27. Will Your Child Be Fat?: How to Prevent Obesity— for Babies on Up

28. Are We Setting the Stage for Obesity and Poor Oral Health?
29. Cancer: How Extra Pounds Boost Your Risk
30. The World Is Fat

Organic

1. Mission Organic 2010: Healthy People, Healthy Planet
7. Schools Can Taste Good
8. The Potential of Farm-to-College Programs
48. 10 Reasons Why Organic Can Feed the World

Supplements

12. Confusion at the Vitamin Counter: Too Little or Too Much?
32. Shaping up the Dietary Supplement Industry
33. Why People Use Vitamin and Mineral Supplements
34. "Fountain of Youth" Fact and Fantasy
37. The Benefits of Flax

Nutrition and sustainability

1. Mission Organic 2010: Healthy People, Healthy Planet
7. Schools Can Taste Good
8. The Potential of Farm-to-College Programs
9. Produce to the People
44. In Search of Sustainability
45. A Question of Sustenance
47. Draining Our Future: The Growing Shortage of Freshwater
48. 10 Reasons Why Organic Can Feed the World

Vitamins

10. Color Me Healthy: Eating for a Rainbow of Benefits
11. Antioxidants: Fruitful Research and Recommendations
12. Confusion at the Vitamin Counter: Too Little or Too Much?
33. Why People Use Vitamin and Mineral Supplements

Weight/weight control

3. Fast Food: Would You like 1000 Calories With That?
4. Smarter—and Healthier—Supermarket Shopping Made Simple
17. Food for Thought: Exploring the Potential of Mindful Eating
24. Why We Overeat

Internet References

The following Internet sites have been selected to support the articles found in this reader. These sites were available at the time of publication. However, because websites often change their structure and content, the information listed may no longer be available. We invite you to visit www.mhhe.com/cls for easy access to these sites.

Annual Editions: Nutrition 10/11

General Sources

American Dietetic Association
www.eatright.org

This consumer link to nutrition and health includes resources, news, marketplace, search for a dietician, government information, and a gateway to related sites. The site includes a tip of the day and special features.

The Blonz Guide to Nutrition
www.blonz.com

The categories in this valuable site report news in the fields of nutrition, food science, foods, fitness, and health. There is also a selection of search engines and links.

CSPI: Center for Science in the Public Interest
www.cspinet.org

CSPI is a nonprofit education and advocacy organization that is committed to improving the safety and nutritional quality of our food supply. CSPI publishes the Nutrition Action Health Letter, which has monthly information about food.

Institute of Food Technologists
www.ift.org

This site of the Society for Food Science and Technology is full of important information and news about every aspect of the food products that come to market.

International Food Information Council Foundation (IFIC)
www.FoodInsight.org

IFIC's purpose is to be the link between science and communications by offering the latest scientific information on food safety, nutrition, and health in a form that is understandable and useful for opinion leaders and consumers to access.

U.S. National Institutes of Health (NIH)
www.nih.gov

Consult this site for links to extensive health information and scientific resources. Comprised of 24 separate institutes, centers, and divisions, the NIH is one of eight health agencies of the Public Health Service, which, in turn, is part of the U.S. Department of Health and Human Services.

UNIT 1: Nutrition Trends

Food Guide Pyramid
www.mypyramid.gov

Visit this website and find out your daily needs for kilocalories and for protein intake.

Food Science and Human Nutrition Extension
www.fshn.uiuc.edu

This extensive Iowa State University site links to latest news and reports, consumer publications, food safety information, and many other useful nutrition-related sites.

Mediterranean Diet
www.webmd.com/diet/features/the-mediterranean-diet

Web MD reviews the popular diets of the world. This link reviews the principles and foods of the Mediterranean diet and offers medical explanation of the health benefits.

Organic Food
www.mayoclinic.com/health/organic-food/NU00255

Mayo Clinic addresses whether organic foods are safer and/or more nutritious, reviews the differences between conventional versus organic farming, and the often confusing labels on organic products.

Slow Food International
www.slowfood.com

Slow Food International is the official website of the Slow Food Movement. It can be viewed in nine languages.

Slow Food USA
www.slowfoodusa.org

Slow Food USA provides basic information on the slow food movement in the United States, programs, events, and how you can get involved at the local level.

UNIT 2: Nutrients

Dole 5 a Day: Nutrition, Fruits & Vegetables
www.dole5aday.com

The Dole Food Company, a founding member of the "National 5 A Day for Better Health Program," offers this site to entice children into taking an interest in proper nutrition.

Food and Nutrition Information Center
www.nal.usda.gov/fnic

Use this site to find dietary and nutrition information provided by various USDA agencies and to find links to food and nutrition resources on the Internet.

NutritionalSupplements.com
www.nutritionalsupplements.com

This source provides unbiased information about nutritional supplements and prescription drugs, submitted by consumers with no vested interest in the products.

U.S. National Library of Medicine
www.nlm.nih.gov

This site permits you to search databases and electronic information sources such as MEDLINE, learn about research projects, and keep up on nutrition-related news.

UNIT 3: Diet and Disease

American Cancer Society
www.cancer.org

Open this site and its various links to learn the concerns and lifestyle advice of the American Cancer Society. It provides information on alternative therapies, tobacco, other Web resources, and more.

Internet References

American Heart Association (AHA)

www.americanheart.org

The AHA offers this site to provide the most comprehensive information on heart disease and stroke as well as late-breaking news. The site presents facts on warning signs, a reference guide, and explanations of diseases and treatments.

The Food Allergy and Anaphylaxis Network

www.foodallergy.org

The Food Allergy Network site, which welcomes consumers, health professionals, and reporters, includes product alerts and updates, information about food allergies, daily tips, and links to other sites.

Heinz Infant & Toddler Nutrition

www.heinzbaby.com

An educational section full of nutritional information and mealplanning guides for parents and caregivers as well as articles and reviews by leading pediatricians and nutritionists can be found on this page.

LaLeche League International

www.lalecheleague.org

Important information to mothers who are contemplating breast feeding can be accessed at this website. Links to other sites are also possible.

National Eating Disorders Association

www.nationaleatingdisorders.org

Offers information on the different types of eating disorders, programs, events, research, resources, insurance coverage, and a support line.

UNIT 4: Obesity and Weight Control

American Society of Exercise Physiologists (ASEP)

www.asep.org

The goal of the ASEP is to promote health and physical fitness. This extensive site provides links to publications related to exercise and career opportunities in exercise physiology.

Calorie Control Council

www.caloriecontrol.org

The Calorie Control Council's website offers information on cutting calories, achieving and maintaining healthy weight, and low-calorie, reduced-fat foods and beverages.

Shape Up America!

www.shapeup.org

At the Shape Up America! website you will find the latest information about safe weight management, healthy eating, and physical fitness. Links include Support Center, Cyberkitchen, Media Center, Fitness Center, and BMI Center.

UNIT 5: Health Claims

Federal Trade Commission (FTC): Diet, Health & Fitness

www.ftc.gov/bcp/menus/consumer/health.shtm

This site of the FTC on the Web offers consumer education rules and acts that include a wide range of subjects, from buying exercise equipment to virtual health "treatments."

Food and Drug Administration (FDA)

www.fda.gov/default.htm

The FDA presents this site that addresses products they regulate, current news and hot topics, safety alerts, product approvals, reference data, and general information and directions.

National Council against Health Fraud (NCAHF)

www.ncahf.org

The NCAHF does business as the National Council for Reliable Health Information. At its Web page it offers links to other related sites, including Dr. Terry Polevoy's "Healthwatcher Net."

QuackWatch

www.quackwatch.com

Quackwatch Inc., a nonprofit corporation, provides this guide to examine health fraud. Data for intelligent decision making on health topics are also presented.

UNIT 6: Food Safety/Technology

American Council on Science and Health (ACSH)

www.acsh.org

The ACSH addresses issues that are related to food safety here. In addition, issues on nutrition and fitness, alcohol, diseases, environmental health, medical care, lifestyle, and tobacco may be accessed on this site.

Centers for Disease Control and Prevention (CDC)

www.cdc.gov

The CDC offers this home page, from which you can obtain information about travelers' health, data related to disease control and prevention, and general nutritional and health information, publications, and more.

FDA Center for Food Safety and Applied Nutrition

www.vm.cfsan.fda.gov

It is possible to access everything from this website that you might want to know about food safety and what government agencies are doing to ensure it.

Food Safety Project (FSP)

www.extension.iastate.edu/foodsafety

This site from the Cooperative Extension Service at North Carolina State University has a database designed to promote food safety education via the Internet.

USDA Food Safety and Inspection Service (FSIS)

www.fsis.usda.gov

The FSIS, part of the U.S. Department of Agriculture, is the government agency "responsible for ensuring that the nation's commercial supply of meat, poultry, and egg products is safe, wholesome, and correctly labeled and packaged."

UNIT 7: World Hunger, Nutrition, and Sustainability

Food and Agriculture Organization of the United Nations (FAO)

www.fao.org/economic/ess/food-security-statistics/en/

The FAO is the premier site for information on food production, consumption, deprivation, malnutrition, poverty, and food trade of countries around the globe. The FAO hunger map is a tool that

Internet References

is commonly used to demonstrate the areas of the world that suffer from malnutrition and food insecurity.

Population Reference Bureau
www.prb.org

A key source for global population information, this is a good place to pursue data on nutrition problems worldwide.

World Health Organization (WHO)
www.who.int/en

This home page of the World Health Organization will provide you with links to a wealth of statistical and analytical information about health and nutrition around the world.

UNIT 1

Nutrition Trends

Unit Selections

1. **Mission Organic 2010: Healthy People, Healthy Planet,** Carol M. Bareuther
2. **A Burger and Fries (Hold the Trans Fats),** Lindsey Getz
3. **Fast Food: Would You Like 1000 Calories With That?,** Sean Gregory
4. **Smarter—and Healthier—Supermarket Shopping Made Simple,** *Tufts University Health & Nutrition Letter*
5. **Eat Like a Greek,** *Consumer Reports on Health*
6. **The Slow Food Movement Picks up Speed,** Sharon Palmer
7. **Schools Can Taste Good,** Katherine Gigliotti
8. **The Potential of Farm-to-College Programs,** Kathleen A. Merrigan and Melissa Bailey
9. **Produce to the People,** Constance Matthiessen and Anne Hamersky

Key Points to Consider

- Should restaurants be forced to post nutrition information on their menus? Consider this question from the perspective of a restaurant owner, a politician, and a nutritionist.

- How have restaurants eliminated trans fats from their menus?

- Why are Europeans at lower risk for developing chronic diseases such as heart disease, cancers, and type 2 diabetes?

- Why are trans fats considered a "bad fat"? How can you best avoid trans fats in your diet?

- If you would have participated in an edible school yard project when you were in elementary school, how would this experience have changed your views about food as you grew up?

- Where is the best place for a community garden in your neighborhood or city?

- How can you cut the time you spend in the grocery store, avoid reading food labels, and still buy foods that are good for you?

- Envision a farm-to-college program at your college/university. Would this program work at your college/university? Why or why not? What groups or organizations at your college/university would be in greatest support of such an initiative?

Student Website

www.mhhe.com/cls

Internet References

Food Guide Pyramid
www.mypyramid.gov

Food Science and Human Nutrition Extension
www.fshn.uiuc.edu

Mediterranean Diet
www.webmd.com/diet/features/the-mediterranean-diet

Organic Food
www.mayoclinic.com/health/organic-food/NU00255

Slow Food USA
www.slowfoodusa.org

Slow Food International
www.slowfood.com

The hottest trends in nutrition today revolve around a change in how we view our food. Whether it is due to the downturn in our economy, the Green movement, the realization that our healthcare system is broken, or the growing awareness of the daily operations of the food industry, more emphasis is being put on a simpler, more natural existence. This change in perspective is demonstrated in the Slow Food movement, Edible Schoolyard projects, the Locavore movement to eat locally grown agriculture, farm to college programs, gleaning programs, community gardens, and the return in popularity of local farmers markets. These initiatives are gaining momentum among all demographics, especially with the "let's make a difference" millennial generation. Other recent trends that encourage healthier food choices include recent action by city and state municipalities to ban trans fats in restaurants in some cities and require restaurants to post calorie and saturated fat contents of their foods either on the menu or by the register. Thankfully the current trends are moving away from non-nutritious convenience foods to foods with higher nutrient density and quality.

Consumers are showing increased interest in and demand for organically grown foods. However, there is still conflicting information about the benefits of eating organic foods versus conventionally produced foods. The first article, Mission Organic 2010, attempts to answer the common question, "Why eat organic?" by referring to reviews of scientific literature addressing the topics of pesticides, nutrient content, and environmental impact of eating organically. This article also advises when it is best to buy organic versus conventionally grown products.

The food industry has responded to our growing demand for healthy foods by adding nutrients or other substances to foods, thus creating supermarket shelves full of functional foods. The grocery store can be a confusing and time-intensive endeavor for many consumers trying to eat healthfully. Trends in product development and marketing of healthier versions of convenience foods may mislead consumers. Do you really benefit from all of the added nutrients in the foods that you eat? The Smarter and Healthier Supermarket article offers suggestions for how to navigate through the confusion brought about by mass marketing of health claims in the grocery store.

The Slow Food Movement sets out to change our view of food from our dependence on fast food to a more simple, natural way of eating. The guiding concepts of slow food emphasize quality ingredients, simple preparation, and enhancing the incredible natural flavors of foods. Although it originated in Italy in the late 1980s, this movement is now gaining popularity in the United States. Along the same mindset is the highly touted Mediterranean diet. The Mediterranean diet is widely accepted as a healthy way of eating. This acceptance by the medical community and popular press are encouraging Americans to adopt principles and foods of the Mediterranean lifestyle. The easy-to-read article published in *Consumer Reports on Health* leads the reader through practical steps of how to incorporate the Mediterranean lifestyle into daily life.

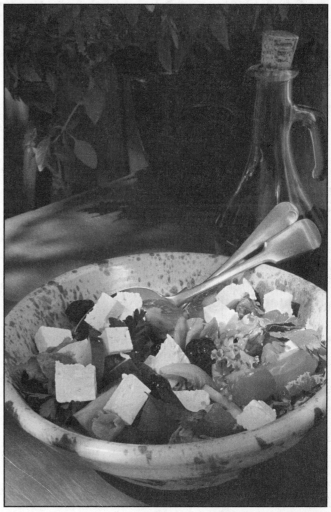

© Jupiterimages/ImageSource

The Edible Schoolyard Project was founded by Alice Waters to prevent malnutrition in at-risk children. It has been a tremendously successful initiative that is enhancing the appreciation and understanding of food by school-aged children across the United States. Edible Schoolyard programs involve creating student-centered school gardens as well as farm-to-school programs.

The premise of eating locally grown, in-season foods, commonly referred to as the Locavore movement, is expanding into higher education through such initiatives as farm-to-college programs. College and University students across the United States are advocating for the purchase of foods that are in season and grown by local farmers. This Locavore movement can be seen in increased use of local farmers markets as well as initiatives such as farm to school programs. This same premise is addressed in one answer to urban food insecurity and lack of accessibility of fresh produce. Community gardens teach homeless teens how to grow fresh produce that offers health benefits and food security.

Mission Organic 2010
Healthy People, Healthy Planet

CAROL M. BAREUTHER, RD

I t's what back-to-earth and Birkenstock-clad consumers have been doing for years. And today, a bushel of compelling and credible scientific evidence suggests that everyone should eat more organically grown and produced foods.

> **"Eating organic is the best way to reduce exposure to toxic agrichemicals, especially in vulnerable populations."**
>
> —Andrew Weil, MD

"Eating organic is the best way to reduce exposure to toxic agrichemicals, especially in vulnerable populations," says Andrew Weil, MD, founder and director of the Program in Integrative Medicine at the University of Arizona in Phoenix and author of 10 books, including *Healthy Aging.* "Of course, there are many other benefits to organic, such as a higher nutrient and antioxidant content in foods and sustainability for the earth."

Mission Organic 2010

In 2002, a group of professionals from many walks of science came together and founded The Organic Center. The group's aim is to collect credible, peer-reviewed scientific information about the benefits of organic farming and to communicate these facts to the public.

Four years after its founding, the center's chief scientist, Charles Benbrook, PhD, the former director of the board on agriculture at the National Academy of Sciences, says, "We knew we had to launch an aggressive communications and education effort in order to get the scientific benefits behind organic out to the masses."

Enter Mission Organic 2010.

Weil, a proponent of the campaign, explains that "the goal of Mission Organic 2010 is to bring organic consumption to 10% of the American market share by 2010. Currently, organic consumption is only about 3%. If it keeps growing at its current pace, it will only be 5% by 2010. In order to get

to the 10%, consumers need to make it happen. It's becoming clear that organic is better both for individuals as well as for the earth. If we can reach 10%, that will be the tipping point persuading farmers, manufacturers, distributors, and stores to convert."

Why Eat Organic?

By definition, organic foods are not treated with synthetic pesticides or fertilizers, and animals raised organically are not given hormones or drugs to promote more rapid growth. Also, genetically modified organisms are not used on any organic farms. As a result, research has indicated that organically produced foods are safer, more nutritious, and earth friendly.

Pesticide Exposure

Scientific evidence backing the need to significantly reduce pesticide levels in the food supply has mounted since the Environmental Protection Agency (EPA) passed the Food Quality Protection Act in 1996. Many believe, however, that progress over the past decade has fallen short. The EPA received a thumbs up for having eliminated most residential uses of organophosphate insecticides, but the agency's efforts to reduce dietary exposures to high-risk organophosphate pesticides received a thumbs down for being few and far between.[1]

This point hit home for Alan Greene, MD, a pediatrician, chairman of the board of The Organic Center, and author of *Raising Baby Green,* when he participated in a study that analyzed the umbilical cord blood of 10 infants born in August and September 2004 in U.S. hospitals. "Of the 287 [industrial] chemicals we detected in umbilical cord blood, we know that 180 cause cancer in humans or animals, 217 are toxic to the brain and nervous system, and 208 cause birth defects or abnormal development in animal tests," according to the study.[2]

Potentially harmful pesticides have also been found in older children, according to results of the study "Dietary Intake and Its Contribution to Longitudinal Organophosphorus Pesticide Exposure in Urban/Suburban Children" published in the

January issue of *Environmental Health Perspectives.* Researchers from the Rollins School of Public Health at Emory University in Atlanta tested the urine of 23 children aged 3 to 11 living in Seattle who consumed only conventional diets except when organic fruits and vegetables were substituted for five-day sampling periods during the summer and fall. Results revealed that urinary metabolite concentrations for target pesticides (malathion and chlorpyrifos) were reduced to nondetectable levels when the children ate organic produce. Interestingly, pesticide levels in the children's urine samples were higher in the winter months when children consumed more imported fruits and vegetables.

This study didn't link pesticide levels to specific fruits and vegetables. However, the Washington, D.C.–headquartered Environmental Working Group has analyzed the results of nearly 51,000 tests for pesticides in domestically grown and imported produce conducted by the USDA and FDA between 2000 and 2005, ranked them, and published the information in its *Shopper's Guide to Pesticides in Produce.* The 10 most contaminated fruits and vegetables were (ranked from most to least): peaches, apples, sweet bell peppers, celery, nectarines, strawberries, cherries, lettuce, imported grapes, and pears. The bottom 10 on this list of 45 items were (ranked from least to most): onions, avocados, frozen sweet corn, pineapples, mangoes, frozen sweet peas, asparagus, kiwi, bananas, and cabbage.

Infants, children, and pregnant women are particularly vulnerable to pesticide exposure because it is at these life stages and ages when critical windows of development occur, some with serious lifelong consequences.

For example, a study published in the October 2007 issue of *Environmental Health Perspectives,* "Maternal Residence Near Agricultural Pesticide Applications and Autism Spectrum Disorders (ASD) Among Children in the California Central Valley," was the first to link children with ASD to mothers who lived near fields treated with pesticides. The study focused on 465 children with ASD born between 1996 and 1998. Maternal pesticide exposures were compared for these children and 6,975 controls (children without ASD living in the same area). Mothers exposed to the organochlorine insecticides dicofol and endosulfan during weeks one through eight of pregnancy (the critical "developmental window" when the central nervous system is first formed) had more than a sixfold higher chance of bearing children with ASD compared with women living away from pesticide applications during pregnancy. The risk of ASD increased with the pounds of pesticides applied near maternal residence and decreased the farther the residence was from fields receiving routine pesticide treatments.

"Endosulfan (Thiodan) remains a widely used insecticide in the U.S. and is found by the USDA in a significant percentage of several fresh fruits and vegetables. It is even more heavily used overseas and often is found in imported foods at levels well above those typically present in domestic produce," says Benbrook.[3]

Other well-documented health risks associated with pesticide exposure include cancer (particularly of the brain and prostate),

birth defects, spontaneous abortion, premature birth, gestational diabetes, insulin resistance, obesity, type 2 diabetes, and neurodevelopmental disorders (learning disabilities). Past childhood, chronic neurodegenerative diseases such as Parkinson's disease and dementia have increased. According to the work of Philip Landrigan, MD, director of Mount Sinai's Center for Children's Health and the Environment in New York, this raises the possibility that pesticide exposures in early life act as triggers of later illness, perhaps by reducing the number of cells in essential regions of the brain to below the level needed to maintain function in the face of advancing age.[4,5]

Nutritious and Delicious

The building blocks of a healthful diet are a variety of nutrient-dense foods. According to a September 2007 report by The Organic Center, "Still No Free Lunch," a large body of research shows that organically grown foods can contain, on average, from a low percent to more than 20% of certain minerals and 30% or more of antioxidants compared with foods grown by conventional agricultural practices.

Researchers at the University of California-Davis were among the most recent to show the superior phytonutrient content of organically grown produce. In the article "Soil Quality From Long-Term Organic Management Nearly Doubles Flavonoids in Organic Tomatoes," published in the July 2007 issue of the *Journal of Agricultural and Food Chemistry,* scientists compared archived dried samples of tomatoes from conventional and organic production systems. Ten-year mean levels of two flavonoids, quercetin and kaempferol aglycones, were 79% and 97% higher, respectively, in organic tomatoes when compared with conventional tomatoes. This is the first study of its kind to demonstrate well-quantified changes in nutrients of tomatoes grown organically over a number of years.

However, Donald G. Davis, Jr, PhD, a former professor at the University of Texas at Austin, showed a well-documented decline in the nutrient content of 43 conventionally grown garden crops over a 50-year period. His landmark article "Changes in USDA Food Composition Data for 43 Garden Crops, 1950 to 1999," published in the December 2004 issue of the *Journal of the American College of Nutrition,* revealed statistically significant declines in six nutrients: protein, calcium, phosphorus, iron, riboflavin, and ascorbic acid.

Davis, in an interview shortly after his work was published, explained: "We concluded that the most likely explanation was changes in cultivated varieties in use today compared to 50 years ago. In the last half century, there have been intensive efforts to breed new varieties that have greater yield, or resistance to pests, or adaptability to different climates. But the dominant effort is for higher yields. Emerging evidence suggests that when you select for yield, crops grow bigger and faster, but they don't necessarily have the ability to make or uptake nutrients at the same, faster rate."

The emphasis on yield and size creates a dilutional effect and plants suffer from a "diabeteslike syndrome," says Benbrook, who first shared this concept via a Webcast for the Institute of Food Technologists on November 29, 2007. "That is, plant crops which are proportionally larger and contain more sugars but fewer nutrients, phytonutrients, and antioxidants. This is a profoundly important new insight. In other words, dietitians should start thinking in a nutrient per calorie basis rather than nutrient per cup or other measure," he says.

The dilutional effect of crops grown by the conventional high-yield system can take a toll on taste. According to The Organic Center's State of Science Review, "Do Organic Fruits and Vegetables Taste Better than Conventional Fruits and Vegetables?" published in December 2006, there have been limited studies published comparing the taste and organoleptic quality of organic and conventional fruits and vegetables such as apples, strawberries, and tomatoes. However, those studies that have been published show that organic produce is often judged to be tastier and more pleasing than conventional produce. This finding appears to be linked to the lower level of nitrates that is usually found in organic produce.

"If organic produce tastes better, consumers will eat more and that's a plus," says Christine McCullum-Gomez, PhD, RD, a Houston-based food and nutrition consultant and member of The Organic Center's Scientific and Technical Advisory Committee.

The nutritional and health benefits of organic also extend to dairy products. Over the last decade, studies from Germany, Italy, and the Netherlands have shown substantially higher levels of conjugated linoleic acid and omega-3 polyunsaturated fatty acid in organic cow's milk compared with conventional milk. Conjugated linoleic acid, a fatty acid found in beef and dairy fats that cannot be produced in the human body, has shown potential anticarcinogenic, antidiabetic, antiobesity, antiatherogenic, and immunomodulatory functions in experimental animals.[6–9]

In August 2007, British scientists reported in the *British Journal of Nutrition* that consumption of organic dairy products was associated with a lower risk of eczema in the first two years of life. This study, "Consumption of Organic Foods and Risk of Atopic Disease During the First 2 Years of Life in the Netherlands," concluded that the mechanism by which organic dairy product consumption may protect against the development of eczema is unknown. "We speculate that a high intake of n-3 fatty acids and/or conjugated linoleic acid from organic dairy products by the child is protective against eczema [independent of atopy] and that also the mother's intake of these fatty acids during pregnancy and lactation contributes to this protection," the authors wrote.

Earth Friendly

There's an urban legend that suggests pesticides are necessary to ensure enough food for the world's population. Ironically, the opposite may be true. In a study published in the June 2007 issue of the *Proceedings of the National Academy of Sciences*, "Pesticides Reduce Symbiotic Efficiency of Nitrogen-Fixing Rhizobia and Host Plants," scientists at the University of Oregon found that a subset of "organochlorine pesticides, agrichemicals, and environmental contaminants induces a symbiotic

---

What Will Increasing U.S. Organic Food Sales to 10% by 2010 Accomplish?

- Eliminate pesticides from 98 million daily U.S. servings of drinking water.
- Ensure 20 million daily servings of milk that are produced without antibiotics or genetically modified growth hormones.
- Ensure 53 million daily servings of pesticide-free fruit and vegetables (enough for 10 million kids to have five daily servings).
- Eliminate the use of growth hormones, genetically engineered drugs and feeds, and 2.5 million pounds of antibiotics used on livestock annually (more than twice the amount of antibiotics used to treat human infections).
- Ensure that 915 million animals are treated more humanely.
- Fight climate change by capturing an additional 6.5 billion pounds of carbon in soil. (That's the equivalent of taking 2 million cars, each averaging 12,000 miles per year, off the road.)
- Eliminate 2.9 billion barrels of imported oil annually (equal to 406,000 Olympic eight-lane competition pools).
- Restore 25,800 square miles of degraded soils to rich, highly productive cropland (an amount of land equal to the size of West Virginia).

Increasing U.S. organic food sales to 10% by 2010 can improve our personal health by:

- Lowering the incidence of neurodevelopmental problems in children, perhaps including attention-deficit/hyperactivity disorder and autism. Abnormal neurodevelopment in children can be caused or worsened by prenatal and early life exposures to pesticides and chemicals that contaminate our food.
- Lowering the number of preterm deliveries each year, which are a leading cause of developmental problems and death in babies.
- Virtually eliminating dietary exposures to insecticides known to be developmental neurotoxins, based on findings reported in two University of Washington studies involving school-age children.
- Reducing unwanted interference with our sex hormones, which should reduce the prevalence of erectile dysfunction, estrogen-related health problems, and the number of people suffering from loss of sexual drive.

Source: The Organic Center.

---

phenotype of inhibited or delayed recruitment of rhizobia bacteria to host plant roots, fewer root nodules produced, lower rates of nitrogenase activity, and a reduction in overall plant yield at time of harvest." Thus, these authors concluded, "The environmental consequences of synthetic chemicals compromising symbiotic nitrogen fixation are increased dependence on synthetic nitrogenous fertilizer, reduced soil fertility, and unsustainable long-term crop yields."

There's an urban legend that suggests pesticides are necessary to ensure enough food for the world's population. Ironically, the opposite may be true.

Furthermore, the paper "Organic Agriculture and Food Security," presented at the International Conference on Organic Agriculture and Food Security in May 2007 in Rome, Italy, states, ". . . organic agriculture has the potential to secure a global food supply, just as conventional agriculture is today, but with reduced environmental impact."

The Bottom Line

Consumers should expand their consumption of organic fresh and processed foods for optimal health. This is especially true for target populations such as infants, children, and pregnant women.

McCullum-Gomez summarizes the following practical suggestions:

- If you can't afford to buy all organic fruits and vegetables, do so for those that are the most contaminated. See the Environmental Working Group's *Shopper's Guide to Pesticides in Produce.*
- Buy in-season, locally grown organic produce, which is often comparable in price to conventional produce. Farmers' markets carry competitively priced organic (and nonorganic) foods. Organic producers are more likely than conventional producers to market their products through farm shops and farmers' markets. To find a farmers' market in your area, visit www .localharvest.org.
- Grow your own organically produced fruits and vegetables. You can freeze and/or can what you harvest for later use (especially in the winter).
- Avoid buying nonorganic imported produce. Organic frozen, canned, and dried fruits make good choices in the winter when there may be a limited selection of domestically grown fresh produce.

Clients who want to learn more about eating organic can register online and download a complimentary Mission Organic

2010 starter kit, which includes information about the program's goal, how to read an organic food label, a pocket guide reference for the 12 most and least contaminated foods, recipes, and a three-point plan outlining how to eat more organics. This plan calls for consumers to purchase one organic food item out of every 10 food items they put in their shopping cart, make one organic meal out of every 10 meals consumed, and ask 10 friends to do the same.

References

1. Benbrook C, Greene A, Landigan P, Lu C. Joint statement on pesticides, infants and children. February 19, 2006. Available at: http://www.organic-center.org/reportfiles/Pesticide_Sym_Joint_Statement.pdf.

2. Environmental Working Group. Body burden: The pollution in newborns. July 14, 2005. Available at: http://archive.ewg .org/reports/bodyburden2/execsumm.php.

3. Greene A, Lu C, Benbrook C, Landrigan P. Successes and lost opportunities to reduce children's exposure to pesticides since the mid-1990s. August 2006. Available at: http://www .organic-center.org/science.pest.php?action=view&report_id=55.

4. Landrigan PJ. Pesticides and polychlorinated biphenyls (PCBs): An analysis of the evidence that impair children's neurobehaviorial development. *Mol Genet Metab.* 2001;73(1):11–17.

5. Landrigan PJ, Sonawane B, Butler RN, et al. Early environmental origins of neurodegenerative disease in later life. *Environ Health Perspect.* 2005;113(9):1230–1233.

6. Jahreis G, Fritsche J, Steinhart H. Conjugated linoleic acid in milk fat: high variation depending on production system. *Nutr Res.* 1997;17(9):1479–1484.

7. Bergamo P, Fedele E, Iannibelli I, Marzillo G. Fat-soluble vitamin contents and fatty acid composition in organic and conventional Italian dairy products. *Food Chem.* 2003;82(4):625–631.

8. Rist L, Mueller A, Barthel C, et al. Influence of organic diet on the amount of conjugated linoleic acids in breast milk of lactating women in the Netherlands. *Br J Nutr.* 2007;97(4):735–743.

9. Adriaansen-Tennekes R, Bloksma J, Huber MAS, et al. Organic products and health. Results of milk research. Publication GVV06. Driebergen, the Netherlands: Louis Bolk Institut; 2005.

CAROL M. BAREUTHER, RD, is a U.S. Virgin Islands-based dietitian and a freelance writer whose articles have appeared in publications such as *Cooking Light, Vegetarian Times, Caribbean Travel and Life,* and *Shape,* as well as in numerous guidebooks. She has also published two books: *Sports Fishing in the Virgin Islands* and *Virgin Islands Cooking.*

A Burger and Fries (Hold the Trans Fats)

Restaurants respond to demand for healthier oils.

Several cities have already put a ban on trans fats. Even if yours isn't one of them, you can still help your patients avoid the danger of these artery-clogging oils.

LINDSEY GETZ

Restaurants across the United States have been slowly making progress toward eliminating trans fats from their menus. Cities such as New York, Philadelphia, and Boston have already placed a ban on the use of these fats in restaurants, while California recently became the first to introduce a statewide ban. It's expected that such bans will continue across the country as consumers begin to recognize the importance of eliminating dangerous trans fats from their diets and demand a change in what restaurants are serving up.

"When California's Gov. Schwarzenegger signed the bill banning trans fats as of January 1, 2010, I think restaurants got the message loud and clear that this change will most likely spread nationwide quickly," suggests Joanne "Dr. Jo" Lichten, PhD, RD, creator of *Dr. Jo's Eat Out & Lose Weight Plan.*

Trans fats are formed when liquid oils are converted into solid fat through hydrogenation. Consuming trans fats can lead to heart disease by raising LDL cholesterol and simultaneously lowering HDL cholesterol. A study published in *The New England Journal of Medicine* in 2006 estimated that approximately 228,000 coronary heart disease occurrences could be avoided by reducing trans fat consumption or eliminating these fats from the American diet. Unfortunately, many popular foods contain them, and many Americans consume these foods in excess. The FDA estimates that the average American consumes approximately 4.7 pounds of trans fats every year.

Trans fats are especially common in baked goods, as they aid with preservation. "I tell my clients that trans fats are essentially a man-made fat," says Sara Shama, RD, director of nutrition for Kingley Health in New Jersey. "It helps Twinkies stay on the shelf for six years without going bad. Baked goods are supposed to go bad!"

Stephanie Dean, RD, LD, coauthor of the book *Fit to Serve,* adds, "While trans fats were created to increase the shelf life of foods, consumers can increase their own 'shelf life' by eliminating trans fats from their diets."

A Change for the Better

Fortunately, many restaurants and chains across the country are making changes—even if they aren't located in a city with a ban. The Cheesecake Factory was one of the leaders pioneering these changes in the industry. "Nearly two years ago, our management team and kitchen staff began partnering with our foodservice manufacturers to work toward the elimination of trans fats from our menu," says Mark Mears, senior vice president and chief of marketing for the company.

The restaurants of Passion Food Hospitality, including DC Coast, TenPenh, Ceiba, and Acadiana, located in Washington, D.C., decided to seek alternatives to trans fats about two years ago. Since losing 125 pounds, chef/owner Jeff Tunks decided to prepare his light dishes even lighter and healthier by eliminating trans fats. "I am the first to admit I would eat a fried shrimp po'boy every day if I could," he says. "But when I take that first bite, it surely sets me at ease to know there is not trans fat in the oil."

Fast-food restaurants, which are one of the biggest culprits of foods high in trans fats, have been quick to follow. Chains such as Burger King, McDonald's, and Hardee's have announced a switch to zero trans fat oils for their cooking. Subway, a chain that had very little trans fats in its food in the first place, has completely eliminated it from its core menu as well. "We always look for ways to improve our products," says Les Winograd, a Subway spokesman. "We have a reputation for offering healthy alternatives to traditional, fatty fast foods. Eliminating even the small amount of trans fats we had was just another way of improving."

Even hotels are recognizing the importance of switching to a healthier alternative. Last year, Carlson Hotels Worldwide announced plans to eliminate shortening containing trans fats at the majority of its hotels. The Radisson Fort McDowell Resort & Casino in Scottsdale, Ariz., was one of the hotels that participated in the pilot program. The resort's restaurant, the Ahnala Mesquite Room, successfully eliminated trans fats from its menu in October 2006 and found that guests actually preferred the flavor of its healthier alternatives and appreciated the restaurant's effort to emphasize good health.

Many restaurants have reported no change in taste after switching to a healthier alternative. Of course, each restaurant has its own alternative formula. McDonald's, for instance, uses a canola oil cooking blend for its fried items, such as French fries, chicken, and its Filet-O-Fish sandwiches. The Cheesecake Factory reports using a blend of olive and canola oils to replace the oils previously used for cooking. "In making the switch to trans fat-free cooking oils, our guests have reported no discernable taste differences to our unique menu items," says Mears, who adds that the switch has not affected menu pricing.

The public has responded positively to increased healthy options—especially those with no trans fat. "Our customers rave about the freshness and selection of ingredients," says Thomas DuBois, CEO and founder of Tomato Tamoto, a new made-to-order salad bar restaurant that recently opened in Plano, Tex.

Of course, that's not to say there haven't been any complaints since these bans first took effect. Much of the initial resistance was due to the high cost of trans fat-free oils, says Lichten. "But as more and more restaurants switch over, this has increased the availability from the oil companies," she adds. "Many restaurants have found that the trans fat-free oils are the same price or even lower."

Some in the restaurant industry have also complained that it's not the government or any other agency's place to ban these fats. Dan Fleshler, a spokesman for the National Restaurant Association, was quoted in 2006 (when New York City's Board of Health voted to make it the nation's first city to ban trans fats) as saying, "We don't think that a municipal health agency has any business banning a product that the Food and Drug Administration has already approved."

However, most restaurants have willingly complied—or even made changes without being placed under a ban—and the general public has been happy with the changes. And dietitians surely agree it's been a change for the better. "Even though it's each person's individual right to choose what they want to consume, as a nation, I believe we should be looking out for the well-being of our people," says Shama. "Everyone's lives are busy and everyone is on the go, and there are times they have to rely on fast or convenient foods. They should be comforted in knowing that whatever they do pick up is something that's not going to give them heart disease because of having trans fats. We have to give people choice, but we still need to look out for their best interest."

Helping Your Patients

Regardless of whether your city has a ban, there seems to be a lot of confusion surrounding trans fats, especially since it's become such a hot news item in the last couple of years. Shama says her patients ask her many questions, but she tries to make it simple. "I call them the artery-clogging, heart disease-causing fats," she says. "That makes it pretty clear."

Elaine Pelc, RD, LDN, of Baltimore, gives patients a visual picture to help them get the point. "I tell my patients to think about what bacon grease does when it cools: It solidifies," she

explains. "I tell them that trans fats do the same thing in your arteries. And when they solidify, they clog up the arteries."

Dietitians can help their patients make wiser choices when dining out, regardless of whether they reside in a city with a trans fat ban. Shama tells clients to check up on places where they plan to eat. "If they know where they're going to eat, they can look up the menu online," she says. "If they take the time to check out the menu beforehand and get a sense of what some of the healthier options are, they'll be less likely to opt for the colossal cheese-burger with fries."

"There are no health benefits of trans fats, and no level is considered to be safe," adds Janel Ovrut, MS, RD, LDN, who is based in Boston. "I tell my clients that when it comes to how much trans fats are in their diet, they should stick to zero."

Ovrut says that Boston's ban on trans fats has taken the guesswork out of which restaurant foods contain them. "Now we can all rest assured that the answer is 'none,'" she says. "I think that Boston residents take pride in the fact that we're part of a health initiative that will hopefully guide other cities and towns to make the same changes. The ban has also created more buzz about the harmful effects of trans fats, and consumers are starting to realize the negative impact after a unanimous vote that forbid trans fats from dining establishments. Consumers take notice and are hopefully making changes in their at-home eating habits as well."

Consumer habits are certainly an issue. Even if people live in an area where a ban is in place, they still may be consuming trans fats at home. That's why it's important to help clients be more proactive about their nutrition, not only when dining out but also when purchasing groceries.

"I advise my clients to read the ingredient list on foods," says Ovrut. "Just because a package says 'zero trans fats' per serving doesn't mean the product is completely void of partially hydrogenated oil. Products can be promoted as trans fat free as long as there is less than 0.5 grams per serving. But once you consume more than one serving of a product—which is easy to do with packaged snacks or baked goods—you're creeping up toward 1 gram or more of trans fats. Some food manufacturers are even decreasing the listed serving size of their product so that it meets the trans fat-free guidelines. Consumers are hungry for more and often eat double or triple the serving size."

However, as a result of consumers' interest in trans fat-free products, some manufacturers—just like many restaurants—have decided to eliminate it, says Lichten. "But remember, trans fat free still does not mean fewer calories. Most trans fat-free products have exactly the same amount of fat and calories as the original," she notes.

A Balanced Diet

Even without reading the ingredient list, patients can have a good idea of which foods might contain trans fat. These include premade desserts, butter spreads, convenience foods, and fried items, says Dean. These are the types of foods that clients should avoid in general.

They also tend to be the products that have a long list of ingredients, adds Stella Lucia Volpe, PhD, RD, LDN, FACSM, an associate professor and the Miriam Stirl Term Endowed Chair of Nutrition at the University of Pennsylvania School of Nursing in Philadelphia. "If you look at a packaged product and it has an extremely long list of ingredients, chances are it's probably not very good for you and may contain trans fats," she explains. "I advise clients to try to make pure food choices. Natural, unprocessed foods like lean meat, fish, fruits, or vegetables are always the best option."

While the increased awareness surrounding the dangers of trans fat has been wonderful, one potential problem with the focus on switching to "healthier alternatives" is that consumers may start to believe that certain foods are healthy just because they don't have trans fat. With or without trans fats, French fries are not a healthy choice. Clients need to know that trans fat-free items may be better for you than those with the dangerous fat, but they still aren't necessarily healthy. "It's important to make healthy choices in general," says Pelc. "People should be limiting their intake of these foods anyway in order to maintain a healthy lifestyle. Choosing trans fat-free foods does not mean that you are choosing healthy foods. It's important for clients to remember that removing trans fat from a food does not necessarily make it a healthy choice."

Most restaurants have willingly complied—or even made changes without being placed under a ban—and the general public has been happy with the changes.

"Just because it says they have zero trans fat still doesn't mean those potato chips or French fries were the best option on the menu," adds Volpe. "I typically try to work on portion control with my clients. If they really love something like potato chips and won't give them up, we can at least work on limiting their portion."

The bottom line? Getting clients to eat a healthy, well-balanced diet may not happen overnight, but helping them eliminate or even simply cut down on trans fat is definitely a step in the right direction.

LINDSEY GETZ is a freelance writer based in Royersford, Pa.

Fast Food: Would You Like 1000 Calories With That?

The Senate wants to make chains post this info front and center, but will that make us eat less?

SEAN GREGORY

How sloppy is that triple whopper with cheese? It has 1,250 calories, or 62.5% of the recommended 2,000-calories-per-day diet. The Fried Macaroni and Cheese from the Cheesecake Factory? Try 1,570 calories—according to health experts, you're better off eating a stick of butter.

If public-health advocates, and now the Senate, get their way, when you look at a menu from a chain restaurant, those calorie counts will be staring you down. "Order me if you dare," the mighty Quesadilla Burger from Applebee's (1,440 calories) may entreat. Spurred by the passage of a slew of state and local menu-labeling laws, on June 10 the Senate reached a bipartisan agreement to include a federal menu-labeling law as part of comprehensive health-care reform. Of course, who knows when that hornet's nest will come up for a vote. But in the meantime, health proponents are likening the Senate provision to legal requirements for a clothing label—i.e., what it's made of. "Isn't information that can help you avoid obesity and diabetes as important as knowing how to wash your blouse?" says Margot Wootan, director of nutrition policy for the non-partisan Center for Science in the Public Interest.

Until recently, the restaurant industry had been pushing a federal bill that would require chains with 20 or more restaurants nationwide to post calorie information somewhere near the point of purchase but not on the menu itself. The industry claimed menu postings would be a costly logistical burden and would clutter valuable real estate on the menus. Not surprisingly, chains won't voice the most obvious argument against high-profile calorie counts. "They're concerned that consumers will be turned off by what they see," says Tom Forte, restaurant analyst at the Telsey Advisory Group, a consulting firm.

In the end, the industry backed the Senate's on-the-menu provision in an effort to pre-empt a patchwork of state and local statutes (13 have passed, and 30 or so more have been introduced). Such legislation would prevent a municipality from requiring both calories and, say, saturated fat to be tallied on menus. (The fried macaroni and cheese at the Cheesecake

---

Stealth (Calorie) Bombers. Tasty? Yes. But Would Full Disclosure Steer Us Away?

1,440 CALORIES QUESADILLA BURGER

A signature item at **Applebee's,** this bacon cheese-burger comes with 4,410 mg of sodium, nearly twice the recommended daily limit

2,140 CALORIES AUSSIE CHEESE FRIES

Yes, it's meant to be shared, but this **Outback Steak-house** appetizer has more calories than you should eat all day

980 CALORIES OREO SUNDAE SHAKE

Order a medium with strawberry ice cream, and **Burger King** will serve up 21 g of saturated fat (more than a day's worth)

700 CALORIES CHICKEN BOWL

Surprise! This **KFC** ensemble has only a third of the rec-ommended daily calories

Sources: Nutrition Action Healthletter; Outback Steakhouse; BurgerKing.com; KFC.com; USDA.

Factory has a staggering 69 grams of saturated fat—more than you should eat in 3½ days.)

As the menu-labeling momentum keeps surging, will such policy really improve eating habits? Well, it can do no worse than what's out there. In a study published in the May issue of the *American Journal of Public Health,* researchers observed 4,311 patrons of McDonald's, Burger King, Starbucks and Au Bon Pain to see if they accessed in-store nutrition data. The info was not on the menu board but in a pamphlet, on a wall poster or an on-site computer. Only six, or 0.1%, of the patrons looked at the numbers. Sure, a few more may have already studied the information. But six out of 4,311? If restaurants are sincere about health, they need to put calorie counts on the menu, straight in the customers' sight lines.

So far, mandatory on-the-menu calorie counts have been implemented in only three localities: Washington's King County (which includes Seattle), New York City and Westchester County, a suburb of New York. And since none of these provisions have been in place for more than a year, nutritionists have yet to gather empirical proof that they work. But some science suggests that prominently displayed calorie counts steer purchases. In 2007, researchers in New York City examined consumer eating habits at Subway, which voluntarily posted calorie info in its stores. This study, also published in the *American Journal of Public Health,* reported that Subway patrons who pondered the calorie information purchased 52 fewer calories than those who didn't. Further, according to a survey conducted in February by Technomic, a food-industry consultancy, 82% of New York City residents said the new highly visible nutrition information has affected their ordering. Of those people, 71% said they sought out lower-calorie options, and 51% said they no longer ordered certain items.

While such statistics are promising, menu counts are no silver bullet. Martin Lindstrom, the noted consumer psychologist and author of *Buyology: Truths and Lies About Why We Buy,* fears that consumers will tune out the numbers long term. "Eventually, calorie counts will just be wallpaper," he says.

82% of New Yorkers said the new in-your-face nutrition data have affected their ordering.

But forced disclosure could lead more restaurants to change their offerings. A report by New York City health officials noted that since menu-labeling went into effect last summer, some chains have lowered the calorie counts on certain items. For example, in March 2007, a Chicken Club sandwich at Wendy's was listed as being 650 calories. In June 2008, as the New York law kicked in, the item was 540 calories—a 17% drop. (Wendy's used a lower-calorie mayo to reduce the count, but a spokesman insists menu-labeling played no part in the move. Call it a happy coincidence.)

Meanwhile, Yum! Brands, parent company of Kentucky Fried Chicken, Pizza Hut and Taco Bell, has promised to post calorie information on its menus by January 2011. If the creator of KFC's Famous Bowls—fried chicken, mashed potatoes, corn, gravy and shredded cheese packed together for your gut-busting pleasure—volunteers to share these numbers, what excuse can other chains claim for not following suit, particularly if Washington lags in forcing them to do so? The writing is on the wall. And perhaps, as a result, fewer calories will be in your stomach.

Smarter—and Healthier—Supermarket Shopping Made Simple

With all the health claims on packaged goods these days and the countless news stories about "super foods," it would be easy to start thinking of your local supermarket as a sort of annex to your doctor's office. Just fill up your cart with "100% Whole Grain Goodness" and "Cholesterol-Fighting Power!" and you can skip that trip to the drugstore, right?

Well, not exactly. While you can find plenty of nutritious foods at your neighborhood supermarket, most grocery stores don't make it easy. Many packaged-goods health claims are confusing or misleading, and may paper over products that are also packed with sugar or sodium. And since supermarkets are designed to make you spend money, after all, your grocery cart's path of least resistance is more likely to lead to soda pop than to broccoli.

Marion Nestle, PhD, MPH, a professor of nutrition, food studies and public health at New York University, recently spent a year studying America's supermarkets, armed with a notebook and calculator, to research her new book, *What to Eat: An Aisle-by-Aisle Guide to Savvy Food Choices and Good Eating* (North Point Press, $30). As she's been interviewed to promote her book, Nestle regularly makes the point that supermarkets want customers to spend as much time as possible wandering their aisles. The more products you see, the more you are likely to buy.

But supermarkets don't necessarily give prominent placement to the healthiest foods, Nestle adds: "Products in the best locations—eye level, ends of aisles, cash registers—sell best. So companies pay the supermarkets to slot their products in prime real estate. These products are mostly junk because they are the most profitable and most heavily advertised."

Food companies spend $12 billion a year on direct media advertising, according to Nestle. Kellogg spends $32 million annually just on advertising its Cheez-Its snack crackers. For every dollar spent on ads, companies spend another two on trade shows, couponing and other promotions.

A typical 48,000-square-foot supermarket might contain 50,000 different items for sale. On average, a quarter of that store space is devoted to products that have added sugar, Nestle says.

In a *Washington Post* interview, Nestle recounted one of her supermarket research trips: "I was in an enormous one in Los Angeles. I couldn't help noticing that soft drinks were everywhere—a wall of them when you first walk in the store.

Making a List

To make your own grocery list of foods certified as heart-healthy by the American Heart Association, go online to checkmark.heart.org. You can build your list searching by manufacturer or food category. A handy "My Items" feature lets you type in household items like soap or cat litter that you also need to buy. Then simply select "Print List" and head for the store. (Be aware, though, Marion Nestle points out, that the heart association seal signifies only that a product is low in fat and cholesterol; it could still contain lots of added sugar.)

Five aisles end with enormous soft-drink displays. Soft drinks next to the fish counter, near the garden furniture. You couldn't possibly go through the store without buying soft drinks."

Even if you're just popping in to buy a gallon of milk, Nestle says, you have to run a gauntlet of sweetened, salty and fatty treats to get to the dairy case—which savvy supermarkets strategically place all the way in the back.

Patrol the Perimeter

So what's a health-conscious supermarket customer to do? In their book *Strong Women, Strong Hearts* (Putnam's, $25.95), Miriam E. Nelson, PhD, and Alice H. Lichtenstein, DSc, both on the faculty of Tufts' Friedman School, advocate "keeping the emphasis on the whole foods available on the perimeter of the supermarket (the produce and dairy aisles, for instance) rather than on the boxed, bagged, canned and other packaged goods lining all the center aisles. Those choices often contain too little fiber, too many refined carbohydrates that lack certain nutrients, and frequently too much in the way of sugar, saturated and trans fats and salt."

Demand Nutrient Density

Look instead for foods that are "nutrient dense." Eileen Kennedy, DSc, RD, dean of Tufts' Friedman School, explains, "They're the foods that are loaded with the nutrients we need to thrive. Think about choosing a potato instead of potato chips, or a banana instead of a soda. Opt for a plate with lots of vegetables, and skip the dinner roll. Ignore the cake and go for the fruit.

"If Americans choose foods based on nutrient density," Kennedy adds, "they will, essentially, be choosing foods based on quality." A food item that is nutrient-dense is generally a better choice than a less nutrient-dense item with the same number of calories.

As a rule, whole-grain breads and cereals are more nutrient-dense than their "white" counterparts. Many fruits and vegetables are nutrient-dense because, in addition to providing some basic carbohydrates, they are low in fat and packed with fiber, vitamins and minerals. Candy and sweetened beverages, in contrast, provide the carbohydrates (and maybe fats) without the other nutrients.

Read and Decode Nutrition Labels

Those "Nutrition Facts" food labels can be a grocery shopper's best friend, if you know how to read them. US law requires food labels on all processed foods; products with little nutritional value, such as coffee, don't have the labels, but do get freshness labels ("sell by" date). In a series of programs including "Supermarket Tour for Elders: No Cart Required!" at Tufts' Jean Mayer USDA Human Nutrition Research Center on Aging, speakers bureau coordinator Jean Bianchetto, RD, LDN, MS, goes through the Nutrition Facts label, line by line. The top section lists substances that Bianchetto says you should limit, such as fat, cholesterol and sodium. The bottom part lists minerals, such as calcium and iron, and vitamins that you should try to include in your diet. The daily value percentages on the label are based on a daily intake of 2,000 calories. Bianchetto notes that 5% of the daily value is considered low, while 20% or more is considered high.

Center-Aisle Survival Tips

If you do stray into the packaged-goods aisles in the center of the supermarket, Nestle has a litany of "rules" that can help:

- Don't buy anything with more than five ingredients.
- If you can't pronounce the ingredients on the package label, don't buy it.
- Don't buy anything with a cartoon on it—it's being advertised directly to your kids or grandkids.
- If you don't want your kids eating junk food, don't have it in your house.
- Don't buy artificial anything—it's just disguising bad taste.

She also cautions against buying foods that seem like health foods—but really aren't. Just because candy comes covered with yogurt, for example, doesn't make it good for you. Also skip the "power bars" and "energy drinks" that purport to help athletes refuel; they're loaded with sweeteners and extra calories. "And don't buy anything with claims for health benefits.

Super Ideas for the Supermarket

Get a jump start on groceries with this list of recommended pantry staples and other basics of healthy food shopping from the National Heart, Lung and Blood Institute:

Fat-free or low-fat milk, yogurt, cheese and cottage cheese
Eggs/egg substitutes
Breads, bagels, pita bread, English muffins (whole grain)
Low-fat flour tortillas
Cereal (whole-grain)
Rice (such as brown rice, or other whole grains)
Pasta (look for whole-grain pasta)
White meat chicken or turkey (remove skin)
Fish and shellfish (fresh or frozen, not battered)
Beef: round, sirloin, chuck arm, loin and extra-lean ground beef
Pork: leg, shoulder, tenderloin
Dry beans and peas
Fresh, frozen, canned fruits in light syrup or juice
Fresh, frozen or no-salt-added canned vegetables
Low-fat or nonfat salad dressings
Herbs and spices

These are out of context and you need to search for the qualifying statements in tiny print."

Of course, it is possible to buy foods that are good for you in those temptation-packed center aisles. That's where you'll usually find whole-grain products, for example, as well as frozen and canned fruits and vegetables. But be careful and scrutinize labels to make sure that grains and healthy produce are all that you're buying.

Consider the aisle where many supermarkets sell not only rice and sometimes specialty grains but also packaged rice dishes. You probably already know that brown rice—a whole grain—is better for you than white rice. But what about those tasty-looking boxes of "rice pilaf"? Though they might sound like a good source of grain, a cup contains a mere 1 gram of fiber—along with 9 grams of total fat, 2 grams of saturated fat and a whopping 1,180 milligrams of sodium, almost half your daily total. Plus you're piling more than 300 calories onto your plate.

Similar cautions apply over in the cereal aisle, where you can buy a box of oatmeal that's all whole grains and nothing but. You might be tempted, though, by the Peanut Butter Toast Crunch cereal—after all, the box says in huge letters, as big as the words "Toast Crunch," "Whole Grain." Sure enough, the first ingredient listed is whole grain wheat. But keep reading, remembering that ingredients are listed in order by weight: Sugar comes next, followed by "creamy peanut butter" made with, yes, sugar, then rice flour and then fructose (another kind of sugar), and a bit farther down is dextrose (yet another kind of sugar). A serving has 10 grams of sugars in all. What about Maple Pecan Crunch cereal, "inspired by the taste of home-baked maple pecan muffins" and an "excellent source of Whole Grain"? It lists oats and then brown sugar, with plain sugar sixth on the ingredients list. Despite the whole-grain claims and homey-goodness appeal, a bowl contains 13 grams of sugars and 6 of fat.

Nothing says you can't indulge in an occasional muffin—or a cereal that tastes like a muffin. Just don't be fooled into thinking it's health food.

Pick Produce with Care

Frozen and canned fruits and vegetables found in supermarket center aisles can be affordable, convenient alternatives to fresh produce, but here too you need to give products a checkup before they go into your cart. Frozen produce is less likely to have added salt or sugar, and fruits and vegetables generally lose fewer nutrients in freezing than canning. Stick to canned goods that are as close to the whole, unprocessed original as possible, without added salt or sugar. The more food preparation and flavoring that a packager does for you, the more likely you're buying ingredients you may not want, at least in such quantities: A serving of canned barbecue baked beans, for instance, has 510 milligrams of sodium and 13 grams of sugars—in fact, sugar is the third ingredient listed, after water and beans.

Now take another look at that can of beans: The serving size is a half-cup. When you have baked beans, how much do you really put on your plate? A typical soup ladle (not heaping) serves about a half-cup. If you take two or three ladles of beans, you need to adjust your thinking accordingly when studying labels at the store.

Even vegetarian meals from those center aisles can be nutritionally iffy. A serving of frozen fettucini alfredo, for example, though meatless, nonetheless has 450 calories, 12 grams of saturated fat and 910 milligrams of sodium—more than a three-ounce lean hamburger including the bun.

So stick to the edges of the supermarket when possible, and always look at labels. Before you check out, remember to give your grocery cart a checkup.

Eat Like a Greek

Want flavor plus good health? The Mediterranean style of dining has it all.

Diets are often doomed to fail because they focus more on what you can't eat than what you can. Don't eat bread. Don't eat sugar. Don't eat fat. On some diets, even certain fruits and vegetables are forbidden. After a few weeks of being told "no," our inner toddler throws a tantrum and runs screaming to Krispy Kreme.

That's what is so appealing about the Mediterranean diet, which isn't really a diet at all but a style of eating that focuses on an abundance of delicious, hearty, and nutritious food. Just looking at the pyramid at right, developed by Oldways Preservation Trust, a nonprofit organization that encourages healthy food choices, may be enough to make you look forward to the next meal.

"What I like about this approach to food is that it's very easy," says Sara Baer-Sinnott, executive vice president of Oldways. "It's not a fancy way of eating, but you'll never feel deprived because the foods have so much flavor."

The best part is that eating like a Greek not only satisfies your need to say yes to food, but has been scientifically proven to be good for your health. Decades of research has shown that traditional Mediterranean eating patterns are associated with a lower risk of several chronic diseases, including the big three—cancer, heart disease, and type 2 diabetes. Most recently, a systematic review of 146 observational studies and 43 randomized clinical trials published in the April 13, 2009, issue of the Archives of Internal Medicine found strong evidence that a Mediterranean diet protects against cardiovascular disease. Other recent research has linked the eating style to a lower risk of cognitive decline and dementia.

So, where do you start? Your next meal is as good a place as any. Just walk through our guide for menu planning.

Stepping into a Mediterranean Lifestyle

Although a trip to southern Italy or Greece would be nice, you needn't go farther than your local supermarket. If your menu planning usually begins with a meat entrée, then adds a starch and a vegetable side dish as an afterthought, you'll want to reprioritize your food choices. "Think about designing a plate where a good half of it is taken up with vegetables, another one-quarter is healthy grains—whole-grain pasta, rice, couscous, quinoa—and the remaining quarter is

lean protein," says Katherine McManus, R.D., director of nutrition at Brigham and Women's Hospital in Boston and a consultant on the most recent version of the Mediterranean pyramid. "Of course, you needn't physically separate your foods in that fashion, but it gives you a good idea of the proportions to aim for."

STEP 1: Start with plant foods. Build your menus around an abundance of fruits and vegetables (yes, even potatoes); breads and grains (at least half of the servings should be whole grains); and beans, nuts, and seeds. To maximize the health benefits, emphasize a variety of minimally processed and locally grown foods.

STEP 2: Add some lean protein. The Mediterranean diet draws much of its protein from the sea, reflecting its coastal origins. Fish is not only low in saturated fat but can also be high in heart-healthy omega-3 fatty acids. Aim for two servings of fish a week, especially those, such as salmon and sardines, that are high in omega-3s but lower in mercury. You can also include moderate amounts of poultry and even eggs.

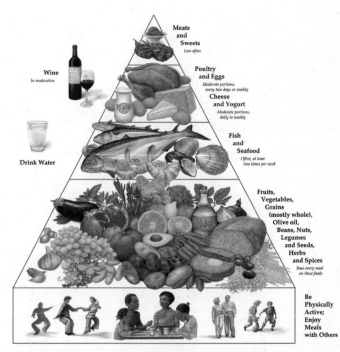

© 2009 Oldways Preservation Trust, www.oldwayspt.org

A Day in the Mediterranean Life

Breakfast

It's hard to go wrong with whole-grain cereal, fruit, and low-fat milk. Variations on the theme include low-fat yogurt with fresh berries and granola, or meaty steel-cut oats topped with fresh fruit, applesauce, whipped yogurt, or a sprinkle of nuts. Enjoy eggs? Try sautéing vegetables or greens in a bit of olive oil until soft and then scramble in a beaten egg. Go Greek with chopped olives and feta, or top with salsa and avocado for a Tex-Mex flair.

Lunch

Whether you're at home or brown-bagging, a Mediterranean lunch is tastier and healthier than drive-through fare and often faster and cheaper, too. Bagged salad greens provide a base for whatever you have on hand—fruit, vegetables, nuts, cheese, or a bit of leftover grilled chicken or fish. Consider topping it with a low-fat ranch dressing, an olive-oil vinaigrette, or just a drizzle of flavorful oil and a squeeze of fresh lemon. Or fill a whole-wheat pita pocket with hummus and as much fresh lettuce, peppers, cucumbers, and tomatoes as you can stuff in. If you're really pressed for time, heat up a can of low-sodium lentil, minestrone, or vegetable soup.

Snack Time

Keep a ready supply of fruit and veggies on hand so you'll grab them at snack time. Hummus, low-fat yogurt, and salad dressings pair nicely with them. If you don't want to invest the prep time, buy pre-cut. It's also a good idea to keep some nonperishable snacks at your desk or in your car—raisins or other dried fruit, nuts, and whole-grain crackers or pretzels.

Dinner

This is when many of us lose sight of nutrition goals because it's so easy after a long day to fall into old, comfortable habits. Fortunately, Mediterranean-style dining emphasizes simple foods and cooking methods.

While your pasta boils, for example, you can sauté a variety of vegetables in olive oil and garlic, then toss in a few shrimp and cook until they turn pink. Mix it all with a sprinkle of cheese, pour yourself a glass of wine, and you're sitting down to a relaxing dinner in less than 20 minutes.

In much the same manner, you can put together a quick stir-fry with slices of chicken breast, vegetables, and rice. Fresh fish is the simplest of entrées because it cooks quickly and doesn't take much dressing up. Spritz it with olive oil and your favorite seasonings and broil it, or coat it in bread crumbs and pan fry in a bit of olive oil. Squeeze on fresh lemon juice and adorn with parsley just before serving.

Two things you should have on hand for your evening meal: frozen vegetables, which are usually just as nutritious as fresh, and a plastic container of salad, preferably filled with a variety of greens. It's also a good idea to stock your crisper with seasonal fruit. A bowl of ripe berries, a chunk of melon, or a soft, farm-fresh peach is a delicious and satisfying end to any meal.

Oldways Preservation Trust, a nonprofit organization that promotes healthful eating, has more recipes and menu ideas on the two Web sites it sponsors: www.oldwayspt.org and www.mediterraneanmark.org.

Or substitute with vegetarian sources of protein, such as beans, nuts, or soy products. Limit red meat to a couple of servings a month, and minimize consumption of processed meats.

STEP 3: Say cheese. Include some milk, yogurt, or cheese in your daily meal. While low-fat versions are preferable, others are fine in small amounts. A sprinkle of high-quality Romano or Parmesan, for example, adds a spark to vegetables and pasta. Soy-based dairy products are fine, too, if you prefer them or are lactose intolerant.

STEP 4: Use oils high in "good" fats. Canola oil is a good choice, but many Mediterranean recipes call for olive oil. Both are high in unsaturated fat. Minimize artery-clogging saturated fat, which comes mainly from animal sources, and avoid the even more heart-harming trans fat, which comes from partially hydrogenated vegetable oil.

STEP 5: End meals with the sweetness of fruit. Make sugary and fatty desserts just an occasional indulgence.

STEP 6: Drink to your health. A moderate amount of alcohol—especially red wine—may help protect your heart. But balance that against the increased risks from drinking alcohol, including breast cancer in women. A moderate amount is one drink a day for women, two for men.

STEP 7: Step out. "The Mediterranean lifestyle is built around daily activity," McManus says. Go for a walk after dinner. And choose leisure activities that keep you moving.

The Slow Food Movement Picks up Speed

Forsake fast food and convenience cuisine. Savor the enjoyment of ripe, locally grown produce and freshly prepared foods that have made a short, simple field-to-plate journey.

SHARON PALMER, RD

There's a slower, gentler food movement afoot. People are talking about slowing down our food supply and enjoying the pure taste of food that isn't weighed down with processing and chemicals. They are buying fresh, ripe produce from local farms that wasn't picked green, polished with wax, and trucked across the country. People are remembering the way their grandparents and great-grandparents ate, when they harvested apples in the fall and made jars of applesauce for the winter. The buzz is about wondering how your lunch was produced instead of inhaling a burger in the car while fielding cell phone calls. It's essentially the antithesis of fast food. Welcome to the slow food movement.

Food professionals, chefs, and foodies are embracing this concept and now dietitians are joining their ranks. It's no surprise, as slow food includes the message that dietitians have been preaching for decades—a focus on whole foods, such as fruits, vegetables, whole grains, nuts, and legumes. The slow food philosophy digs deeper into the food system, tracing foods all the way back to the very soil in which they were grown. According to Melinda Hemmelgarn, MS, RD, columnist and a Kellogg Foundation Food and Society Policy fellow, the message of slow food is about "thinking beyond your plate."

As the food supply became increasingly centralized and mega food companies started feeding a growing percentage of American bellies, people lost touch with the food supply and the flavors of real food. These days, it's easy to find food products that boast maltodextrin as the first ingredient and families gathered around the dinner table for a packaged, convenience meal with a long list of ingredients from all over the country. Ask a classroom of urban kids whether they've ever picked a fresh strawberry and let the juice run down their chins. Then, for extra credit, ask them how strawberries are cultivated.

"With the globalization of food, we are no longer eating food in season or fresh. We want to bring it back to people's consciousness.

We don't want our palates dulled, we want to eat only when it's ripe and at its fullest," said Alice Waters recently at the Association of Food Journalists conference in San Francisco. Founder and owner of Chez Panisse in Berkeley, Calif., Waters is widely regarded as the mother of the local, sustainable food movement.

The Birth of Slow Food

Slow Food, an international organization, was founded in 1986 in Italy by Carlo Petrini, who maintained that the industrialization of food was standardizing taste and leading to the extinction of thousands of food varieties. With 83,000 members worldwide, the network is organized into local groups called *convivia* that are engaged in organizing dinners, tastings, and promoting campaigns. Slow Food's mission is to help motivate people to come back to kitchens and tables to nurture culture and community. By doing so, the organization hopes to invigorate regional and seasonal culinary traditions and celebrate taste while promoting ecologically sound food production.

"Carlo Petrini, the father of Slow Food, spoke at the Food and Society Policy conference last spring. He described quality food as meeting three criteria: 1) It tastes great; 2) It is produced sustainably, with care for the environment; and 3) The food is produced in a humane and socially just manner," explains Hemmelgarn. "For example, a food may be delicious and grown organically, but if the people working in the fields are treated like slaves, then it doesn't fit with the Slow Food philosophy. Individuals who embrace the concept of Slow Food believe it is important to critically question the food we eat and ask, Who grows or produces it and under what conditions? Where was the food produced and how many miles did it have to travel to reach my plate? How were the animals treated in life and in death, and how will the growing practices impact our environment?"

Measuring Food Miles

In the slow food world, people throw around the term *food miles* almost as frequently as dietitians use the word *calories*. A food mile is the distance food travels from where it is grown or raised to where it is ultimately purchased by the consumer. In the United States, food typically travels 1,500 to 2,500 miles to get to our plates, according to a recent study by the Worldwatch Institute.[1]

Most Americans don't realize that much of food production and processing happens far from where they live and rarely consider the costs of food related to production, processing, storage, and transportation. The environmental costs are the increased amount of fossil fuel used to transport food long distances and the increase in greenhouse gas emissions resulting from the burning of these fuels. According to USDA Agricultural Marketing Service produce arrival data from the Chicago terminal market, produce arriving by truck traveled an average distance of 1,518 miles. Data from three Iowa local food projects where farmers sold to institutional markets found that the food traveled an average of 44.6 miles to reach its destination. A conventional system used four to 17 times more fuel and released five to 17 times more carbon dioxide from the burning of the fuel than the Iowa-based regional and local food systems.[2]

Fresh from the Farm

Slow food has helped save small farms that may have been swept up by the big food industry. By supporting local farms, proponents help preserve the bucolic scenery of faded barns and patchwork farms that have been woven into the American landscape, as well as genetic diversity in crops.

In Marin County, California, 25 years ago dairy woman Ellen Straus and biologist Phyllis Faber sensed that agriculture was in danger of being lost forever to non-agricultural land development. They set out to protect the land through the Marin Agricultural Land Trust, which is now a model for farmlands across the country. This preservation compensates farmers and ranchers for the development value of their land while permanently protecting the land for agriculture. Now the region is studded with small farms and ranches, such as the James Grossi Ranch and the McEvoy Olive Ranch.

One of the best ways to support slow foods is to frequent farmers' markets, which promote locally grown, organic fruits and vegetables, and small family farms. The number of farmers' markets has doubled in the last five years. A recent study from the Leopold Center for Sustainable Agriculture showed that farmers' markets produced $20.8 million in sales and more than 325 jobs for the Iowa economy, turning out to be the No. 1 marketing channel for Iowa's vegetable and fruit growers.[3]

Artisan Foods Move in Quickly

The artisan movement, in which purveyors craft foods on a small scale with a dedication to quality ingredients, is walking hand in hand with slow foods, creating a whole new market.

People are willing to pay a higher price for food not prepared by the food giants. With 38 workers, The Straus Family Creamery (Marin County, Calif.) sells 27 million pounds of milk per year for as much as 50% more than major brands. Stores like Whole Foods Market and Wild Oats, whose philosophies support slow food, have seen double annual revenue in the past five years. Whole Foods not only stocks a plethora of specialty foods, they have started their own Authentic Food Artisan program in which foods are labeled with a special sticker indicating artisan status. Chefs in elegant restaurants now spell out artisanal products and sources of food ingredients on their menus by name.

Laura Chenel, founder and owner of Laura Chenel's Chevre, Inc., credits her affinity for goats as motivation for starting her artisan goat cheese production company, considered to be the originator of American goat cheese. Chenel claims that she is extremely involved with her herd of 500 goats, even down to calling them by name. "For me, an artisan is a craftsperson. It is all about care and attention to detail, pride, and ownership," says Chenel. Her goats are on a healthy schedule of grain and alfalfa feedings intermixed with grazing and play times in the pasture that may put mothers of human kids to shame.

Even meat purveyors are becoming part of the slow and artisan food movements. Oregon Country Natural Beef raises their meat without antibiotics and hormones. At Marin Sun Farms in Northern California, David Evans watches over his family's herd of Hereford-Angus cows and more than 1,000 laying hens, becoming known for his innovative and humane ranching techniques.

Seasonal Celebration

One tenant of slow foods is eating seasonally, the way people did generations ago. Our ancestors never dreamed of eating raspberries in January. Preservation was necessary and traditional dishes evolved that celebrated the seasons. Celebrity chefs and Martha Stewart have helped make the lost art of preservation en vogue again. A slow food advocate before it had a name, Waters says, "This is an idea that has been around since the beginning of time. We rigidly follow seasons. When we got into winter vegetables, we discovered the flavor and varieties of the winter palette."

Simply in Season (*World Community Cookbook*) [Herald Press, 2005], cowritten by Mary Beth Lind, RD, and Cathleen Hockman-Wert is packed with inspiration for eating seasonally. The book lists six reasons to eat simply in season, which include freshness, taste, nutrition, variety, environment, and local health, as farmers' markets support the local economy.

Slow Roots in Culinary Arts

Slow food gained momentum in the culinary arts community. Waters opened Chez Panisse in 1971 with a dedication to local, seasonal products. Today's chefs follow in her footsteps by boasting their own organic gardens to supply their kitchens, even picking fresh salad greens on their way to work. They frequent farmers' markets and change their menus daily to incorporate the

Out of Africa

Dietitians such as Stacia Nordin, RD, nutrition consultant in sustainable food and nutrition security specialist, have found ways to fit the slow food philosophy into their careers. Nordin has been working in Malawi, Africa, to improve food and nutrition security, partly through reviving the knowledge of indigenous foods and integrating them into modern diets. In the past, the diet of the people of Malawi revolved around a variety of local fruits, vegetables, nuts, seeds, millets, sorghums, roots, and animal foods. But such foods began to vanish because of the push to supply year-round maize and the interest in western foods. With more than 90% of people living in Malawi fulfilling their nutrition needs through subsistence agriculture, if the environment around them doesn't supply the necessary food, there is nothing to eat.

—SP

latest harvest. They are starting to develop personal relationships with farmers. Dishes on restaurant menus have become simpler so they celebrate the flavor of one particular food, whether it's a fresh peach or Neiman Ranch beef. Slow food followers are searching Web sites to discover which restaurants are slow food-friendly before they make a reservation. Hemmelgarn reports that she asks waiters which foods on the menu are local before ordering.

Chefs Collaborative is an organization directed to chefs and the food community with a mission to foster local foods and a sustainable food supply. With their Seafood Solutions, Meat of the Matter, and Farmer-Chef Connection programs, Chefs Collaborative offers helpful information about making decisions in the food supply and hopes to be a catalyst for change in the country. "We provide tools for purchasing decisions for chefs and guidelines for sustainable, healthful food," says Nancy Civetta of Civetta Comunicazioni, the public relations company for Chefs Collaborative.

Edible Gardens for Kids

As it becomes painfully clear that our kids do not have enough face time with real food, slow food has started to take root in school gardens. Dan Desmond, 4-H Youth Development Advisor in El Dorado County, California, says, "In recent years with poor nutrition seen in children, the garden offers one solution. Early research shows that when children garden, they include fruits and vegetables more regularly into their diet." The National Farm to School Program is listed as a resource in the School Wellness Policy Web site.

"We need to develop the relationship between the child and food products. Taking junk food out of schools is great, but you need to change the whole culture. If you want to change the culture, you have to start with children," says Desmond. He reports that the school garden is alive and well in many parts of

the United States and that there are approximately 3,000 school gardens in California, ranging from half wine barrels to 20-acre farms. Desmond believes California First Lady Maria Shriver will probably jump on the school garden bandwagon to help promote the Live Deliciously campaign.

Waters created the Chez Panisse Foundation, which started the Edible Schoolyard, a garden and kitchen classroom at Berkeley's Martin Luther King, Jr. Middle School. Last year, the Berkeley Unified School District signed an agreement with the Chez Panisse Foundation to create a formal curriculum that includes organic gardening, cooking, and eating healthy lunches for the district's 9,000 students. "We're trying to reach kids who aren't eating with their parents and don't know about food," says Waters. "I want them to come to foods and fall in love, to have a whole new relationship with food that is connected to nature, tradition, and culture."

The Food Project in Massachusetts has a mission to help grow a community of youth and adults from diverse backgrounds to work together to build a sustainable food system. Since 1991, the Food Project built a model of getting young people to change through sustainable agriculture. They work with hundreds of teens and thousands of volunteers to farm on 31 acres of rural Lincoln and on several lots in urban Boston, growing nearly a quarter-million pounds of food without chemical pesticides, one-half of which is donated to local shelters.

Dietitians Move Slow

It seems that dietitians can benefit from learning more about slow food, whether they work in wellness or manage a school foodservice program. "The philosophy behind slow food is part of my DNA, a part of how I was raised, but the principles of slow food have not generally been a part of the dietetic curriculum. Many dietitians need help understanding these ideas and translating them into practical recommendations," says Amanda Archibald, RD, founder of Field to Plate, a company that aims to teach the principles of local, seasonal, and regional foods. Archibald reports that her workshops reveal that dietitians are often curious and hungry for new ideas in food and nutrition education and are becoming more motivated to learn about slow food. "There are Dietary Guidelines for Americans, but I believe that we are ready for something more sustainable in our approach to nutrition education. We're ready to 'green' the guidelines," says Archibald, who recommends that dietitians join the Hunger and Environmental Nutrition Dietetic Practice Group, whose motto is that all people should have access to food from a healthy, sustainable environment.

"There is growing interest and awareness in the importance of how local agriculture methods are impacting our food system and the health of our region and the people in it, from an economic, environmental, and medical perspective. This interest and awareness does not originate from the conventional healthcare community, sadly enough. It comes from the general public recognizing the impact and interconnection of their medical concerns with what is happening in the greater world," says Lynn Mader, MBA, RD, food system consultant. Mader is involved with a farm-to-school initiative to identify local, seasonal foods that can be used by schools.

Slow Food Is Moving

Slow food is inching its way across the country, even though it currently resides mostly in the well-educated, high-income strata of society. Since slow food typically costs more, plenty of people simply can't afford it. "Slow food remains an amazing philosophy, but it's out of reach to so many people," adds Archibald. Some experts predict that slow food will trickle down to all walks of life, as do many trends.

Some food professionals argue that slow food is not realistic, as consumers are still just as pressed for time as ever. After all, new products keep rolling out that conveniently fit into car cup holders. But new companies are proving that slow foods may not be just a pipe dream. Take Burgerville, a chain of 39 fast-food restaurants in the Pacific Northwest that features a McDonald's-like menu, but most ingredients come from local farms. Sodexho is starting to offer regionally sourced meals to their university and corporate clients and Kaiser Permanente is hosting farmers' markets at some facilities. It looks like the future of food may be moving more slowly for a change.

References

1. Halweil B. Homegrown: The Case for Local Food In A Global Market, November 2002. Available at: http://www.worldwatch .org/pubs/paper/163

2. Pirog R, Van Pelt T, Enshayan K, et al. Food, Fuel, and Freeways: An Iowa perspective on how far food travels, fuel usage, and greenhouse gas emissions. Leopold Center for Sustainable Agriculture. June 2001. Available at: http://www .leopold.iastate.edu/pubs/staff/ppp/food_mil.pdf

3. Study Shows Positive Economic Impact of Iowa Farmer's Markets, 5-10-05, Leopold Center for Sustainable Agriculture. Available at: http://www.leopold.iastate.edu/news/ newsreleases/2005/markets_051005.htm

SHARON PALMER, RD, is a freelance food and nutrition writer in southern California.

Schools Can Taste Good

A chef leads the way in making good nutrition a required part of the school day.

KATHERINE GIGLIOTTI

If you build it, they will come. . . . But if you plant squash and Swiss chard, will kids eat it? Some people think so. Alice Waters, a well-known California chef at Chez Panisse launched her "Edible Schoolyard" 10 years ago. Now her pilot program is going district-wide in Berkeley, Calif., to help kids make the connections between food and table, good planting and good eating.

The idea behind the Edible Schoolyard—to address hunger and nutrition by helping children learn about agriculture and farming—is not unique to Berkeley. School gardens and farm-to-school programs are popping up in urban schools across the country. Districts from Harlem, N.Y., to Compton, Calif., are recognizing that partnerships with farmers, hospitals and other community institutions can support programs to reduce hunger and improve nutrition in low-income, urban settings.

"No sector—government, foundation, private or nonprofit—can do it all," says Kansas Representative Melvin Neufeld. "Addressing hunger challenges requires collaboration between all these partners."

An Edible Schoolyard?

In 1995, before public concern about America's obesity epidemic became widespread, Waters recognized the growing problem of poverty in public schools—deteriorating buildings, overworked teachers and undernourished kids. In her home town of Berkeley, Calif., students attending a middle school located just down the street from the prestigious University of California attended class in buildings with peeling paint and no hot water. Forty percent of the students qualified for free or reduced price lunch, and 64 percent were from an ethnic minority. Waters viewed these challenges as "a very good test case" to see if her program could be successful.

Waters began with an unused, abandoned acre on the side of Martin Luther King Jr. Middle School and planted it with seasonal produce, herbs, vines, berries, flowers and fruit trees. The garden now also includes a seed propagation table, tool shed, wood-fired oven, picnic area and chicken coop. Two teachers, the chef teacher and the garden teacher and manager, run the program. Throughout the school year, sixth, seventh and eighth grade students are involved in the garden and kitchen, preparing the beds, sowing the seeds, transplanting, composting, watering, weeding and harvesting. Kitchen activities include preparing the recipe of the day, setting the table, eating, cleaning up and preparing scraps for compost.

> **"It is amazing that something so simple could have so many benefits . . . it is a great way to teach science, to teach nutrition, and it also produces healthy food."**
>
> —California Assemblywoman Wilma Chan

Students come for 90-minute sessions several times a week for lessons that weave gardening with other subjects. Math classes measure the garden beds, science classes study drainage and soil erosion. History classes learn about pre-Columbian civilizations from grinding maize. English classes write recipes.

"It is amazing that something so simple could have so many benefits . . . it is a great way to teach science, to teach nutrition, and it also produces healthy food," says California Assemblywoman Wilma Chan, who has sponsored legislation to promote healthy eating and physical activity in schools.

Although teaching children how to eat right is only one goal of the program, administrators have learned that when children grow it, harvest it, and cook it, they want to eat it. It is "great to see the kids working in the garden, and being excited about gardening and eating nutritious food," says Chan.

A study conducted by Harvard Medical School in the Edible Schoolyard's fifth year of operation found that not only were kids eating more fruits and vegetables, they were getting better grades. Parents report that, to their amazement, children are asking to re-create recipes at home and eating squash and even Swiss chard.

The Next Step

Chef Waters has another vision. She wants to make school lunch an academic subject. She says it's a logical next step that can be built on the successful Edible Schoolyard project. Her new

Establish Partnerships

A variety of public, private and nonprofit groups has an interest in reducing hunger and obesity and improving nutrition among school children, including hospitals, environmental and conservation groups, farmers and businesses.

Establishing partnerships with local farmers can be a particularly effective way to reduce the barriers of bringing fresh produce into schools. Two pilot projects funded by the federal government support these types of partnerships.

Legislators can also maximize federal nutrition programs—school breakfast, school lunch, summer food and food stamps—by providing supplemental funding and outreach initiatives.

"Maximizing the use of government funding for school meals to purchase nutritious locally produced food benefits the health of students and our local economies," says New York Assemblyman Felix Ortiz. He says these projects "provide new opportunities for city and rural residents to support each other."

Federal pilots that may soon be expanded include:

- Fresh Fruit and Vegetable Pilot Program. Established by the 2002 Farm Bill, the Fresh Fruit and Vegetable Pilot Program helps pay for fresh and dried fruits and vegetables for schoolchildren. During the 2004–2005 school year, $9 million was made available. The program is available to selected schools in Indiana, Iowa, Michigan, North Carolina, Ohio, Pennsylvania and Washington. Congress is currently working to expand the program.
- Department of Defense Fresh Produce Program. This pilot program established in 1994 and operated by the U.S. Department of Defense allows school food service directors to use federal commodity money to purchase state-grown produce from the Department of Defense, which purchases the products from small- and mid-sized family farmers. The program currently operates in Florida, Georgia, Kentucky, Michigan, Mississippi and New Mexico. Illinois and New York are in the process of developing programs. Legislatures can provide start-up funds or direct the appropriate state agency to establish a partnership with the Department of Defense.

NCSL's Hunger and Nutrition Partnership

Current efforts to reduce hunger and improve nutrition are fragmented across disciplines—WIC in the health department, food stamps in the human services agency, and child nutrition programs in state and local education authorities—and in the private and nonprofit sectors through food banks and community kitchens. The Hunger and Nutrition Partnership is an NCSL initiative, supported by The UPS Foundation, that works across public and private sectors and across disciplines to enhance the ability of state policymakers to alleviate hunger and improve nutrition in their communities. For the latest publications from the Hunger and Nutrition Partnership, including the newly released Promising Practices Guide Bringing Legislators to the Table and Addressing Hunger and Nutrition: A Tool Kit for Positive Results, please visit: www.ncsl.org/statefed/humserv/hunger.htm. Additional information can be found at: www.ncsl.org/programs/health/publichealth/foodaccess/index.htm.

idea, called the School Lunch Initiative, is already underway in the Berkeley Unified School District. Students and teachers are involved in preparing healthy meals using local, seasonal ingredients from sustainable farms. A new school cafeteria is the focal point for everyday, hands-on experiences that link learning opportunities in kitchen classrooms and instructional gardens with academic and physical education programs. The Berkley pilot includes a new set of school cafeteria menus that make the connection between farms, schools and the environment by using fresh, seasonal, locally produced food. Funding for the School Lunch Initiative comes from the school district, the Chez Panisse Foundation and the Center for Ecoliteracy.

State lawmakers can help duplicate successful models such as the Edible Schoolyard through startup funds or pilot programs. In 1999, the California Legislature established the Instructional School Gardens Program. Through this grant, administered by the State Department of Education, local school districts and county offices of education help pay for the start-up of school gardens.

Building partnerships between local nonprofits, foundations, the health community and businesses can help establish a pilot school garden program in an at-risk school. According to Waters, in the case of Berkeley's Edible Schoolyard, the Children's Hospital Oakland proved to be a valuable partner because they recognized that there were "4,000 kids at risk in Berkeley, and their clinic could care for only 150." Supporting the Edible Schoolyard was a way to reach at-risk children while they were still forming their eating habits and before they reached an unhealthy weight.

The Potential of Farm-to-College Programs

Colleges and universities across the United States are increasingly sourcing the food for their dining halls from local farms through farm-to-college (FTC) programs. Although participation in FTC programs may increase the visibility of the school to prospective students and parents, support the local economy, and introduce new options into campus eateries, FTC programs face a number of operational barriers. Inadequate student support, institutional procurement policies, and seasonality limit the reach of FTC efforts. This article discusses these barriers in detail through the perspective of New England higher education institutions and uses Tufts University as a case study in the challenges and potential for FTC programs to become mainstream in college and university food service.

KATHLEEN A. MERRIGAN, PHD AND MELISSA BAILEY, MS

The demand for local food has been stimulated, among other things, by Michael Pollan's best-selling book *Omnivore's Dilemma,* food safety scares, and advocacy organizations seeking to support family farms. As a result, the share of food spending that US consumers put toward the purchase of local farm products is increasing as individual households, K-12 school systems, and, more recently, university and college dining halls join the "buy local" food movement.[1] Many institutions of higher education now have procurement managers and food service directors who specifically work toward connecting the consumer (the students frequenting their dining facilities) to the producer of the food served (local farmers) through what are called "farm-to-college" (FTC) programs. The implementation of FTC programs is meant to support the goals of the broader buy-local movement. These include preservation of farmland from development pressure by keeping farmers in business, support of local economies within a community via retention of dollars spent at local farms and grocers, improved freshness and flavor through minimizing food travel time, and reductions in energy used in trucking and shipping to transport foods to their destination.[2]

Regardless of the specific goals that a given FTC program strives to meet, it is often the implementation of the FTC program itself that proves difficult for both farmers and universities. These difficulties can be further complicated in the northeastern United States because of its short farm season and relatively small agricultural base. This article uses Tufts University as a case study to demonstrate the barriers faced by New England higher educational institutions in their journey to start and maintain a successful FTC effort. Data from the National FTC

Survey conducted by the Community Food Security Coalition (CFSC) confirm that the Tufts experience is common to many New England universities and colleges and that food service providers in the Northeast share similar motivations, barriers, and opportunities while participating in the FTC movement.

What Motivates the Creation of FTC Programs?

Each college that participates in FTC programs has different operational characteristics that influence its ability to adopt the practice of local food sourcing. In the case of Tufts University, the main campus, which is located in Medford, Massachusetts, has 2 main dining halls that serve an undergraduate population of 4,900 students. In a sense, Tufts has a "captured" consumer who must purchase from the dining facilities because all freshmen and sophomores at Tufts are required to participate in a meal plan, although it is optional for juniors and seniors. In general, Tufts' meal plans combine dining hall meals with "Dining Dollars" that can be used elsewhere on campus (eg, vending machines) or at a number of other on-campus eateries (eg, grab-n-go service, campus convenience store). Graduate students, staff, and faculty also use the various on-campus eateries, although far less frequently than do the undergraduate students. All of the eateries are self-operated by Tufts University Dining Services (TUDS). Food suppliers/vendors are in a contractual relationship for their services with the university.

The FTC program at Tufts began in 1994, prompted by a graduate student project that brought together students and

TUDS staff to investigate the potential of substituting apples sourced from New England orchards for those imported from Washington State. In this case, the FTC program succeeded because of student involvement and demand for produce from local farms. In fact, from 1994 through 2007, the amount of FTC programming undertaken by TUDS ebbed and flowed with the falling and rising student interest in having such a program. For a number of years, Tufts' FTC efforts were minimal because of the lack of student inquiries requesting more locally sourced foods. This experience highlights what we consider to be the most important factor motivating and enabling FTC programs to succeed: student support and demand. It is reasonable to think of the university's dining service as a business and the students as its clientele who drive the current and future direction of the business. Unless the clientele request a service such as FTC and support it through their spending habits, it is less likely for a self-operating dining service to take on the added logistical and financial burden of sourcing from local farms.

Student support and demand for the program are essential.

Although student demand may be the strongest motivator for a university dining service to implement a FTC program in its daily operations, there are a number of alternate rationales that engage food service in higher education institutions to work toward sourcing more of their food supply locally. These motivators range from philosophical reasons (eg, a college wants to be a good citizen) to reasons that are grounded in business strategy, institutional policy, and government incentives. As can be demonstrated from the Tufts experience and evidence from local universities, it is often a convergence of these motivators, combined with student interest, that prime higher education institutions for FTC programs.

Tufts has a strong history of citizen action and public service. By establishing a university-wide environmental policy and a Dining Services policy that embraces sustainability, Tufts has set a goal of being an environmentally responsible institution. Because of the need to work toward these goals, Tufts became ripe for embracing changes in facilities and operations, such as the implementation of a FTC program. However, in the case of business strategy, Tufts has not capitalized on implementing a FTC program as a way to add value in its marketing approaches to attract new students. A well-positioned public relations campaign on the successes of Tufts' FTC program to date may stand out and draw new students and their parents to Tufts as a progressive competitor in elite higher education. In contrast, Yale University appears to have used its position as an early innovator of a FTC approach, which includes a vegetable farm and a hugely popular dining hall that uses only local ingredients as a marketing tool to gain some degree of competitive advantage in the Ivy League marketplace.

Various local, state, and federal agencies that mandate or encourage education institutions to source local foods have proliferated in recent years, providing yet another motivator for establishing FTC programs. At the federal level, a partnership between the US Department of Defense and the US Department of Agriculture allows a portion of purchases under the National School Lunch Program in K-12 schools to go toward provision of locally produced fruits and vegetables. This ability to source local foods for school food service was further emphasized in the 2002 Farm Bill, which directed the Secretary of Agriculture to encourage institutions in the school lunch and breakfast programs to purchase locally produced foods for school meal programs, to the maximum extent practicable and appropriate.[3,4] Federal action has not yet begun, however, to influence FTC programs because directives have been limited to public K-12 school systems via required nationwide school lunch and breakfast programs.

In contrast, regulations at the state level have been relevant to higher education. The Massachusetts legislature, for example, passed a local purchasing provision in 2006 as part of an economic stimulus package, directing purchasing agents of the Commonwealth, including agents at state colleges and universities, to give preference to sourcing local agricultural products:

> To effectuate the preference for those products of agriculture grown or produced using locally grown products, the state purchasing agent responsible for procuring the products on behalf of a state agency or authority shall: (1) in advertising for bids, contracts, or otherwise procuring products of agriculture, *make reasonable efforts to facilitate the purchase of such products of agriculture grown or produced using products grown in the commonwealth;* and (2) *purchase the products of agriculture grown or produced using products grown in the commonwealth,* unless the price of the goods exceeds, by more than 10 percent, the price of products of agriculture grown or produced using products grown outside of the commonwealth (emphasis added).[5]

Farm-to-college programs may be good publicity for participating colleges.

Similar efforts are under way in other states to allow preferential purchasing of agricultural goods in public education institutions, both K-12 and state-funded universities.[6] These kinds of regulations can serve as stimuli for state colleges and universities to establish and grow FTC programs. The Massachusetts procurement provision, coupled with a strong local farm economy in western Massachusetts, for example, has enabled the University of Massachusetts in Amherst to expand its FTC effort. The university established a goal of purchasing 30% of its food from local farms in the 2007–2008 academic year; this is a 5% increase in local farm product purchases from the last academic year (Ken Toong, e-mail communication, October 15, 2007).

Understanding the Barriers to Successful Implementation

FTC programs face varying challenges given the differing operational structures in which they function (eg, "all you can eat" vs "pay as you go" dining halls). However, data from a recent FTC survey effort show that there are commonalities, especially when regional/geographical differences such as those in the Northeast are taken into account. In 2004, the CFSC began collecting data on FTC programs around the United States via a self-administered Web survey.[7] A senior member of the Dining Services staff of each college or university was targeted to fill out a survey that included information on how their FTC program started, the degree of student involvement, the percentage of the overall dining budget allocated for local purchases, and the barriers and solutions faced in implementing their program. As of May 2007, a total of 117 self-selected surveys have been submitted to this database since the fall of 2004. Overall, the CFSC survey identified coordination and seasonality as the most significant barriers to FTC programs nationally. However, the CFSC analysis does not break down respondents by region to look for any differences in the barriers faced by FTC programs in New England as compared to the national survey results.

To understand the context and challenges faced by FTC programs in New England, publicly available data from CFSC were aggregated by the authors to include only respondents from New England institutions. Of the 117 surveys available when the CFSC database was accessed, a total of 20 surveys sent in by New England institutions were included in this aggregate. This aggregate provides a good summary of the challenges and barriers faced by FTC programs in the northeastern United States.

As shown in Figure 1, the coordination of purchasing and delivery for procuring from local farms was identified by 11 of the 20 New England schools as a key challenge. Practical examples from Tufts' FTC program confirm this sentiment. If the university is to purchase directly from a farmer (which gives the farmer the highest proportion of each dollar in sales as profit), then a new vendor relationship must be established through the purchasing system. This requires an adaptation of the ordering software, a relatively easy accommodation. More significantly, it means that the farmer must have a certain amount of liability insurance to be eligible to enter into an agreement as a vendor with the university, but many farmers do not. College administrators are also leery of heavy truck traffic on campus. Direct farmer deliveries mean increasing traffic on loading docks and complicating the timing of staffing to help unload trucks and stock supplies. Furthermore, it means increased traffic where students expect to stroll and enjoy the beauty of campus with little regard to vehicular interference.

Direct buying from the farmer has been fraught with inventory problems. Managers of dining halls place orders in anticipation of receiving the goods they specified to meet the large volume and quick turnover of meals in their facilities. In a number of instances, farmers will substitute items when they run short. This is not because these farmers are poor planners or irresponsible, but because the nature of farming itself is unpredictable. Farmers may deliver different vegetables from

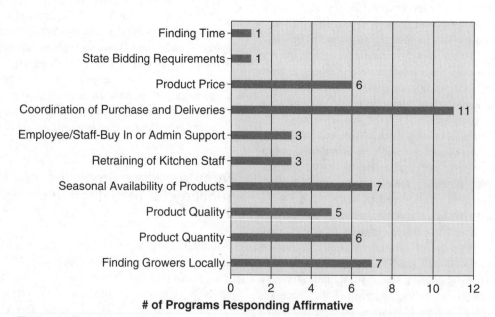

Figure 1   Barriers in 20 Farm-to-college programs in New England. Most frequently cited barriers by New England farm-to-college (FTC) programs. Data from the following Community Food Security Coalition FTC survey respondents: Colby College, Bates College, Bowdoin College, Clark University, College of the Atlantic, Dartmouth College, Harvard University, Massachusetts Institute of Technology, Middlebury College, St Joseph's College (Maine), St Joseph's College (Connecticut), Smith College, Sterling College, Trinity College, Tufts University, University of Connecticut, University of Massachusetts, University of New Hampshire, Williams College, and Yale University.

what was ordered because bad weather delayed maturation of the desired vegetable (whereas a distributor would simply fill the order with the desired vegetable from a different region). This has had negative consequences. The dining manager must revise the meal for that particular day, if possible, and if the substituted vegetable requires unexpected processing (eg, peeling, chopping), labor must be found to undertake the task. Such a situation leaves the manager frustrated with the ordering and receiving process and cites lack of time to "deal with" coordinating an FTC program.

One way to ease these problems is to work with produce distributors who are able to serve as the middleman between local farms and the institution. The advantage from an institutional perspective is that many of these distributors are already vendors with contracts and liability coverage with the university. Another option is to work with dining hall managers over the years, securing a great deal of "relationship capital." This approach, however, does have its own coordination problems similar to those when buying direct from farmers. For example, a box of apples may arrive with the expectation that they have been sourced from a local Massachusetts orchard only to discover that the apples are from Washington state. In this scenario, dining hall managers are not as frustrated as with farmer substitutions because, in a sense, they have the same product (ie, do not have to adjust the menu for the day). However, representing to students that the university buys local and then serving apples with stickers declaring "Grown in Washington State" easily erode the spirit of the FTC program. With improved tracking and traceability throughout local supply chains and a better understanding between distributors and dining staff, this kind of mix-up could be avoided, making the use of distributors a feasible approach in institutional sourcing of local foods. Conversely, some distributors may place demands on the institution, imposing contractual terms that establish themselves as sole distributor of certain products, thus preventing FTC programs altogether.

Another major barrier to FTC programs in New England is the seasonal availability of local products. Figure 1 shows that almost half of CFSC survey participants from the New England region identified this as a challenge for their dining operations; this is similar to the national survey results. Currently, Tufts' regular purchases of locally grown produce are limited to apples, pumpkin, squash, pears, peaches, nectarines, Swiss chard, and tomatoes. The tomatoes are sourced from a Maine farm that uses greenhouses to extend their vegetable season. Special events featuring local foods do bring more variety (eg, locally raised beef). Despite significant effort, however, Tufts' purchases of local produce account for about $85,000—less than 2% of what is spent on all food procurement at the university (Julie Lampie, e-mail communication, October 15, 2007). This accounts only for Tufts' produce purchases and does not include the amount spent on other local farm products (eg, dairy); there is much more potential to be realized.

One reason why most purchasing goes to nonlocal fruits and vegetables is a mismatch in the academic year (September–June) with the New England peak harvest season (June–September). For example, stone fruits from local orchards

would be a great alternative to the usual offering of bananas and apples in the dining halls; however, Tufts can only catch the tail end of local peach, plum, and pear production when the fall semester kicks off. One way to address this is through an annual "Summer Fruit Extravaganza" at the start of the academic year, but this 1-day event does not translate into huge economic benefits for the farmers and may not be worth their time for a 1-day sale. Cold storage could extend the season for these locally grown products. But most farmers need to sell their product within days of harvest because they lack cold storage facilities to maintain product quality for extended periods. Universities typically face the same constraint, so there is limited ability to keep food on-site for more than a few days. To add to these challenges, dining staff and students are largely unaware of production regions and seasons for fresh produce because they, along with the general population, have grown accustomed to an international flow of goods that has erased these previously known food facts. This lack of sensitivity translates in low expectations for farm fresh food.

Dining room consumers are not always knowledgeable about local sources.

Finding local growers is a significant barrier identified in the New England aggregate of the CFSC survey. Oftentimes, the burden of locating good sources for locally produced products falls upon a dining service staff member who has embraced the FTC program as a pet project. This means that there is little time to devote to seeking out the best quality and pricing that will truly fit the institution's needs. Quantity is a challenge in New England, where typical farms are small and diversified. This may make a distributor who is able to consolidate product from various farms attractive. However, the bundling of products from various farms may create problems of uniformity, as one farmer may grow Roma tomatoes while his neighbor grows Brandywine. Large-scale farming operations may provide some processing before delivery to the distributor or institution, meaning less labor for dining staff. For example, most large producers of California lettuce harvest, wash, and bag lettuce before distribution, whereas small New England growers do not. To overcome some of these barriers, a small working group was established at Tufts to help find new sources of goods from local farmers and facilitate conversation. Similarly, others have recognized the need for a "matching service" of sorts to connect farmers with institutions. A new online program, for example, Farm Fresh Rhode Island, allows farmers to post what will be harvested soon, allowing colleges to order in advance to fulfill their dining hall needs.[8]

A Strategy to Increase Student Demand

The most critical barrier to implementing a FTC program is not an operational characteristic but rather the drive of current students to demand and support the FTC effort. This was not mentioned explicitly in the barriers section of the CFCS survey; however, it has been voiced repeatedly by FTC leaders in New England at buy-local and related meetings. As discussed, the "good citizen" mission of our university has enabled the development of a modest FTC effort on campus. However, this "do good" motivator only goes so far and cannot compensate for the lack in student support for a buy-local program. Recognizing this reality, advocates of FTC programs have refocused their efforts on educating and mobilizing the student body. Activities have included developing a Web site on food options and sustainability initiatives, establishing an annual 1-day farmers' market on campus, serving an all locally grown menu during freshmen orientation events for subpopulations of likely supporters (eg, fitness club orientation), and a poster campaign.

The series of fun posters may be the most innovative effort. The posters display students endorsing alternative food choices, specifically locally grown, organic, and fair trade options. Students were chosen to be poster celebrities, with a calculation for diversity (eg, different academic majors, years, sex, ethnicity, sports, and club interests). In one, a senior biochemical engineering student juggles local fruits and vegetables and comments on why he supports buying local foods. In another example, a junior international relations major holds homemade pizza made from local ingredients. These and other posters are a new intervention, and the extent to which they have succeeded in raising awareness is unknown.

It may be prudent for FTC champions at colleges and universities to take a step back and reflect on the kind of student body and culture evident at their school. Campaigns should be tailored based on this information. The predominant undergraduate major at Tufts is international relations. Given this, events such as "Multicultural Night" should be targeted for FTC education. The university also has an immigrant farmer training program, providing the school an opportunity to feature ethnic dishes in dining halls made with items such as locally grown bitter melon and Chinese broccoli grown on satellite farms.

The Future of FTC Programs in New England

Institutional purchasing direct from farmers is catching on. According to CFSC, more than 768 school districts in 34 states have farm-to-school programs.[9] Regional supermarkets such as Hannaford Brothers and national retailers, ranging from "natural food" stores such as Whole Foods to the largest retailer in the world, Wal-Mart, have instituted varying degrees of buy-local in their operations. Healthcare management companies (eg, Kaiser Permanente) are beginning to partner with local hospitals to bring farmers markets and local produce to medical institutions. And now, more than 100 colleges and universities have begun or are seriously considering FTC programs.

But direct farm purchasing programs require serious effort. A solid foundation for FTC programs in the Northeast has been set, but much more must be done to ensure their success. The next steps range from revising institutional policies (eg, making terms of payment for direct purchases from farmers less than the 90 days and more in line with their needs of 30-day terms) to inspiring students to demand local products in their dining halls.

References

1. Shartin E. Movement toward more sustainable food systems is growing. *Boston Globe,* third edition. July 26, 2006:E2.
2. Hinrichs CC. The practice and politics of food system localization. *J Rural Stud.* 2003; 19:33–45.
3. The Public Health and Welfare. School lunch programs. Chapter 13. 42 USC §1758.
4. Caplan R. Memo to the Harrison Institute for Public Law on Preemption of Geographic Preferences in School Food Procurement. http://www.foodsecurity.org/HarrisonPreemptionAnalysis.doc. Accessed September 30, 2007.
5. Section 23B of Massachusetts General Law. Mass Stat Chap 7 §23*B*.
6. Section 5-60.4 of Oklahoma Statues. Oklahoma Stat Title 2 §5-60.4 on the development of nutrition plans using locally grown farm-fresh products in state school districts.
7. Community Food Security Coalition. http://www.farmtocollege.org/survey.htm. Accessed May 14, 2007.
8. Farm Fresh Rhode Island. RI fresh Network. http://www.farmfreshri.org/about/freshnetwork.php. Accessed October 15, 2007.
9. Community Food Security Coalition. National Farm to School program Web site. http://www.farmtoschool.org/. Accessed October 22, 2007.

KATHLEEN A. MERRIGAN, PhD, is an assistant professor and director of the Agriculture, Food, and Environment Program at the Friedman School of Nutrition Science and Policy at Tufts University. **MELISSA BAILEY,** MS, is a PhD candidate in the Agriculture, Food, and Environment Program at the Friedman School of Nutrition Science and Policy at Tufts University.

From *Nutrition Today,* August 2008, pp. 160–165. Copyright © 2008 by Lippincott, Williams & Wilkins/Wolters Kluwer Health. Reprinted by permission.

Produce to the People

Community gardens and farmers' markets challenge convenience stores and fast-food joints.

CONSTANCE MATTHIESSEN AND ANNE HAMERSKY

The United States may be the land of plenty, but in many parts of the country—particularly the low-income neighborhoods—fresh fruits and vegetables are hard-to-find luxury items. Grocery chains resist opening stores where sales of high-markup gourmet products can't be guaranteed, and they often close existing supermarkets in poor areas. For residents of these neighborhoods, the choice comes down to traveling long distances to buy groceries or shopping at expensive corner stores that sell high-fat, high-sugar convenience food and little or no fresh produce. The consequences are the wages of poverty: diabetes, obesity, and heart disease.

A quiet but powerful movement is tackling the problem by building "food security"—the ability to obtain safe, nutritious, high-quality food—in some of the poorest corners of the country. Inner-city kids get hands-on experiences of nature by turning trash-strewn vacant lots into bountiful community gardens. Parents campaign to get junk food out of public schools, and local farmers are invited to sell their produce directly to eager customers. Communities are determining for themselves how best to meet their food needs and, in doing so, are reaping benefits that go beyond the health effects of greens and fresh fruit. Here's how the food-security movement has blossomed in four California communities.

Fresno, California, is in the middle of one of the world's most abundant agricultural regions, the great Central Valley, which provides a quarter of the U.S. food supply. Still, many residents worry about their next meal. A 2005 report by the Brookings Institution found that Fresno has the highest concentration of poverty of any large city in the nation, and more than 85 percent of the children in its school system qualify for subsidized lunches. Food insecurity shows itself not in the lack of calories so much as in the overabundance of poor food choices: In Fresno County, 46 percent of ninth-graders and nearly two-thirds of adults are overweight.

Fresno Metro Ministry, an interfaith social-justice organization, is trying to reverse these trends by providing low-income people access to healthy food. "It's pretty basic," says Edie Jessup, FMM's Hunger and Nutrition Project coordinator. "Food, housing, healthcare—so many have to struggle to fulfill these basic needs. If they aren't met, people can't learn and grow and contribute."

Jessup and FMM recently worked with the local school district to adopt a "wellness policy" that promotes healthier school meals, bans soda from campuses, teaches nutrition, and encourages physical education. The group also helped expand the district's free-lunch program to the summer months. And after learning that weekly flea markets are a major source of produce for many of Fresno's poorest residents, FMM wrangled permission for them to use food stamps to buy directly from area farmers.

The centerpiece of FMM's efforts has been establishing community gardens throughout Fresno. These are particularly prized by the city's large population of Hmong refugees, rural people from the Laos area who sided with the United States in the Vietnam War and migrated here afterward. In Fresno, many Hmong live crowded into small apartments, barely scraping by on public assistance. Depression and other psychological problems are common, and childhood obesity and type 2 diabetes (often associated with poor diets) are on the rise.

But just give these former farmers access to some land. In small patches of ground tucked behind churches and strip malls, Fresno is blooming with lush, immaculate gardens of not only corn and beans but also lemongrass, ginger, and medicinal plants. The gardens allow Hmong families to exercise, work beside friends, and reconnect to the land, something many have missed since leaving their native country.

Still, waiting lists are long, and the gardens are impermanent. One was paved over by a local church to build, yes, a parking lot. "Where will my grandmother grow her food?" Jessup overheard one Hmong child ask. "And where will the butterflies go?"

Thirty-four acres of the former naval air base in Alameda, California, have made the transition from swords to plowshares and now provide a refuge for formerly homeless families. The architecture on the sprawling base on San Francisco Bay is serviceable, though military drab, and few trees interrupt the flat, wind-scoured landscape. But on a sunny spring day, the corner maintained by the Alameda Point Collaborative (APC) is idyllic. At one end of a street of scrubbed and neat cookie-cutter houses, a color-splashed flower bed flourishes; at the other, a community garden.

Not far away, APC's community center buzzes with activity as some of the 500 residents (half of them children) gather for the monthly group dinner, prepared in part from produce grown in the garden. The center offers classes in parenting, cooking, and gardening, as well as job training and childcare. Teens gather in front, talking excitedly. Dressed in T-shirts, sweatshirts, and baggy pants, they would fit in on any urban street corner—except, perhaps, for the topic of their conversation. Farell Williams, a tall 16-year-old with a cherubic face, is showing the others a tremendous cabbage he just picked from the garden, explaining how he's going to cut it up for a stir-fry. Williams wants to be a chef and plans to take cooking classes over the summer.

Williams's dreams are due in large part to Kate Casale, who directs APC's Growing Youth Project and clearly loves her job. She supervises the teens with respect, affection, and occasional exasperation. They are adolescents, after all, many of whom grew up in the Bay Area's toughest neighborhoods. Their families lived on the streets and in shelters, and some kids were victims of domestic violence.

Casale is impressed by how hard the teens work—and how much they've learned. "Half of what we teach them is about turning in a time sheet, being on time, showing up," she says. "It's been amazing to watch how much they've grown."

Seventeen-year-old Dawn Caraway was homeless for four years before she and her mother moved to Alameda. "I was never able to let go or let my guard down before I came here," she says. "I always lived in cities before; I had no experience of nature. Now I found out I like growing things, working in the garden. To me, this is heaven on Earth."

Neelam Sharma got involved in food security over lunch—her son's, to be precise. Ten years ago, Sharma and her family moved from England to South Central Los Angeles. Even though her son, Lawrence, qualified for the free-lunch program at his middle school, she noticed that he was always hungry after school. The meals were awful, he told her, so awful that he couldn't eat them.

Sharma, who is small and intense and speaks with an elegant British accent, went to Lawrence's school to see for herself. "The food was all heavily processed and unpleasant-looking," she recalls. "Kids were taking one or two bites and throwing the rest away. The only fresh fruit were these tasteless apples, all mangly and waxy-skinned."

Working with several other parents, Sharma started the Healthy School Food Coalition to improve the district's nutrition programs. It was clear to Sharma that the problem of food quality in South Central extended beyond the schools. "I had to leave my community to find quality, affordable produce," she says. "Few grocery stores choose to locate here, so it's no wonder people in South Central are disproportionately plagued with diet-related diseases—diseases that are striking at younger and younger ages."

Today Sharma works with an organization called Community Services Unlimited, overseeing its food-security program. CSU has built gardens at two South Central schools and runs five more mini urban farms, plus a produce market.

CSU found that two-thirds of the merchants who own corner stores in the neighborhood would be willing to sell fresh produce if the group handled the logistics. So CSU purchased an old school bus, converted it to run on biodiesel, and plans to use it to deliver produce later this year.

Even though her program struggles financially—Sharma gives most of her small salary to the youth she's hired—she isn't discouraged. "From the kindergartner who beams when she sees that her radish seed has germinated to the adult who jumps up and down when his bean seeds sprout—every reconnection to the earth makes it all worthwhile."

On a sunny spring day in Oakland, California, food security has the sound, taste, and smell of a really great party. The Mo' Better farmers' market is small, with just a dozen vendors, but vibrant: Old-school soul music competes with the latest rap, and the air is scented by barbecue and grilled vegetables. Making sure everything runs smoothly is teacher and community activist David Roach, who helped establish the market in 1998 through the Mo' Better Food program.

"Black farmers are losing land at five times the rate of other farmers," Roach says. "Part of the problem is that there are so few markets for their food in black communities." Roach and Mo' Better are trying to change that by running this farmers' market, distributing fresh produce to corner shops, and establishing two local grocery stores.

When he was a kid, Roach says, Oakland's black community had more of a connection to the land. Many people had gardens, and friends who stopped by for a visit seldom left without a bag of greens or plums from the backyard tree.

"If you lose something," Roach says, "you want to get it back." As activists work to bring fresh, nutritious produce to neighborhoods around the country, they are creating not just food security but stronger, healthier communities as well.

CONSTANCE MATTHIESSEN is a San Francisco writer and journalist. ANNE HAMERSKY'S last feature for Sierra was *"Who Grows Your Food? (And Why It Matters)"* (November/December 2004).

Veggies In The Hood—The Community Food Security Coalition, based in Venice, California, is the umbrella organization for food-security efforts across the country. The coalition has 325 member groups in the United States and Canada, including social-justice, religious, environmental, labor, and antipoverty organizations. It provides education and training and holds an annual conference. For more information, visit foodsecurity.org.

UNIT 2
Nutrients

Unit Selections

10. **Color Me Healthy: Eating for a Rainbow of Benefits,** Julian Schaeffer
11. **Antioxidants: Fruitful Research and Recommendations,** Pamela Brummit
12. **Confusion at the Vitamin Counter: Too Little or Too Much?,** Bonnie Liebman
13. **Minerals Matter: The Wrong Amounts Can Harm You,** *Consumer Reports on Health*
14. **Fiber Free-for-All,** *Nutrition Action Health Letter*
15. **The Fairest Fats of Them All (and Those to Avoid),** Sharon Palmer
16. **Omega-3 Madness,** Bonnie Liebman

Key Points to Consider

- What color is your diet? List foods that you eat that are naturally dark orange, red, yellow, green, and purple. Think of ways that you can improve the color quality of your diet.

- Identify the four nutrients that function as antioxidants. Then identify the best sources of these nutrients in foods that you commonly eat.

- Why do Americans consume so many supplements rather than getting their nutrition from foods?

- Identify the three bad fats and food sources of each.

- Which fats and oils are highest in monounsaturated fats?

Student Website

www.mhhe.com/cls

Internet References

Dole 5 a Day: Nutrition, Fruits & Vegetables
www.dole.com/#?superkids.com

Food and Nutrition Information Center
www.nal.usda.gov/fnic

NutritionalSupplements.com
www.nutritionalsupplements.com

U.S. National Library of Medicine
www.nlm.nih.gov

As the greatest segment of the U.S. population ages, demand for health and nutrition information, supplements, and magic bullets is at an all time high. Because of this increased awareness and interest in health and disease prevention, the media meets this demand for stories of a late breaking, new ideas about nutrition and health. Media outlets often report sensational, even erroneous, data, which confuses the public and creates misunderstandings. Preliminary reports of nutrition and health research have to undergo rigorous testing in cell and animal models and then clinical trials before they are accepted and implemented by the scientific community. This is a difficult situation considering information is so readily available to the U.S. public. The time that is required to produce sound scientific findings contradicts the expectation of Americans being able to get the correct answer within a mouse click.

The articles of this unit have been selected to present current knowledge about macronutrients, micronutrients, and phytochemicals. Articles addressing the function of nutrients and bioactive food components and their effects on chronic disease are also included. Many of these articles provide the best food sources and compare the bioavailability of these nutrients in supplement versus natural form.

Historically, the health benefits of foods have been explained by vitamins, minerals, fiber, and protein. Research on other bioactive food components, such as phytochemicals, provides yet another aspect to the benefit of eating a variety natural colors of plant-based foods. The first two articles in this unit discuss antioxidants and the best food sources for these naturally occurring promoters of health. The second article simplifies the message of variety by encouraging us to eat a rainbow of natural colors (not the artificial colors that are found in most processed foods with color).

The importance of vitamins is of great interest to consumers since vitamins have been touted to cure and/or prevent disease. As the baby boomers are aging, diseases that affect their bones, immune system, and predispose them to diabetes and cancer are of great concern. With more than 40 percent of Americans taking supplements, and the exponential scientific evidence as to their functions, consumers are confused as to which vitamin and how much of it to take. Since foods have been recently fortified with folic acid, consumers need to be cautious of high folic acid consumption.

Mineral nutrition has been associated with the development and progress of many diseases. The mistaken thoughts of "more must be better" does not apply to mineral consumption. There is confusion about daily doses for prevention versus therapeutic doses for diseases. Inadequate, excessive, and adequate intake of calcium, magnesium, potassium, sodium, iron, selenium, zinc, and chromium are presented and discussed in this section.

The beneficial effects of naturally occurring fibers on cardiovascular disease, diabetes, colon cancer, obesity, and regularity have been documented. The food industry is responding to consumer demand by adding isolated fiber in foods that do not naturally contain fiber even though there is scant evidence of beneficial effects of this form of fiber on degenerative disease.

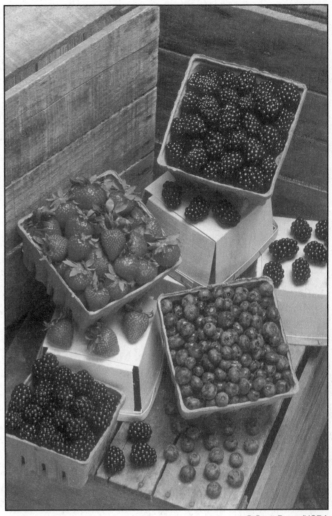

© Scott Bauer/USDA

One of the main health messages elicited in the 1990s was "fat is bad." The next decade ushered in the "carbs are bad" era, and thankfully we now consider the nutrient density or quality of a food rather than just eliminating an entire macronutrient group. The article by Sharon Palmer addresses the difference in bad fats and good fats and provides an Oil Primer that reviews the different oils available in the U.S. market, their fatty acid components, and practical information about the oils that will help you add the healthier oils to your diet.

Another topic of current interests is omega-3 fatty acids and the best source for these beneficial fats. Demand for supplements and fortified foods containing omega 3s has culminated in a vast number of products on the market. Since the metabolic pathways of these PUFAs are complex, there is a great deal of confusion when it comes to information presented on the label and in the media. One of the articles in this section provides advice on how to intelligently interpret the claims about omega-3 fatty acids. Another article discusses the difference between omega 3s from flax seed oil versus fish oil.

Color Me Healthy
Eating for a Rainbow of Benefits

Got the blues? Not your mood, your food! While you're at it, make sure you also have reds, yellows, and other bright colors on your plate.

JULIANN SCHAEFFER

Beige may be a mainstay in many wardrobes because of its versatility, but when it relates to diet, simply beige is all the rage for all the wrong reasons. Americans' affinity for all that is quick, cheap, and convenient is directing many to the cracker, cereal, and cookie aisles, leading to a high-fat and highly processed "beige diet" that is nutrient impaired.

According to Susan Bowerman, MS, RD, CSSD, a lecturer in the department of food science and nutrition at Cal Poly San Luis Obispo and coauthor of *What Color Is Your Diet?* a purely beige diet may fill Americans up now, but it could cost them later.

"We eat foods primarily based on their taste, their cost, and how convenient they are," she notes. "The food manufacturers have done a great job of creating many foods that are easy to eat, inexpensive, and rich in sugar, fat, and salt so that they taste good. Starches, fats, and sweets are the least expensive foods in the diet, so it's easy to see why we lean toward these 'brown/beige' foods. They fill us up for very little monetary cost, but there are significant health costs to a diet that is so high in refined carbohydrates and devoid of the vitamins, minerals, fiber, and phytochemicals that are so abundant in plant foods."

Americans' fondness for foods lacking color also reflects a metaphor of what else is lacking in processed foods: phytochemicals. While some processed foods may reincorporate key nutrients during processing, "Many of the flavonoids, tannins, etc are not replaced during processing," says Susan Kasik-Miller, MS, RD, CNSC, a clinical dietitian at Sacred Heart Hospital in Eau Claire, Wis. "The metaphor also holds for the look of our diet. Literature references bland beige swill as the only food offered to suffering people. A colorful, balanced diet is associated with good health and prosperity."

Phytochemical-Filled Produce

So what does color have to do with diet anyway? One word: phytochemicals. These substances occur naturally only in plants and may provide health benefits beyond those that essential nutrients provide. Color, such as what makes a blueberry so blue, can indicate some of these substances, which are thought to work synergistically with vitamins, minerals, and fiber (all present in fruits and vegetables) in whole foods to promote good health and lower disease risk.

According to information from the Produce for Better Health Foundation (PBH), phytochemicals may act as antioxidants, protect and regenerate essential nutrients, and/or work to deactivate cancer-causing substances. And while research has not yet determined exactly how these substances work together or which combination offers specific benefits, including a rainbow of colored foods in a diet plan ensures a variety of those nutrients and phytochemicals.

"Plant products are sources for phytochemicals of which there are thousands that have been identified," explains Kasik-Miller. "These chemicals are known to have disease-preventing properties, but the color of a food does not necessarily mean it contains one particular phytochemical class. Foods contain multiple phytochemicals, as well as vitamins and minerals, and it is not known how many other phytochemicals await to be identified and what functions they have with health."

Kathy Hoy, EdD, RD, nutrition research manager for the PBH, says eating a variety of foods helps ensure the intake of an assortment of nutrients and other healthful substances in food, such as phytochemicals, noting that color can be a helpful guide for consumers. "Nutrients and phytochemicals appear to work synergistically, so maintaining a varied, colorful diet with healthful whole foods is a pragmatic approach to optimal nutrition."

"Tomatoes help support the health of prostate and breast tissue," adds Bowerman.

And although some nutrients, such as vitamin C, are diminished with the introduction of heat, Hoy says, "The benefits of eating produce are not dependent on eating raw foods. In fact, cooking enhances the activity of some phytochemicals, such as lycopene. Obtaining optimal benefit from the nutrients in food, especially produce, depends on proper selection, storage, and cooking of the produce."

Cooked tomato sauces are associated with greater health benefits compared with the uncooked version because the heating process allows all carotenoids, including lycopene, to be more easily absorbed by the body, according to information from the PBH.

"In addition to vitamin C and folate, red fruits and vegetables are also sources of flavonoids, which reduce inflammation and have antioxidant properties. Cranberries, another red fruit [whose color is due to anthocyanins, not lycopene], are also a good source of tannins, which prevent bacteria from attaching to cells," says Kasik-Miller of more reasons to relish red.

Examples: Tomatoes and tomato products, watermelon, pink grapefruit, guava, cranberries.

Yellow/Orange

Behind the color: "We had an orange/yellow group representing beta-cryptoxanthin and vitamin C," says Bowerman. "Our orange group foods are also rich in beta-carotene, which are particularly good antioxidants."

Beta-cryptoxanthin, beta-carotene, and alpha-carotene are all orange-friendly carotenoids and can be converted in the body to vitamin A, a nutrient integral for vision and immune function, as well as skin and bone health, according to information from the PBH.

"These foods are commonly considered the eyesight foods because they contain vitamin A. Beta-carotene, which can be converted into vitamin A, is a component of these foods as well. In addition, they may have high levels of vitamin C, and some contain omega-3 fatty acids," says Kasik-Miller.

Since eyesight is dependent on the presence of vitamin A, Kasik-Miller notes that it is considered the "vision vitamin." "Other [phyto]chemicals typically found in yellow/orange fruits and vegetables protect our eyes from cataracts and have anti-inflammatory properties. They also help with blood sugar regulation," she adds.

Tsang notes that the beta-carotenes in some orange fruits and vegetables may also play a part in preventing cancer, particularly of the lung, esophagus, and stomach. "They may also reduce the risk of heart disease and improve immune function," she says.

```
┌─────────────────────────────────────────────┐
│ Menu                                         │
│ ▬▬▬▬▬▬▬▬▬▬▬▬▬▬▬▬▬▬▬▬▬▬▬▬▬▬▬▬▬▬▬               │
│                                              │
│ Breakfast                                    │
│ Cereal with dried fruit and low-fat milk     │
│ Glass of 100% fruit juice                    │
│ Whole grain toast with fruit spread          │
│                                              │
│ Lunch                                        │
│ Vegetable soup                               │
│ Sandwich with lettuce, tomato, peppers, and  │
│   olives                                     │
│ Fresh fruit in season (or canned fruit in    │
│   juice)                                     │
│ Low-fat milk                                 │
│                                              │
│ Snack                                        │
│ Fruit muffin, dried fruit, or whole wheat    │
│   bagel with peanut butter                   │
│                                              │
│ Dinner                                       │
│ Black bean burritos with avocado slices and  │
│   lettuce                                    │
│ Brown rice with tomatoes Fruit salad         │
│                                              │
│ —Menu Provided By Susan Kasik-Miller, MS,    │
│   RD, CNSC.                                   │
└─────────────────────────────────────────────┘
```

Examples: Carrots, mangos, cantaloupe, winter squash, sweet potatoes, pumpkins, apricots.

No Color? No Problem

While color can give clients a general idea about what lies beneath eggplant's exterior, a food's hue does not tell all, and it is certainly not an exclusive indicator of phytochemical content. While some phytochemicals are pigments that give color, others are colorless.

"The largest class of phytochemicals are the flavonoids, which for the most part are colorless," explains Bowerman. "Flavonoids are powerful antioxidants, and these help the body to counteract free-radical formation. When free-radical damage goes unchecked, it can cause significant damage to body cells and tissues."

There are more than 4,000 different flavonoids, and according to information from the PBH, they are classified into the following categories:

- flavonols:
  -myricetin (in berries, grapes, parsley, and spinach);
  -quercetin (in onions, apples, broccoli, cranberries, and grapes);
- flavones:
  -apigenin (in celery, lettuce, and parsley);
  -luteolin (in beets, bell peppers, and Brussels sprouts);

- flavanones:
  -hesperetin and naringenin (both in citrus fruits and juices);
- flavan-3-ols:
  -catechin (in tea, red wine, and dark chocolate);
  -epicatechin, gallate, epigallocatechin, and epigallocatechin gallate (in teas, fruits, and legumes); and
- anthocyanidins (in blue/purple and red fruits and vegetables).

Although not enough research has been conducted to definitively match specific phytochemicals with particular benefits, researchers are currently investigating flavonoids' effect on lowering the risk of cardiovascular disease and several types of cancer and their role in promoting lung health and protecting against asthma.

Eat Your Colors

The concept of suggesting that clients eat a certain color ratio of foods may be premature, but Hoy says the take-away message is that including a variety of colors in one's diet seems to equal better overall health, especially in relation to produce. "Epidemio-logical research suggests that food patterns that include fruits and vegetables are associated with lower risk for some diseases, and a recent article suggested that more variety in fruit and vegetable intake was associated with a lower risk for pharyngeal and laryngeal cancers, suggesting that variety may also be another important factor to consider. However, it is not known if there is an optimal ratio of colors to be consumed or what that is," says Hoy.[2,3]

Kasik-Miller agrees: "At this time, scientists are not sure what proportion of phytochemicals is the right balance for disease prevention. There have been studies where specific antioxidants were given and there was an increase in the disease rate. To make recommendations to eat a specific number of servings of beets or blueberries is premature; eat what looks good and you can afford. Foods of the same color do not necessarily contain the same vitamins, minerals, or phytochemicals, so recommendations to eat specific amounts of colored foods is impossible."

And considering that the majority of individuals are not meeting current recommendations for fruit and vegetable intake, encouraging consumers to use color as a guide for increasing produce consumption is a good strategy, Hoy says.[1]

What's the best way to convey this message to clients? Instead of delving into a complex and complicated conversation about phytochemicals, Molly Morgan, RD, CDN, owner of Creative Nutrition Solutions, says the more matters idea can easily be tweaked to more color matters. "I believe consumers can do better by consciously trying to include many different colors in their eating plan rather than getting stuck on what colors do what. Each color provides various health benefits and no one color is superior to another, which is why I believe a balance of all colors is most important," she says.

"I think the color approach that we used in *What Color Is Your Diet?* resonated well with people because intuitively they knew that colors equal health and that the more colors that were eaten, the better it probably was to overall health," says Bowerman of getting this message out to the masses. "Educating people as to the health benefits is a start, but they also have to be willing to try new foods or new varieties of foods—or maybe to prepare unfamiliar foods in a way that will make them taste good—so that they will be willing to add more plant foods to their diet."

Once people are aware of this dietary color concept, Hoy says creativity can go a long way. "Creatively including fruits and vegetables at meals will help them to include a wide range of different foods. In addition to simple things like adding fruits or vegetables to casseroles, cereal, or sandwiches, being open to trying new foods, recipes, or meal patterns will help to increase variety," she says. "Other ways to increase variety would include making fruits and vegetables more center of the plate when planning meals, including a fruit and/or vegetable at every eating occasion, adding an extra fruit and/or vegetable side dish to meals, and substituting fruits, vegetables, and beans for other ingredients such as meat in recipes."

Planning ahead is Morgan's mantra, and she recommends challenging clients to take notice of color when grocery shopping. She says to tell clients, "Challenge yourself to look at your cart when leaving the produce section, and if you have all red items, head back and swap something out for another color. For example, if you had strawberries, watermelon, and tomatoes, swap the strawberries for some oranges."

And since winter is fast approaching and the season is swinging away from some of the colorful foods familiar to consumers, such as blueberries and strawberries, Kasik-Miller says a trip to the farmers' market may be warranted. "Also, people need to get into the habit of cooking at home," she says. "If you are not sure about what to do with a colorful food or are looking for a new way to eat it, go to the grower's association Web site to get recipes and new ways to eat foods. I think people need to be more creative with how they prepare foods. People know they need lots of color in their diet but find it hard to change food habits. They need to make small changes over a period of time to achieve success."

While there may not be much to compare between dinner and Dior, it seems this much is true: There appears to be more reason to eat the spectrum of colors than to wear them.

Notes

1. Cook AJ, Friday JE. *Pyramid Servings Intakes in the United States 1999–2002, 1 Day.* Beltsville, Md.: USDA, Agricultural Research Service, Community Nutrition Research Group. 2005. Available at: http://www.ars.usda.gov/sp2UserFiles/Place/12355000/foodlink/ts_3-0.pdf

2. Garavello W, Giordano L, Bosetti C, et al. Diet diversity and the risk of oral and pharyngeal cancer. *Eur J Nutr.* 2008;47(5):280–284.

3. Garavello W, Lucenteforte E, Bosetti C, et al. Diet diversity and the risk of laryngeal cancer: A case-control study from Italy and Switzerland. *Oral Oncol.* 2008; Epub ahead of print.

Resource

Produce for Better Health Foundation:
www.pbhfoundation.org, www.fruitsandveggiesmorematters.org

JULIANN SCHAEFFER is an editorial assistant at *Today's Dietitian.*

Antioxidants: Fruitful Research and Recommendations

PAMELA S. BRUMMIT, MA, RD/LD

Free radicals, which are produced during food metabolism and by external factors such as radiation and smog, can damage cells and may contribute to some diseases—notably heart disease and cancer—and many experts believe antioxidants can help prevent this damage.

The body's immune system helps defend against oxidative stress. As we age, this defense becomes less effective, which contributes to poor health. Clinical studies hypothesize that when we consume antioxidants, we provide our bodies with protection and health benefits.

Antioxidants Defined

The USDA identifies beta-carotene (vitamin A), selenium, vitamin C, vitamin E, lutein, and lycopene as antioxidant substances.

Lycopene is a pigment that gives vegetables and fruits such as tomatoes, pink grapefruit, and watermelon their red hue. Several studies suggest that consuming foods rich in lycopene is associated with a lower risk of prostate cancer and cardiovascular disease. Lycopene is better absorbed when consumed in processed tomato products rather than in fresh tomatoes.

Selenium is a trace mineral that is essential to good health but required only in small amounts. Its antioxidant properties help prevent cellular damage from free radicals. Plant foods are the major dietary sources of selenium, but the content in a particular food depends on the selenium content of the soil where it's grown. Soils in the high plains of northern Nebraska and the Dakotas have very high levels of selenium.

Lutein is found in large amounts in the lens and retina of our eyes and is recognized for its eye health benefits. It may also protect against damage caused by UVB light and is a critical component to overall skin health. Lutein is found naturally in foods such as dark green, leafy vegetables and egg yolks.

The antioxidant function of beta-carotene (precursor to vitamin A) is its ability to reduce free radicals and protect the cell membrane lipids from the harmful effects of oxidation.

In addition, beta-carotene may provide some synergism to vitamin E.

As a water-soluble antioxidant, vitamin C reduces free radicals before they can damage the lipids. These antioxidant properties fight free radicals that can promote wrinkles, age spots, cataracts, and arthritis. Also, the antioxidants in vitamin C have been found to fight free radicals that prey on organs and blood vessels.

As an antioxidant, vitamin E may help prevent or delay cardiovascular disease and cancer and has been shown to play a role in immune function. DNA repair, and other metabolic processes.

Fruits and vegetables, nuts, grains, poultry, and fish are major sources of antioxidants.

Research

Researchers have studied antioxidants and disease processes for years. Some studies have found that an increased intake of beta-carotene is associated with decreased cardiovascular mortality in older adult populations. Studies on the effects of vitamin E on aging have shown potential relationships between the vitamin and the prevention of atherosclerosis, cancer, cataracts, arthritis, central nervous system disorders such as Parkinson's disease, Alzheimer's disease, and impaired glucose tolerance. Studies on vitamin C suggest that it may help protect against vascular dementia, and studies on selenium point to its potential role in cancer prevention.[1-3] Beta-carotene, vitamin C, and vitamin E showed a positive improvement in muscle strength and may improve physical performance in older adults.[4]

One lycopene study found that eating 10 or more servings per week of tomato products was associated with up to a 35% reduced risk of prostate cancer. Another study suggested that men who had the highest amount of lycopene in their body fat were one half as likely to suffer a heart attack as those with the least amount. Numerous studies correlate a high intake of lycopene-containing foods or high lycopene serum levels with reduced incidence of cancer, cardiovascular disease, and macular degeneration. However, estimates of lycopene consumption have been based on reported tomato intake, not on the use of lycopene supplements. Since tomatoes are sources of other nutrients, including vitamin C, folate, and potassium, it is unclear whether lycopene itself is beneficial.[5-7]

Some researchers suggest that eliminating free radicals may actually interfere with a natural defense mechanism within the body. Large doses of antioxidants may keep immune systems from fighting off invading pathogens.

Three out of four intervention trials using high-dose beta-carotene supplements did not show protective effects against cancer or cardiovascular disease. Rather, the high-risk population (smokers and asbestos workers) showed an increase in cancer and angina cases. It appears that beta-carotene can promote health when taken at dietary levels but may have adverse effects when taken in high doses by subjects who smoke or who have been exposed to asbestos.[8]

Results from one study indicate that antioxidant supplementation may not be beneficial for disease prevention. This study showed no consistent, clear evidence for health effects. However, the preliminary studies suggest antioxidants may block the heart-damaging effects of oxygen on arteries and the cell damage that might encourage some kinds of cancer.[9]

There remains a lack of knowledge regarding the safety of long-term mega-doses of vitamins. Research continues to be inconclusive and the data incomplete. Research has not been able to validate a link between oxidative stress and chronic disease. As with all research, the studies have been too diverse to provide conclusions.

Recommendations

The American Dietetic Association and the American Heart Association (AHA) recommend that people eat a variety of nutrient-rich foods from all of the food groups on a daily basis because this provides necessary nutrients, including antioxidants. Some researchers believe antioxidants are effective only when they are consumed in foods that contain them.

The recognized beneficial roles that fruits and vegetables play in the reduced risk of disease has led health organizations to develop programs encouraging consumers to eat more antioxidant-rich fruits and vegetables. The AHA and the American Cancer Society recommend that healthy adults eat five or more servings per day. The World Cancer Research Fund and the American Institute for Cancer Research report that "evidence of dietary protection against cancer is strongest and most consistent for diets high in vegetables and fruits."

Given the high degree of scientific consensus regarding the benefits of a diet high in fruits and vegetables—particularly those that contain dietary fiber and vitamins A and C—the FDA released a health claim for fruits and vegetables in relation to cancer. Food packages that meet FDA criteria may now carry the claim, "Diets low in fat and high in fruits and vegetables may reduce the risk of some cancers." The FDA also released a dietary guidance message for consumers: "Diets rich in fruits and vegetables may reduce the risk of some types of cancer and other chronic diseases." The 2005 Dietary Guidelines for Americans states, "Increased intakes of fruits, vegetables, whole grains, and fat-free or low-fat milk and milk products are likely to have important health benefits for most Americans."

Antioxidant research continues to grow and emerge as researchers discover new, beneficial components of food. Reinforced by current research, the message remains that antioxidants obtained from food sources, including fruits, vegetables, and whole grains, may reduce disease risk and can benefit human health.

Using the latest research technologies, USDA nutrition scientists measured the antioxidant levels in more than 100 different foods, including fruits, vegetables, nuts, dried fruits, spices, and cereals. The top 20 ranked foods that interfere with or prevent damage from free radicals are artichokes (cooked), black beans, black plums, blackberries, cranberries, cultivated blueberries, Gala apples, Granny Smith apples, pecans, pinto beans, plums, prunes, raspberries, Red Delicious apples, red kidney beans, Russet potatoes (cooked), small red beans, strawberries, sweet cherries, and wild blueberries.

How can we encourage older adults to eat more fruits and vegetables, especially those high in antioxidants? Share this helpful list with your older adult clients and patients.

1. Try one new fruit or vegetable per week. Variety is key!
2. Keep washed, ready-to-eat fruits and vegetables on hand and easily accessible. On the run? Take a bag of fruits or vegetables with you to munch on.
3. Serve fruits and vegetables with other favorite foods.
4. Add vegetables to casseroles, stews, and soups and puréed fruits and vegetables to sauces. Include vegetables in sandwiches and pastas.
5. Sprinkle vegetables with Parmesan cheese or top with melted low-fat cheese or white sauce made with low-fat milk.
6. Experiment with different methods of cooking fruits and vegetables.
7. Enjoy vegetables with low-fat dip for a snack.
8. Try commercial prepackaged salads and stir-fry mixes to save time.
9. Drink 100% fruit juice instead of fruit-flavored drinks or soda.
10. Serve fruit for dessert.
11. Keep a bowl of apples, bananas, and/or oranges on the dining room table.
12. Choose a side salad made with a variety of leafy greens.
13. Bake with raisin, date, or prune purée to reduce fat intake and increase fiber consumption.
14. Order vegetable toppings on your pizza.

15. Sip fruit smoothies for breakfast or snacks. Blend papaya with pineapple for a cool afternoon treat, or sip on a glass of fresh tomato juice at dinner.

16. Make a fruit salad to try many different types of fruit at once.

17. Learn to recognize a serving of fruits and vegetables: a medium-sized piece of fruit or ½ cup of most fresh, canned, or cooked fruits and vegetables.

18. Start your day with fruit. For example, add fruit to cereal or yogurt or pile on waffles. Or add vegetables—tomatoes, onions, potatoes—to an omelet or scrambled eggs.

19. Top meat and fish with salsa made from tomatoes, onions, corn, mangos, or other fruits and vegetables.

20. Try vegetarian choices: Vegetable stir fry, bean burrito, etc.

PAMELA S. BRUMMIT, **MA, RD/LD**, is the founder and president of Brummit & Associates, Inc, a dietary consulting firm. She has held more than 20 board positions in local, state, and national dietetic associations and is past chair of Consultant Dietitians in Health Care Facilities dietetic practice group.

Confusion at the Vitamin Counter
Too Little or Too Much?

BONNIE LIEBMAN

Forty percent of Americans take vitamins. Odds are, 95 percent of them are confused about exactly what to take.

That's partly because the marketplace is a riot of come-ons and claims that have no relationship to the science. And it's partly because the science keeps changing. Here's the latest on three nutrients that aren't what scientists expected.

The Risk of Too Much
Folic Acid

Up until the last few years, nearly all the news about folic acid was good.

In the late 1990s, the evidence was clear: The B vitamin could lower the risk of neural tube birth defects like spina bifida (an open spine) and anencephaly (no brain).

But the defects occur before most women know that they are pregnant. To protect the one-out-of-two pregnancies that are unplanned, the Food and Drug Administration required bakers to add enough folic acid to "enriched" white flour to raise the average intake by an estimated 70 to 120 micrograms a day.

It worked.

"In the U.S., fortification has prevented 1,500 to 2,000 kids from being born with devastating neural tube defects per year," says Joel Mason, director of the Vitamins and Carcinogenesis Laboratory at the Jean Mayer U.S. Department of Agriculture Human Nutrition Research Center on Aging at Tufts University in Boston.

Meanwhile, researchers launched trials to see whether high doses of folic acid could cut the risk of cancer, heart attacks, and strokes, as studies suggested.

They didn't.

Folic acid didn't prevent heart disease, according to an analysis of 12 trials, though it seemed to lower stroke rates in one study.[1,2] And last December, the news got worse.

Researchers reported on the follow-up of a three-year trial that had given either a placebo or 1,000 micrograms a day of folic acid to roughly 1,000 people who had already had a precancerous polyp (adenoma) removed from their colon or rectum.

"We saw what looked like an increased risk of advanced adenomas in people who got folic acid," says co-author John Baron, a professor of medicine at Dartmouth School of Medicine in Hanover, New Hampshire. And more folic acid takers (10 percent) than placebo takers (4 percent) had at least three new adenomas.[3]

What's more, more folic acid takers (11 percent) than placebo takers (6 percent) were diagnosed with a cancer outside the colon or rectum. Most were in the prostate.

"In a sample of 600 people, that's the only cancer—other than non-melanoma skin cancer—that's common enough to look at," says Baron.

Joel Mason wasn't entirely surprised.

"We have pretty compelling data that *adequate* folic acid protects against certain cancers, particularly colorectal cancer," he explains. "But eight to ten years ago, we started seeing that an *abundant* quantity of folic acid might accelerate carcinogenesis in animal studies, and now data from human studies is starting to emerge."

In fact, the first hints showed up decades earlier. "In the 1940s, Sidney Farber gave high doses of folic acid to leukemia patients," says Mason. Instead of curbing the abnormal proliferation of the cancer cells, "he got a tremendous expansion of the leukemia cells."

(Farber went on to test a drug that blocks folic acid, launching the first successful treatment of childhood leukemia.)

Folic acid's impact on cancer makes sense. "It's necessary for the synthesis of DNA," explains Mason. In fact, our bodies use folic acid to make thymidine, the building block of DNA that's in shortest supply.

"Cells need to produce DNA every time they divide," he adds. "So it's no surprise that folic acid can accelerate carcinogenesis in people who harbor cancer or precancerous cells."

Mason recently published data showing that colorectal cancer rates rose soon after companies started adding folic acid to foods.[4] "The increase meant 15,000 extra cases of colorectal cancer per year," he notes. "But it's just a hypothesis. We have yet to prove that folic acid fortification was responsible for the upswing in the 1990s."

Among the other explanations: "It's possible," says Mason, "that a surge in the use of colonoscopies meant that more cancers were found," not that there were more cancers.

And Baron's trial raises the specter that folic acid may promote other cancers. "A very large proportion of elderly men are harboring indolent prostate tumors that slowly churn along over decades," says Mason. Most die of other causes and don't know they have the tumors.

"If you give large quantities of folic acid to individuals with existing cancers, it may get the cancers revved up."

A recent study found a higher risk of advanced prostate cancer in men who took multivitamins more than seven times a week, though another study found no higher risk among men who got at least 640 micrograms of folic acid a day.[5,6]

Another worry: The Prostate, Lung, Colorectal, and Ovarian Cancer Screening Trial (PLCO) recently found a 19 percent higher risk of breast cancer in postmenopausal women who were taking at least 400 mcg a day of folic acid from supplements.[7]

In contrast, a recent Swedish study found a lower risk of breast cancer in women who consumed the most folic acid. But "the most" is much less in Sweden, where flour isn't fortified.[8]

"The Swedish women with the highest intake were consuming only about 380 to 400 mcg per day," says Mason. "But in the PLCO study, the group taking the most folic acid averaged 850 mcg a day. Maybe folic acid only enhances the growth of tumors when you exceed a threshold."

If so, older people should be most concerned. "Colorectal, prostate, and breast cancer occur as we age," says Mason. "I'm concerned that older people are harboring precancerous lesions and that folic acid may accelerate their growth."

That has left experts unsure about the wisdom of adding folic acid to flour, especially when some advocates of reducing birth defects want those levels raised.

"The worst possible case is where involuntary intake of folic acid benefits some people and harms others," says Baron. "But we don't know if we're there yet."

Two more trials that gave folic acid to people with adenomas should be published soon. "In one trial, it wasn't good or bad, and the second hasn't released any results publicly," says Baron. But both trials lasted only three years. Baron's trial found no harm until people were followed for six years.

What to do in the meantime? "People shouldn't be concerned about foods—like leafy green vegetables—that are naturally rich in folate," says Mason. Folate is absorbed less efficiently than the folic acid that's added to pills and fortified foods.

That's where the micrograms start to add up, especially in fortified breakfast cereals and in multivitamins, which usually have 400 mcg of folic acid. "If you take a supplement, it's not that difficult to reach 800 mcg a day," says Mason.

Neither Mason nor Baron has urged people to stop taking a multi.

"I think it's reasonable to say don't go overboard," says Baron. "My guess is that taking 400 mcg a day in a multivitamin is probably safe."

But, he adds, "when we're exposing people to something that could be harmful, it's not a time to be guessing."

THE BOTTOM LINE
If you take a daily multivitamin with 400 mcg of folic acid (100% of the Daily Value), don't eat (on a daily basis) a cereal, energy bar, or other food that contains 400 mcg (in the serving *you* eat).

Selenium

The Nutritional Prevention of Cancer Study (NPC) has been full of surprises.

The trial, which started in 1983, was designed to test whether selenium supplements (200 micrograms a day) could lower the risk of squamous and basal cell skin cancers in 1,312 people who lived in areas of the Southeast where selenium intakes are often low.[9]

It didn't work. "In 2003 we reported a slight *increase* in squamous cell skin cancers with selenium," says James Marshall of the Roswell Park Cancer Institute in Buffalo, New York, who now heads the study.[10] But that wasn't the end of the story.

"The original study found that selenium protected against prostate, colon, and lung cancer," says Marshall. That led to a flurry of new trials on selenium and cancer.

Meanwhile, researchers recently went back to see if selenium takers in the NPC had a lower risk of other illnesses. "There was a belief that as an antioxidant, selenium would protect against heart disease," says Marshall. "But the data was absolutely flat. We found no protection."

Next came diabetes. Marshall's team analyzed the data "because of the theory that oxidative stress could increase the risk of diabetes." This time, they found something. But it wasn't what they expected.

After nearly eight years, more selenium takers (10 percent) than placebo takers (6.5 percent) had been diagnosed with diabetes.[11]

"I wouldn't say that the findings raise alarms," says Marshall. "But they're another cautionary tale that it's not a good idea to take high doses of nutrients."

Adding to the uncertainty: a recent study of nearly 9,000 U.S. residents found that diabetes was more common among those with higher blood selenium levels, though selenium was linked to a lower risk of diabetes in an earlier study.[12,13]

But it will take more evidence to know if selenium promotes diabetes. "It could be a fluke," cautions Marshall.

By 2012, we should have results from the SELECT trial, which is testing whether selenium (200 mcg) and/or vitamin E

(400 IU) every day can lower the incidence of prostate cancer in 35,000 men.

"SELECT will be a more definitive trial because it's huge," notes Marshall. And it's encouraging that the trial is still under way, because studies are halted if researchers find that a treatment is causing harm. "I'm sure the data monitoring board is looking at interim analyses, and it hasn't stopped the trial," says Marshall.

In the meantime, he adds, "I don't recommend that people take selenium supplements. If there's enough doubt that we need to do a clinical trial, there's not enough reason to take it."

On the other hand, he isn't worried about the lower doses of selenium in multivitamins. (Most have just a fraction of the Daily Value, which is 70 mcg.) "I take a multi, and I wouldn't tell people to stop," he says.

THE BOTTOM LINE
Until we know more, don't take a daily multivitamin with more than 70 mcg of selenium (100% of the Daily Value). The latest recommended intake is 55 mcg a day.

The Risk of Too Little
Vitamin D

Researchers may be worried about high doses of folic acid and selenium, but when it comes to vitamin D, they worry that we're getting too little.

"The vitamin D studies are all coming back with good news," says Reinhold Vieth, a professor of nutritional sciences and of laboratory medicine and pathobiology at the University of Toronto.

Vieth is one of a growing number of experts who argue that the current Recommended Dietary Allowances for vitamin D should be higher.[14] The RDAs for adults range from 200 IU (if you're 50 or younger) to 600 IU (if you're over 70). Most multivitamins have 400 IU (the RDA for people 51 to 70).

"I flat-out recommend that people take 1,000 IU a day all the time," says Vieth. "There's no downside."

(Vieth helped develop a liquid vitamin D supplement called Ddrops.)

Bones & Muscles

The strongest evidence for higher intakes comes from trials that gave older people vitamin D (often with calcium) to prevent bone fractures or falls or to boost muscle strength.

"Trials that gave people only 400 IU a day did not show an effect," says Bess Dawson-Hughes, director of the Bone Metabolism Laboratory at the Jean Mayer U.S. Department of Agriculture Human Nutrition Research Center on Aging at Tufts University.

"Trials that had positive results gave people bigger doses."

How much vitamin D is enough? "For the average older person, it's 800 to 1,000 IU a day," says Dawson-Hughes, who is also past-president of the National Osteoporosis Foundation. "That's the average amount needed to get the 25-hydroxy vitamin D blood level up to 75 nanomoles per liter."

That's the level that lowers the risk of breaking a hip or other bone (but not the spine, which isn't affected by vitamin D).[15] "It's also the ballpark minimum for improving muscle performance and preventing falls," adds Dawson-Hughes.

It's easy to see how vitamin D could prevent fractures. Researchers have long known that it boosts bone mineral density, in part by helping the body absorb calcium from foods. But muscle?

"Biopsies show enlarged fast-twitch muscle fibers in people who are treated with vitamin D," explains Dawson-Hughes.

Stronger muscles helps explain why trials have found a 35 percent lower risk of falls in older people who are given 800 IU a day of vitamin D.[15] But that's not the whole story.

"Vitamin D may also be affecting balance because we know it has effects in the brain," suggests Dawson-Hughes. "There are vitamin D receptors just about everywhere you look in the brain."

Vitamin D's impact on bone and muscle is backed by the strongest evidence, and that's enough to recommend that people take 1,000 IU a day. In the meantime, studies examining the vitamin's impact on other diseases are coming fast and furious.

"The whole field is blowing open," says Dawson-Hughes. "It's very exciting."

Beyond Bones

A month doesn't go by without new reports that vitamin D may lower other risks:

Cancer. So far, there's some evidence that people with higher blood levels of vitamin D have a lower risk of cancers of the breast and prostate.[16–18] But overall, says Dawson-Hughes, "there's much more evidence for colon cancer."

For example, men in the Health Professionals Follow-Up Study and women in the Nurses' Health Study who had higher blood vitamin D levels in 1993 had roughly half the risk of colon cancer over the next 8 to 11 years than those with lower blood levels.[19]

But in 2006, the Women's Health Initiative reported that the roughly 18,000 women who were randomly assigned to take vitamin D (400 IU a day) for seven years had no lower risk of colon cancer than the 18,000 who took a placebo.[20] End of discussion? No.

"The dose wasn't high enough and people weren't taking their pills enough," says the University of Toronto's Reinhold Vieth. Virtually all of the women had blood vitamin D levels lower than 75 nanomoles per liter (nmol/L).

In fact, when researchers looked at all the women, whether they were told to take vitamin D or the placebo, those with levels under 31 nmol/L had 2½ times the risk of those with at least 58 nmol/L.

"There was a substantial reduction in colon cancer as blood levels of vitamin D went up," Vieth notes. But the drop wasn't related to whether women were told to take vitamin D, he adds, because "the dose was trivial and people weren't compliant enough."

Diabetes. After reviewing a number of studies, experts estimated that people with higher blood levels of vitamin D had a 64 percent lower risk of diabetes than people with lower levels.[21]

"Vitamin D is needed for optimal insulin secretion," says Tufts' Bess Dawson-Hughes. "And vitamin D may also influence responsiveness to insulin."

Periodontal disease. When researchers used probes to poke around more than 77,000 teeth in 6,700 people aged 13 to 90, the gums of those whose blood vitamin D levels averaged 100 nmol/L were 20 percent less likely to bleed than the gums of those whose levels averaged 32 nmol/L.[22]

"The evidence on gingivitis and tooth loss suggests that vitamin D influences oral health by decreasing inflammation," explains Dawson-Hughes.

And in a trial that gave 145 older people a placebo or 700 IU a day of vitamin D—enough to raise their blood levels from 71 to 112 nmol/L—the vitamin D takers had a 60 percent lower risk of tooth loss.[23]

Mental function. A few small studies have suggested that low vitamin D blood levels are linked to poor scores on thinking and memory tests.[24]

"It's looking like low vitamin D contributes to poor mental function in the elderly," says Dawson-Hughes.

Arthritis. In 1996, researchers reported that people who had osteoarthritis in their knees were three times more likely to get worse if they had low blood vitamin D levels.[25] But a recent study didn't find a link.[26]

"There's a large vitamin D trial at Tufts to see what happens to osteoarthritis of the knee," says Dawson-Hughes. Scientists are putting 144 people with arthritis in their knees on either vitamin D (2,000 IU a day) or a placebo for two years.

Multiple sclerosis. When researchers compared blood vitamin D levels of 257 Army and Navy recruits who were later diagnosed with multiple sclerosis to the blood levels of 514 recruits who remained free of the disease, the risk of MS was 62 percent lower in those with the highest vitamin D levels (they averaged 99 nmol/L).[27]

"There's research on a number of auto-immune diseases, but so far, multiple sclerosis is the most highly linked to vitamin D," says Dawson-Hughes.

Why would one vitamin affect so many systems?

"A lot of different tissues have the ability to make the vitamin D hormone because it's a signaling molecule," explains Vieth. "The quality of communication between cells is determined by the vitamin D because it's the raw material for the message."

In contrast, there's no shortage of raw material to make other hormones.

"Testosterone and estrogen, for example, are made from cholesterol, which circulates in the bloodstream in abundance, so you don't have to worry about supply," says Vieth. "Circulating levels of cholesterol are about 5 million nanomoles per liter, but for vitamin D, they're about 100 nanomoles per liter."

It's plausible that vitamin D could matter so much because the body can make it from the sun's ultraviolet light, which was never scarce when humans were evolving. "Throughout most of evolution we lived in the tropics," explains Vieth.

Still, what researchers are learning about folic acid and selenium raises the question: Should people worry about taking too much vitamin D?

"If you're talking about vitamin D toxicity, you're talking about gross excess," says Vieth. "I tend to be pretty blasé about vitamin D toxicity because it has always been industrial scale goof-ups when somebody makes a mistake and adds a milligram instead of a microgram to foods or supplements."

Vieth recently gave megadoses ranging from 4,000 to 40,000 IU a day of vitamin D to 12 patients with multiple sclerosis.[28] After 28 weeks, their blood levels rose to an average of 386 nmol/L, but extensive blood tests found no problems. "We raised the vitamin D to very high levels and nothing happened," says Vieth.

Vitamin D only causes toxicity if it raises levels of calcium in the blood.

THE BOTTOM LINE

Shoot for a total of 1,000 IU a day of vitamin D$_3$ (cholecalciferol) from your multivitamin plus an extra vitamin D supplement combined. Vitamin D$_2$ (ergocalciferol) is only about half as potent.

If you want to know your blood vitamin D level, make sure your doctor tests 25-hydroxyvitamin D. The levels should be at least 75 nmol/L (or 30 ng/L) and ideally 90 to 100 nmol/L (36 to 40 ng/L).

"But for that to happen, you have to saturate all the vitamin D carriers in the bloodstream," explains Vieth. "Less than one-fortieth of the carrier proteins are normally occupied, so you have to throw in huge excesses to overwhelm the system."

Could vitamin D have some unexpected adverse effect at lower doses?

So far, the only cloud on the horizon comes from a study of Finnish smokers in which men with higher blood levels of vitamin D had a higher risk of pancreatic cancer.[29] But those results might not apply to non-smokers. For example, a study of roughly 46,000 U.S. men and 75,000 U.S. women found that higher vitamin D intakes were linked to a lower risk of pancreatic cancer.[30]

And Finland is so far north that it may be unusual. "Vitamin D levels go up and down in Scandinavia," notes Vieth. "They're never in a steady state, as they should be."

And, he adds, studies show lower overall cancer rates and death rates in people with higher vitamin D levels in their blood.[31,32]

In any case, Vieth has urged the National Academy of Sciences' Institute of Medicine to raise the Upper Level—the highest safe dose to take regularly—for vitamin D. "The UL should be 10,000 IU, rather than the current 2,000 IU," he contends.

In the meantime, says Vieth, taking 1,000 IU a day would raise the average person's blood level of vitamin D to 75 nmol/L.

"Forget cancer, forget everything—the evidence on bone alone directs people to get 1,000 IU a day," he argues. "How many reasons do you need?"

Notes

1. *J. Am. Med. Assoc. 296:* 2720, 2006.
2. *J. Am. Med. Assoc. 298:* 1212, 2007.
3. *J. Am. Med. Assoc. 297:* 2351, 2408, 2006.
4. *Cancer Epidemiol. Biomarkers Prev. 16:* 1325, 2007.
5. *J. Natl. Cancer Inst. 99:* 754, 2007.
6. *Am. J. Epidemiol, 163:* 989, 2006.
7. *Am. J. Clin, Nutr. 83:* 895, 2006.
8. *Am. J. Clin, Nutr. 86:* 434, 2007.
9. *JAMA 276:* 1957, 1996.
10. *J. Natl. Cancer Inst. 95:* 1477, 2003.
11. *Ann. Intern. Med. 147:* 217, 2007.
12. *Diabetes Care 30:* 829, 2007.
13. *J. Am. Coll. Nutr. 24:* 250, 2005.
14. *Am. J. Clin. Nutr. 85:* 649, 2007.
15. *Am. J. Clin. Nutr. 84:* 18, 2006.
16. *Am. J. Clin. Nutr. 85:* 1586, 2007.
17. *Cancer Epidemiol. Biomarkers Prev. 15:* 1427, 2006.
18. *PLoS Med. 4:* e103, March 2007. doi: 10.1371/journal.pmed.0040103.
19. *J. Natl. Cancer Inst. 99:* 1120, 2007.
20. *N. Engl. J. Med. 354:* 684, 2006.
21. *J. Clin. Endocrinol, Metab. 92:* 2017, 2007.
22. *Am. J. Clin. Nutr. 82:* 575, 2005.
23. *Am. J. Med. 111:* 452, 2001.
24. *Arch. Biochem. Biophys. 460:* 202, 2007.
25. *Ann. Intern. Med. 125:* 353, 1996.
26. *Arthritis Rheum. 56:* 129, 2007.
27. *JAMA 296:* 2832, 2006.
28. *Am. J. Clin. Nutr. 86:* 645, 2007.
29. *Cancer Res. 66:* 10213, 2006.
30. *Cancer Epidemiol. Biomarkers Prev. 15:* 1688, 2006.
31. *J. Natl. Cancer Inst. 98:* 451, 2006.
32. *Arch. Intern. Med. 167:* 1730, 2007.

Minerals Matter
The Wrong Amounts Can Harm You

The ever-shifting messages from advertisements and news reports have made it increasingly difficult to know which minerals you need and in what amounts. A generation ago *Geritol* ads touted iron tonics; today, many people are still worried about "iron poor" blood. Moreover, television and the Internet are swarming with pitches for megadoses of less-familiar minerals such as chromium, selenium, and zinc. Even the seemingly rock-solid advice to get plenty of calcium is now under attack: In February 2006, headlines reported that the mineral doesn't prevent fractures or colon cancer after all.

To put that information in perspective and determine your requirements for various minerals, it helps to divide them into three groups, based on typical consumption in the United States:

- **Inadequate intake.** A close reading of the clinical trial that sparked the February 2006 headlines reveals that calcium is still a vital nutrient. However, the average person consumes substantially less than the recommended amounts of calcium and two other bone-bolstering minerals, magnesium and potassium, all of which work synergistically to fight osteoporosis as well as high blood pressure. Moreover, they may each offer additional benefits, such as helping to prevent diabetes, premenstrual syndrome, or kidney stones.

- **Excessive intake.** Some 75 percent of women and nearly all men consume amounts of sodium that can undermine the benefits of calcium, magnesium, and potassium. And most people consume slightly more than the recommended amount of iron, a potential risk to the hundreds of thousands of Americans with a relatively common but often undetected genetic disorder that can cause dangerous iron buildup in the body.

- **Adequate but possibly not optimal intake.** Extra doses of three minerals in this group deserve special attention: chromium, because weight-loss and diabetes-prevention claims have made it a top seller; selenium, because studies suggest that supplemental doses may ward off prostate cancer; and zinc, marketed for treating the common cold,

because it may have serious adverse effects. The zinc evidence includes the results of our Freedom of Information Act request submitted to the Food and Drug Administration for this report that link zinc nasal sprays to impairments in the sense of both taste and smell.

Calcium: Still Worthwhile

The February 2006 calcium trial, involving some 36,000 post-menopausal women, failed to conclusively show that supplemental calcium plus vitamin D—which may also contribute to bone health and cancer prevention—fended off either fractures or colon cancer. The strongest finding: a slight increase in the risk of kidney stones.

However, the study had several flaws that may have impaired its ability to detect any benefits: lower initial colon-cancer risk than in previous studies, unusually high calcium intakes apart from the assigned pills, poor compliance with the treatment, widespread use of bone-building estrogen, and possibly inadequate study length and vitamin-D doses.

Despite those limitations, when researchers zeroed in on the women who actually adhered to the prescribed regimen, they found significant support for calcium: a 29 percent reduction in the risk of hip fracture, the most debilitating and deadly kind.

That finding indicates that calcium is still essential for skeletal health. But the mineral has other important benefits as well. Observational studies have generally linked low calcium intakes with excess fat or body weight. Several small trials of low-calorie diets have found that calcium-rich regimens lead to more loss of weight or fat than those with little calcium, possibly because the mineral binds with ingested fat and ferries it out of the body.

The reduction in artery-clogging fats may also explain why calcium slightly reduces levels of the "bad" LDL cholesterol. Finally, consuming 1,000 to 1,200 milligrams (mg) of calcium per day may reduce symptoms of premenstrual syndrome—such as mood swings, water retention, and food cravings—by some 50 percent, according to the largest study performed so far.

Iron: Meat vs. Plant Sources

Some plant foods, such as soybeans and lentils, contain even more iron than meat generally does—though the body absorbs the mineral slightly better from meat.

Combined Mineral Power

Research increasingly shows that potassium and magnesium play important, complementary roles along with calcium—and not just for the bones. Several observational studies have linked a high dietary intake of those two minerals, both of which improve calcium absorption, with increased bone density. Results from a large clinical trial, published in 2003, showed that a healthful diet rich in all three

Salt: Where You Least Expect It

Salty-tasting snacks may contain less sodium per serving than many foods that don't taste salty. For example, Wise Potato Chips and Planter's Salted Peanuts have much less sodium than Aunt Jemima's Original Pancake Mix or a Burger King Spicy Tendercrisp Chicken Sandwich.

nutrients improved bone structure more than the expected bolstering from calcium alone.

Moreover, that study, called the Dietary Approaches to Stop Hypertension (DASH) trial, has documented that the mineral trio provides an even greater effect on blood pressure. The reductions in pressure were especially large in individuals who need them the most: black people, who face an above-average risk of stroke, and those who already have hypertension. The minerals may lower blood pressure by blunting the effect of sodium (see above), at least in part by flushing it out of the body.

In addition, magnesium and, to a lesser extent, potassium provide their own unique benefits.

- **Magnesium:** Beyond its effect on blood pressure, magnesium may further protect the heart by helping to prevent abnormal heart rhythms and blood clots, and to ward off or control type 2 diabetes. The evidence is particularly strong for diabetes. Three large observational studies, including one published in March 2006, have shown that people who consume the most dietary magnesium have a reduced risk of developing either diabetes or a crucial contributing factor called insulin resistance. Other research hints that magnesium supplements improved long-term blood-sugar control in people who already have the full-blown disease.
- **Potassium:** Adequate intake of this mineral can help prevent muscle cramps and kidney stones.

How to Get Enough

Less than one-third of Americans regularly consume the recommended amounts of calcium or magnesium or potassium. To boost your intake, it's best to focus on foods rather than supplements. Foods rich in those minerals tend to be high in other substances—such as B vitamins, vitamins C, D, and K, and fiber—that may also help prevent osteoporosis, hypertension, heart disease, or even cancer.

And getting too much of those minerals, which is easy to do with supplements, can cause problems: diarrhea from excessive magnesium; kidney stones and blocked absorption of other nutrients from too much calcium; and kidney damage from potassium overload in people who take certain drugs, notably potassium-retaining diuretics, or who have kidney or heart failure.

Note that while some observational studies have linked high calcium intakes with increased prostate-cancer risk, the first randomized trial to study that question, published in March 2005, suggested that the mineral may actually protect against the malignancy, though the results were not consistent.

For advice on the recommended intakes of these three minerals plus good dietary sources of each, see the accompanying table, "Foods Rich in Three Neglected Minerals." In addition,

the DASH eating plan is available free online at www.nhlbi.nih .gov/health/public/heart/hbp/dash.

Too Much Salt and Iron

Americans' craving for salt can have significant consequences. In addition to raising blood pressure in susceptible people, excess sodium increases the excretion of calcium into the urine, which may contribute to osteoporosis and the risk of kidney stones. High sodium intake may also raise the risk of stomach cancer by damaging the protective mucus membrane, and of asthma by making the lungs more susceptible to irritants.

Excess iron intake is far less common but sometimes even more serious. While many people still assume they need as much iron as possible, the average man and postmenopausal woman actually get more than they need from diet alone. Even premenopausal women, who need more iron than other people, can usually get enough from diet alone, unless they have unusually heavy menstrual bleeding or are elite athletes.

More important, about 1 in 250 Americans has an inherited disorder called hemochromatosis, which causes gradual accumulation of damaging iron in the body's organs. That can lead to liver or heart failure, premature menopause in women, and impotence in men. And diagnosis is often dangerously delayed, in part because many doctors don't connect the signs of organ damage with hemochromatosis, which was considered a rare disorder just two decades ago.

Here's how to avoid consuming too much of those minerals:

- **Sodium.** The strongest evidence that slashing sodium intake helps lower blood pressure comes from the DASH study. It showed that reducing daily intake to about 1,500 mg, the recommended amount for people age 50 and under, reduced blood pressure in all groups, especially blacks and those with hypertension. Limiting consumption to 2,400 mg—slightly higher than the government-recommended ceiling but still well below the average U.S. intake of about 3,500 mg—likely helps somewhat and prevents blood pressure from creeping up with age.

However, cutting back on sodium, which comes mainly from salt, poses practical problems. Taste is the least of them, since salt craving usually disappears after a few weeks. Adopting the DASH diet, which is loaded with fruits and vegetables, will likely get you down to about 2,400 mg. But to reach 1,500 mg you'll have to cook nearly all your food at home from scratch, since about three-fourths of the average American's sodium intake comes from processed or restaurant food.

Aiming for 1,500 mg is definitely worthwhile if you have blood pressure above the optimal limit for normal, 120/80 millimeters of mercury, or risk factors for hypertension. For other people, 2,400 mg is a more realistic goal. Since some individuals respond dramatically to sodium, you don't necessarily have to reach 1,500 mg to see a meaningful decline, though the less sodium you consume, the lower your blood pressure will likely go. Conversely, evidence suggests only about half of people with high blood pressure respond to a low-sodium diet. So you may not need to maintain the extra effort if you see no improvement after several months.

- **Iron.** Our medical consultants say all adults should have a one-time, $250 blood test for hemochromatosis, which measures levels of iron and transferrin, an iron-transporting protein. Although many people with hemochromatosis never develop iron-related problems, the consequences for those who do are serious and irreversible.

Foods Rich in Three Neglected Minerals

Most people get less than the recommended amounts of each of the minerals listed below. Eating lots of the foods in our table can help you reach the target amounts for your age and gender. Some people may also need calcium pills, though the intake from all sources should stay below the safe upper limit of 2,500 mg a day. Extra doses of the other two minerals are generally unnecessary and potentially harmful. Supplemental magnesium can cause diarrhea. Moderately high potassium intake can cause kidney problems in people who take potassium-retaining diuretics, angiotensin-receptor blockers (ARBs), or ACE inhibitors, or who have diabetes or heart or kidney failure. They should talk with their doctor before increasing even their dietary intake of potassium.

Good Dietary Sources | Amount (mg)[1]

Calcium

Yogurt: Plain, low fat (8 oz.)	415
Sardines: With bones, canned (3 oz.)	325
Milk: Skim (8 oz.)	300
Tofu: Firm, made with calcium sulfate (1/2 cup)	205
Cheese: Cheddar, mozzarella (1 oz.)	185 to 205[2]
Pink salmon: With bones, canned (3 oz.)	180
Greens, cooked: Kale, spinach, turnip greens (1/2 cup)	50 to 120
Beans, boiled: Great northern, navy, white (1/2 cup)	60 to 80
Nuts: Almonds, Brazil (1 oz.)	45 to 70
Orange (1 medium)	60

Recommended daily intake

- Men under age 50 and premenopausal women: 1,000 mg
- Men 50 to 65: 1,200 mg
- Men over 65 and postmenopausal women: 1,200 mg to 1,500 mg, depending on bone density.

Magnesium

Halibut (3 oz.)	90
Nuts: Almonds, cashews, peanuts (1 oz.)	50 to 80
Spinach, cooked (1/2 cup)	75
Potato, baked: With skin (1 medium)	50
Yogurt: Plain, low fat (8 oz.)	45
Beans: Baked, kidney, pinto (1/2 cup)	35 to 40
Avocado (1/2 cup)	35
Banana (1 medium)	30
Cereal: Oatmeal (1/2 cup), no milk	30
Milk: Skim (8 oz.)	30

Recommended daily Intake

- Men: 420 mg
- Women: 320 mg

Potassium

Potato, baked: With skin (1 medium)	
Avocado (1/2 cup)	585
Yogurt: Plain, low fat (8 oz.)	575
Beans, boiled: Black, lentils, lima, kidney, pinto (1/2 cup)	305 to 485
Greens, cooked: Spinach, Swiss chard (1/2 cup)	420 to 480
Orange juice (8 oz.)	475
Squash: Winter (1/2 cup)	450
Artichoke (1 medium)	425
Banana (1 medium)	420
Milk: Skim (8 oz.)	410

Recommended daily intake

- Men and women: 4,700 mg

[1] All amounts rounded to the nearest 5. [2] Hard cheeses tend to have more calcium than soft cheeses.

Fiber Free-for-All

Not all fibers are equal.

How much fiber do you need?

According to food labels, 25 grams is a day's worth. That's right for women 50 and under, but men of the same age need 38 grams, says the National Academy of Sciences. And the targets drop to 21 grams for women and 30 grams for men over 50.

It's not that people need fiber less as they get older. "The advice is to get 14 grams of fiber per 1,000 calories, and older people need fewer calories," explains Thomas Wolever, a fiber researcher and professor of nutritional sciences at the University of Toronto.

Most Americans consume half the recommended levels. A typical woman gets about 13 grams of fiber a day, while the average man hovers around 17 grams.

What's the harm in falling short of the target? Here's a rundown of the key links between fiber and health.

Heart Disease

The daily fiber targets "are based on data that fiber prevents cardiovascular disease," notes Joanne Slavin, a University of Minnesota researcher who served on the National Academy of Sciences Panel on the Definition of Dietary Fiber.

The NAS relied heavily on studies that found a lower risk of heart disease in people who reported eating the most fiber (about 29 grams a day for men and 23 grams a day for women).[1,2] In each of those studies, the fiber that seemed to protect the heart came from cereals, breads, and other grains, not from fruits or vegetables.

But it was never absolutely clear that it was the fiber that mattered. Several inconsistencies have always troubled scientists:

Fiber or whole grains? It's hard for researchers to know if it's the fiber, or something else in whole grains, that matters.

"Whole grains also have phytoestrogens, antioxidants, lignans, vitamins, and minerals, so a lot comes along with the fiber package," says Slavin.

Soluble or insoluble? The kind of fiber that's linked to a lower risk of heart disease isn't the kind that lowers cholesterol.

Although all fruits, vegetables, and grains have both soluble and insoluble fiber, most grains, like wheat, are richer in *insoluble* fiber, which is not broken down by digestive enzymes or by bacteria in the gut.

In contrast, a few grains (oats and barley, for example) are richer in viscous (gummy) *soluble* fibers, which *are* broken down by bacteria in the gut.

"When researchers feed people viscous soluble fiber, it lowers cholesterol, but insoluble fiber doesn't," notes Wolever.

Yet in the large studies that the National Academy of Sciences relied on, a lower risk of heart disease was linked to foods rich in either kind of fiber, not just soluble. "It's a disconnect," says Wolever.

One possibility: even though the mostly insoluble fiber from grains doesn't lower cholesterol, it may protect the heart by reducing blood pressure or the risk of blood clots.

"Insoluble fiber may prevent heart attacks by reducing inflammation," says Wolever. "We don't know how the heck it works."

Fiber or fiber eaters? Researchers can't be sure if it's fiber, or something else about people who eat high-fiber diets, that lowers their risk of heart disease.

"We just don't have a lot of people who eat high-fiber, whole-grain diets and are out there smoking," says Slavin. "Eating fiber goes together with other healthy behaviors."

Fiber was big in the mid-1980s, when President Ronald Reagan was diagnosed with colon cancer and Kellogg ran TV commercials saying that high-fiber foods like All-Bran could "reduce the risk of some cancers."

But the fiber boomlet was soon eclipsed by the (much bigger) oat bran craze, followed by the low-carb bubble, and, most recently, the whole-grain movement (with scattered minifads in between).

Now things have come full circle. Fiber is back. Foods that never had any (yogurt, ice cream, water, juice) sometimes have some, and foods that always had some (cereals, breads, pasta) often have more. Why?

Fiber is showing up in foods because, well, companies have figured out how to put it there. And they know that if they pump up the fiber, people will pull out their pocketbooks.

Here's what you need to know about fiber & and where to get the kinds that matter.

Researchers typically adjust for smoking, weight, exercise, education, alcohol, saturated fat, and other factors that influence heart disease risk, but they could still miss something.

Those inconsistencies didn't matter so much as long as people were getting their fiber from whole grains, fruits, and vegetables, rather than from purified fibers added to foods like ice cream.

"That's why we have always encouraged people to eat fiber from foods like whole grains," says Slavin. That way they're getting both soluble and insoluble fiber and the whole "fiber package."

Diabetes

"There's moderately strong evidence that fiber is linked to a reduced risk of diabetes, and it's based on whole foods like vegetables, fruits, and whole grains," says JoAnn Manson, professor of medicine at Harvard Medical School and chief of preventive medicine at Brigham and Women's Hospital in Boston.

The evidence that fiber prevents diabetes parallels the evidence that it prevents heart disease, as do the inconsistencies.

In two studies—on roughly 65,000 women and 43,000 men—those who reported eating the most fiber *from grains* (8 grams a day) had about a 30 percent lower risk of diabetes than those who reported eating the least fiber from grains (3 grams a day).[3,4]

As with heart disease, it could always be something else about fiber eaters, or something other than the fiber in grains, that matters. "We don't have large-scale trials showing that fiber prevents diabetes," cautions Manson.

But in short-term clinical studies, the gummy *soluble* fibers (in foods like oats and barley) keep a lid on blood sugar.

"There's good evidence that fiber slows the absorption of the carbohydrate in foods, which leads to a less marked increase in blood sugar and less demand for insulin," explains Manson.

If those studies had lasted longer, researchers might have found that *insoluble* fiber also lowered blood sugar.

"When we fed insulin-resistant women a cereal high in insoluble fiber for a year, nothing happened for six months," says Wolever. Then the bacteria in the colon started to change, and the women became more sensitive to insulin.

How? "We think that bacteria in the colon affect gut hormones, which could keep beta-cells in the pancreas from dying," he speculates. Beta-cells produce insulin.

Much of that evidence is preliminary, cautions Wolever. What fiber does to bacteria in the colon "is still pretty much a black box."

Colon Cancer

In the mid-1980s, the evidence made it seem like a slam-dunk that fiber could prevent colon cancer. Then in April 2000, two large studies released unexpected news.

In a three-year trial, roughly 700 people who were told to eat 13 ½ grams of wheat bran a day had no fewer new precancerous colon polyps than 700 others who were told to eat only 2 grams a day.[5]

The Bottom Line

- Whole-grain breads and cereals, which are naturally rich in fiber, are linked to a lower risk of **heart disease** and **diabetes.**
- Foods rich in insoluble fibers, like wheat bran, help prevent **constipation** and possibly **diverticular disease.**
- The evidence that high-fiber foods lower the risk of **colon cancer** is inconclusive.
- Eating fruits, vegetables, and other high-fiber, lower-calorie foods may help slow **weight gain.**
- Isolated inulin, polydextrose, and maltodextrin are soluble fibers but they're not gummy, so they probably don't lower **blood cholesterol** or **blood sugar.**
- Isolated oat fiber and soy fiber are insoluble, so they may help keep you **regular.** Polydextrose may also help, but inulin and maltodextrin don't seem to.

And in a four-year trial, roughly 1,000 people who were told to eat a lower-fat diet rich in fiber (36 grams a day) from fruits, vegetables, and whole grains had no fewer polyps than 1,000 others who were told to eat their usual diet.[6]

"The trials are not ambiguous," says John Baron, a professor of medicine at Dartmouth Medical School who has conducted trials testing calcium and folic acid on the risk of precancerous colon polyps. "They have shown no effect."

Despite the two disappointing trials, the American Institute for Cancer Research concluded last year that fiber-rich foods "probably" prevent colon cancer. Its evidence: studies like the European Investigation into Cancer and Nutrition (EPIC), which tracked more than 500,000 people in 10 countries for five years. EPIC found a 40 percent lower risk of colon cancer in people who reported eating more fiber-rich foods.[7]

So why did the two trials strike out? Maybe it's not fiber, but something else about fiber eaters, that cuts their risk of cancer.

Or maybe the trials found nothing because they looked at polyps, not cancers.

"If fiber keeps polyps from progressing to colon cancer but has no effect at earlier stages, you may not see a connection between fiber and polyps in these trials," offers Manson.

The bottom line: "The jury is still out for fiber lowering the risk of colorectal cancer," says Manson. "The evidence is stronger for coronary heart disease and diabetes than for cancer."

Baron is less optimistic. "The jury may still be out, but it's polling eight-to-four against."

Obesity

Can fiber help keep you slim by slowing the rate at which food exits your stomach, which could make you feel full for longer?

"Fiber might help maintain weight," says the University of Toronto's Thomas Wolever. "But it's not magic. It's not a strong effect."

In a study of roughly 75,000 women, those who boosted their fiber intake by 12 grams a day curbed their weight gain

Bulk Delivery

Here's a sampling of foods that are rich in intact fiber (along with a few lower-fiber foods for comparison). Whole wheat is mostly insoluble fiber, but most fruits, vegetables, beans, and nuts have a mix of soluble and insoluble fiber.

Fruits & Juices	Fiber *(grams)*	Nuts *(number closest to 1 oz., unless noted)*	Fiber *(grams)*
Blackberries *(1 cup)*	8	Almonds *(24)*	4
Pear *(1)*	5	Peanuts *(28)* or Peanut butter *(2 Tbs.)*	2
Apple or Orange *(1)*	4	Cashews *(18)*	1
Figs, dried *(2)*	4		
Kiwi *(2)*	4	**Beans** *(½ cup cooked, unless noted)*	
Apricots, dried *(5)*	3	Black beans or Split peas	8
Banana *(1)* or Raisins *(¼ cup)*	3	Kidney beans	7
Blueberries or Strawberries *(1 cup)*	3	Lentils	7
Prunes *(5)* or Prune juice *(1 cup)*	3	Chickpeas or Pinto beans, canned	6
Peach *(1)*, Avocado *(⅛)*,		Hummus *(2 Tbs.)* or Tofu *(3 oz.)*	2
or Grapefruit *(½)*	2	**Bread & Crackers**	
Cantaloupe *(¼)* or Grapes *(1½ cups)*	1	Finn Crisp Thin Crisps, Original *(4)*	6
Orange juice *(1 cup)*	0.5	Whole wheat bread *(2 slices)*	6
		Nabisco Triscuits *(6)*	3
Vegetables *(cooked, unless noted)*		White bread *(2 slices)*	1
Peas *(½ cup)*	5	**Hot Cereal** *(1 cup cooked)*	
Sweet potato, baked, with skin *(1)*	4	Oat bran	6
Broccoli *(½ cup)* or Green beans *(⅔ cup)*	3	Wheatena	5
Green pepper, raw *(1)*	3	Oatmeal	4
Potato, baked, with skin *(1)*	3	Cream of wheat	1
Asparagus *(6 spears)*	2		
Carrot, raw *(1)*	2	**Cold Cereal**	
Cauliflower *(⅔ cup)* or Corn *(½ cup)*	2	Kellogg's All-Bran, Original *(½ cup)*	10
Romaine lettuce *(1¾ cups shredded)*	2	Post Shredded Wheat 'n Bran *(1¼ cups)*	8
Spinach, Kale, or Brussels		Kellogg's Raisin Bran *(1 cup)*	7
sprouts *(½ cup)*	2	Post Grape-Nuts *(½ cup)*	7
Tomato *(1)*	2	Post Shredded Wheat *(2 biscuits)*	6
		Post Bran Flakes *(¾ cup)*	5
Grains & Pasta *(cooked)*		General Mills Wheaties *(¾ cup)*	3
Bulgur *(¾ cup)*	6	Kellogg's Corn Flakes *(1 cup)*	1
Pasta, whole wheat *(1 cup)*	6	Special K *(1 cup)*	1
Popcorn, air-popped *(4 cups popped)*	4		
Pasta, regular *(1 cup)*	3		
Rice, brown *(¾ cup)*	3		
Rice, white *(¾ cup)*	0.5		

Note: numbers below 1 rounded to the nearest 0,5 gram.
Sources: company information and USDA.
Table compiled by Amy Johnson.

by 8 pounds over the next 12 years.[8] And in a study that tracked 22,000 men for 8 years, those who upped their fiber by 20 grams a day cut their weight gain by 12 pounds.[9]

"We saw less weight gain in women who consumed a higher-fiber diet," says Manson, who was a co-author of the study on women. "It's plausible that fiber leads to satiety and a less calorie-dense diet, but long-term trials are needed."

Of course, if high-fiber foods curb weight gain because people are eating high-fiber, lower-calorie foods like fruits and vegetables, that wouldn't apply to high-fiber, *not*-low-calorie bars, crackers, cereals, and ice cream.

Regularity

A few studies have suggested that people who eat more insoluble fiber have a lower risk of diverticular disease (small pouches that bulge out through weak spots in the large intestine, sometimes becoming inflamed or infected).[10]

But fiber's starring role in the GI tract is in the stool department. Insoluble fiber tends to help "laxation" by adding bulk to stool.

"We know that insoluble fibers like wheat bran are good for stool weight and laxation and soluble fibers like pectin aren't," explains the University of Minnesota's Joanne Slavin.

After dozens of studies, researchers have even estimated how much you can expect stool weight to increase for each gram of fiber you eat. (That's 5.4 grams for wheatbran fiber, 4.9 grams for fruit and vegetable fiber, 3 grams for isolated cellulose, and 1.3 grams for isolated pectin, in case you were wondering.)[11]

Insoluble fiber from bran helps prevent constipation because it bulks up the stool. "The bran fiber is still there at the end of the GI tract, where it binds water, so it's going to increase stool weight," explains Slavin.

In contrast, most soluble fibers, like the pectin in fruits and vegetables, are digested by bacteria in the gut, "so there's nothing left at the end of the GI tract."

But it's not just a question of insoluble vs. soluble. For example, psyllium, the (mostly) soluble fiber in Metamucil, is a laxative. And wheat bran has a bigger impact than cellulose—its purified cousin—even though both are insoluble.

"If you pulverize wheat bran, it has less effect on stool weight," notes Slavin. "The size of the particles or structure of the food may make a difference in how much survives the digestive tract."

Isolated vs. Intact

Companies are now adding a host of isolated fibers—like inulin, maltodextrin, oat fiber, and polydextrose—to foods. And their ads and labels imply that those fibers are equal to the intact, naturally occurring fiber in foods.

But the evidence on isolated fibers is much skimpier. "There's not much out there," says Slavin.

Researchers can divide the new fibers into soluble and insoluble, but that's not enough. To lower LDL ("bad") cholesterol, for example, fiber has to be soluble *and* viscous.

"Inulin, polydextrose, and maltodextrin are soluble fiber, but they're not viscous at all, so they absolutely don't lower cholesterol," says Slavin.

Isolated viscous fibers—like those from oats, barley, or guar gum—would make foods like ice cream and yogurt too gummy. "They'd be almost impossible to consume," explains Slavin.

The new isolated fibers aren't gummy at all, she adds. "That's why you can put them in so many foods."

Each fiber's impact on regularity also goes beyond soluble vs. insoluble. For example, you wouldn't expect inulin to do much for regularity because gut bacteria gobble most of it up.

In contrast, polydextrose might help keep your GI tract moving, at least according to one industry-sponsored study done in China.[12] "It would be nice to have more evidence," notes Slavin.

Unfortunately, both inulin and polydextrose have a downside in large doses.

"Inulin may cause gas or other GI problems at doses above 15 grams a day," says Slavin. "For some people, the gas isn't a big issue, but others are really sensitive."

And foods that contain more than 15 grams of polydextrose per serving must warn consumers that "sensitive individuals may experience a laxative effect from excessive consumption of this product."

On the other hand, "some modified starches have no GI effects at 50 grams a day," adds Slavin.

And yet, despite all the differences among isolated fibers—and between isolated and intact fiber—they all look the same on a food's Nutrition Facts panel.

"On the label, it all looks like good stuff," says Slavin. "But fiber does not equal fiber," she adds.

"If you eat five fiber-fortified yogurts a day, you can meet your fiber goal. But that's not the message we want people to get. It's not the same as getting 25 grams of fiber from a variety of fruits, vegetables, and whole grains."

It won't hurt to eat yogurt, ice cream, or other foods with added fiber. . . . unless it becomes an excuse to eat fiber-rich cookies instead of bran cereal.

"I wouldn't want people to feel that they don't have to eat fruits, vegetables, and whole grains any more because they're eating ice cream with inulin," says Wolever, "especially if it means that instead of one serving of ice cream, they'll have two servings because they think it's healthy."

Notes

1. *JAMA 275:* 447, 1996.

2. *JAMA 281:* 1998, 1999.

3. *JAMA 277:* 472, 1997.

4. *Diabetes Care 20:* 545, 1997.

5. *N. Engl. J. Med. 342:* 1156, 2000.

6. *N. Engl. J. Med. 342:* 1149, 2000.

7. *Lancet 361:* 1496, 2003.

8. *Am. J. Clin. Nutr. 78:* 920, 2003.

9. *Am. J. Clin. Nutr. 80:* 1237, 2004.

10. *J. Nutr. 128:* 714, 1998.

11. *Spiller, GA, ed., CRC Handbook of Dietary Fiber in Human Nutrition* (Boca Raton, FL: CRC Press, 1993), 263–349.

12. *Am. J. Clin. Nutr. 72:* 1503, 2000.

The Fairest Fats of Them All (and Those to Avoid)

The science on fats is changing as rapidly as today's fashions. So work hard to know your fats—from bad to good.

SHARON PALMER, RD

Think you're in step with the latest in fat science? If you're still preaching low fat to your patients, perhaps you need to brush up on your fat knowledge. Low fat is as out of fashion as shoulder pads. Today's nutrition advice should be all about healthy fats.

"I think the fat phobia of the '90s is old school now. Dietitians need to keep up with the research. We should not really be recommending low fat anymore. There is tremendous value in olive oil. Dietitians need to know this concept and to recommend that their patients consume good fats. People can have an enjoyable diet with food that tastes great. Dietitians need to be aware of these issues and incorporate them in their work," says Janet Bond Brill, PhD, RD, LDN, a nutrition and fitness consultant and the author of *Cholesterol Down: 10 Simple Steps to Lower Your Cholesterol in 4 Weeks—Without Prescription Drugs.*

If keeping up with research on fat is challenging for nutrition professionals, you can imagine how confusing it is for the public. First it was low fat, then zero trans fat, and now it's a push toward monounsaturated fatty acids (MUFAs). "Absolutely, there is confusion in the public over fats," says Brill. And it's time to set them straight.

"There is general agreement that about 30% of total calories should come from fat," says Joyce Nettleton, DSc, editor of the *Fats of Life* newsletter and *PUFA Newsletters*. The American Heart Association (AHA) suggests that 25% to 35% of total calories should come from fat. Brill reports that within the total fat intake, 7% of calories or less should come from saturated fats, less than 1% should come from trans fats, at least 10% and up to 20% of calories should come from MUFAs, and the remaining amount (up to 10%) should come from polyunsaturated fatty acids (PUFAs).

Fats to Beware

"The message needs to be made loud and clear that saturated fats, cholesterol, and trans fats need to be avoided. These are the three things that contribute to heart disease, which is our No. 1 killer among men and women," says Brill.

Suggestions for limiting dietary cholesterol and saturated fats have existed for decades. We know that saturated fats increase low-density lipoprotein (LDL) cholesterol levels, thus increasing the risk of heart disease. And during the past few years, the public has been hit over the head with the message that trans fats are the bad guys, since trans fats raise LDL cholesterol and may lower high-density lipoprotein cholesterol.

While saturated fats may not be totally eliminated from the diet because they are found in foods that provide important nutrients, such as animal and dairy products, artificial trans fats can be phased out. Naturally occurring trans fats are found in very small amounts in animal products, but most of the trans fats people consume are found in processed and restaurant foods, which can be produced using healthier oil formulations.

Nettleton points out that food manufacturers and restaurants have made great strides in ridding the food supply of trans fats; however, there are still areas for improvement. Many products, from deep-fried fast foods to microwave popcorns, are still chock full of trans fats, and manufacturers may still list "0 grams" of trans fat on food labels when products contain less than 0.5 grams of trans fat per serving.[1]

"Hopefully, we are getting trans fats out of the food supply. We need legislation like Denmark, where it is banned in the entire country. California state legislation against trans fats is a great step," says Brill, who advises her clients to look for and then avoid sources of hydrogenated oils on all ingredient lists before choosing foods.

Today, we face new challenges with upholding the strategy of lowering saturated fats. The elimination of trans fats from food production has reintroduced saturated fats as a functional solution to food processing. Even home cooks are turning more frequently to butter as a baking alternative in an attempt to avoid trans fats. And although the high-protein diet has lost its initial gloss, it promoted a lingering notion that eating larger portions of animal protein, with their accompanying contribution of saturated fat, is a "lean" way of eating.

The solutions to these issues are not always clear. For example, Nettleton reports that palm oil, an increasingly common fat that food manufacturers use to replace trans fat, is rich in palmitic acid, which for the most part has no effect on blood cholesterol levels. But many experts still recommend avoiding palm oil because it is a source of saturated fat. And when people are reaching for a suitable fat for their favorite chocolate chip cookie recipe, which presents the lesser evil: saturated fat in butter or trans fat in stick margarine?

Navigating these challenges may be best accomplished by analyzing individual lifestyles and making recommendations accordingly—something at which dietitians are skilled. The "budget" approach to saturated fats is an option. How do you want to spend your saturated fat allotment for the day: on really good cheese, filet mignon, or homemade cookies? Trans fat may be a nonissue for someone who enjoys cooking and eating at home, but it can pose difficulties for people who regularly eat out of food packages and from fast-food drive-throughs. "It depends on people's food habits. It comes down to individual food choices and everything in moderation," says Nettleton.

The new shift in fat science focuses on the fact that the Western diet is flooded with the omega-6 fatty acid linoleic acid and is low in omega-3 fatty acids, an eating style that appears to be proinflammatory and conducive to chronic disease. As people were urged to increase their intake of polyunsaturated vegetable oils to reduce blood cholesterol levels in decades past, there was a tremendous increase in the agricultural production of oil seed crops, primarily soybean. Estimates indicate that 20% of the calories in the American diet come from soybean oil alone. The vast majority of liquid vegetable oils used in food processing, such as soybean, corn, and safflower oils, are high in omega-6 fatty acids. "We need to get our omega-6 fatty acids way down. Right now, they are at a ratio of 20 to 30:1 omega-6 to omega-3 fatty acids, and they need to be at a ratio of 4:1 or lower," says Brill.

"At the same time that we need to decrease omega-6, we need to increase long-chain omega-3 fatty acids. Epidemiological studies show overall heart health with high PUFAs, but we need higher levels of long-chain omega-3 fatty acids to offset the high levels of omega-6. If we didn't have such low levels of long-chain omega-3 fatty acids, the high omega-6 intake wouldn't be so problematic," adds Nettleton.

Good Fats to the Rescue

To achieve a healthier fat lineup, the secret is to focus on healthier MUFAs and omega-3 fatty acids. According to the AHA, adding healthy MUFAs and omega-3s can help provide antioxidants such as vitamin E and selenium; foster absorption of important nutrients in fruits and vegetables; prevent and treat diabetes, heart disease, cancer, obesity, musculoskeletal pain, and inflammatory conditions; positively affect cholesterol, blood pressure, blood clotting, and inflammation; and support brain growth and development.[1]

"The best strategy for getting a more positive ratio of omega-6 to omega-3 fatty acids is to eat less linoleic acid and increase omega-3 fatty acids. We need to replace these oils with olive oil as the main fat, which is part one. The No. 1 oil for home use should be olive oil; it can be used in salad dressings and cooking. For baking, canola oil is a good choice," says Brill, who also notes that extra-virgin olive oil is an even better choice than regular olive oil because it has not been treated with excessive heat or solvents. Thus, it offers an added bonus of polyphenols and antioxidants.

"The best strategy for getting a more positive ratio of omega-6 to omega-3 fatty acids is to eat less linoleic acid and increase omega-3 fatty acids."

—Janet Bond Brill, PhD, RD, LDN

MUFAs are found in canola, olive, peanut, and sunflower oils, as well as avocados, seeds, and nuts. But it's difficult to find MUFAs as the main source of fat in processed foods, so focusing on whole foods and cooking at home is paramount. "There should be an emphasis on monounsaturated fats in cooking use, such as canola oil and olive oil. Minimize the use of corn, soybean, and safflower oils, as you'll get mostly linoleic acid," adds Nettleton.

"Part two is bumping up omega-3 fatty acids by getting daily doses of plant omega-3 fatty acids such as flax and walnuts and marine sources of omega-3 fatty acids, DHA [docosahexaenoic acid] and EPA [eicosapentaenoic acid], by eating fatty fish at least two to three times per week. This shifts the physical environment away from a high omega-6 ratio, which promotes a proinflammatory situation conducive to blood clotting and chronic disease," says Brill. Unfortunately, the conversion of the plant form of omega-3 fatty acids, alpha-linolenic acid (ALA), to long-chain omega-3 fatty acids is modest at best. "Plant sources of omega-3 fatty acids are not equivalent to the long-chain omega-3 fatty acids DHA and EPA. People should target 500 milligrams per day of long-chain omega-3s," says Nettleton.

A growing body of evidence is linking increased intakes of long-chain omega-3 fatty acids found in fish and fish oil to decreased risk of cardiovascular disease, arrhythmias that can lead to sudden cardiac death, and thrombosis that can prompt myocardial infarction or stroke; decreased levels of triglycerides; slower growth of atherosclerotic plaque; improved vascular endothelial function; modest blood pressure lowering; and decreased inflammation. The omega-3 fatty acid ALA has benefits of its own, including reduced coronary heart disease risk.[2]

"There is significant research pointing out that ALA has tremendous health benefits. Even though the conversion rate to long-chain omega-3 fatty acids is low, I say get it in the diet anyway. These plant sources of ALA are very healthy foods, and we haven't fully discovered yet how they provide such great value to health. Perhaps there is some other mechanism other than conversion by which they provide benefits," says Brill.

Nettleton points out that ALA can help redress the balance of omega-6 to omega-3. But if people rely on ALA exclusively, they will not get the tremendous benefits specifically linked with long-chain omega-3s.

Oil Primer

"It's time for an oil change in this country," says Janet Bond Brill, PhD, RD, LDN, a nutrition and fitness consultant. Check out this profile on popular cooking oils to see how they rate for their fat ratios and cooking properties.

Oil	Fat Lineup	Properties
Olive	77% mono, 9% poly, 14% saturated	Rich olive taste, low smoke point. Best in dressings, marinades, sauces, sautés, pastas, casseroles, stir-fries, soups, and meat dishes.
Hazelnut	76% mono, 14% poly, 10% saturated	Brown colored with hazelnut flavor, high smoke point. Best used to bring out flavor in baked desserts, dressings, and meats.
Avocado	70% mono, 10% poly, 20% saturated	Light avocado flavor, high smoke point. Best in salad dressings and marinades, sautés, casseroles, pastas, and meats.
Canola	62% mono, 32% poly, 6% saturated	Light color and flavor, moderately high smoke point. Best for baking or in dishes that require a mild flavor.
Peanut	49% mono, 33% poly, 18% saturated	Peanut flavor and aroma, high smoke point. Best in foods that benefit from peanut flavor, such as Asian stir-fries, noodles, rice, and salads.
Sesame	40% mono, 46% poly, 14% saturated	Light and mild sesame flavor, moderately high smoke point. Best in Asian stir-fries, noodles, rice, and salads.
Palm	38% mono, 10% poly, 52% saturated	Red-orange color and unique flavor, high smoke point. May bring out the flavor in Caribbean and South American dishes but is moderately high in saturated fat.
Corn	25% mono, 62% poly, 13% saturated	Light and mild flavor, high smoke point. Best used in baking or deep-frying but is high in linoleic acid.
Soybean	24% mono, 61% poly, 15% saturated	Slightly heavy flavor, high smoke point. Best used in baking or deep-frying but is high in linoleic acid.
Sunflower	20% mono, 69% poly, 11% saturated	Light and flavorless, high smoke point. Best used in baking but is high in linoleic acid.
Walnut	19% mono, 67% poly, 14% saturated	Rich walnut flavor, moderately high smoke point. Best used to bring out flavor in baked desserts, dressings, and meats. High in alpha-linolenic acid.
Grape seed	17% mono, 71% poly, 12% saturated	Mild flavor, high smoke point. Best in sautéing or frying but is high in linoleic acid.
Safflower	13% mono, 77% poly, 10% saturated	Light color and flavor, high smoke point. Best for searing meats, baking desserts, and deep-frying foods but is high in linoleic acid.
Coconut	6% mono, 2% poly, 92% saturated	Solid at room temperature, buttery texture, low smoke point. Popular in Southeast Asian Dishes but is high in saturated fats.

Note: Sorted in descending order of monounsaturated fat level. Fat levels and smoke points may vary depending on variety and oil refinement process.
Adapted from RecipeTips.com. Oils and fats nutritional facts, Available at: http://www.recipetips.com/kitchen-tips/t-153-1194/oils-and-fats-nutritional-facts.asp; The Nibble, Culinary oils glossary, Available at: http://www.thenibble.com/reviews/main/oils/culinary-oil-glossary.asp; What's Cooking America, Questions & answers—Smoking points of various oils. Available at: http://whatscookingamerica.net/Q-A/SmokePointOil.htm

In the end, it seems dietitians have their work cut out for them trying to simplify the complicated science on fats for the public's easy digestion. But it looks like the stars are aligned for doing so. Chefs are warbling their praise for extra-virgin olive oil, the Mediterranean diet is as hot as ever, and there seems to be a newfound respect for healthy food that tastes great.

"The public is slowly but surely realizing the value of adding healthy fats to the diet. You can see it in the popularity of the Mediterranean diet, and the American Heart Association is no longer concentrating on low fat but on healthy fats," says Brill.

Notes

1. American Heart Association. Face the fats. Available at: http://www.americanheart.org/presenter.jhtml?identifier=3046074
2. Linus Pauling Institute. Essential fatty acids. Available at: http://lpi.oregonstate.edu/infocenter/othernuts/omega3fa/index.html

SHARON PALMER, RD, is a contributing editor at *Today's Dietitian* and a freelance food and nutrition writer in southern California.

Omega-3 Madness

Bonnie Liebman

Are omega-3s the latest mega-trend? You can find claims on everything from mayonnaise to margarine, eggs, cereal, milk, yogurt, cookies, frozen pizza, and (naturally) canned fish. You can even buy Iams Smart Puppy dog food with DHA ("just like babies, a puppy's ability to learn depends upon healthy brain development").

But not all omega-3s are created equal. It's largely DHA and EPA, the long-chain omega-3 fats in fish oil, that are linked to a lower risk of heart disease and possibly cancer, Alzheimer's, eye disorders, and other problems.

Yet many claims appear on foods that have ALA (alpha-linolenic acid), an omega-3 fat that may not prevent much of anything (and may raise the risk of prostate cancer). And some labels don't say which omega-3s their food contains.

Here's a sampling of tricks that can trip you up in the search for omega-3s.

Confusing but Not Concise

"Supportive but not conclusive research shows that consumption of EPA and DHA omega-3 fatty acids may reduce the risk of coronary heart disease," says the squished print on the back of StarKist Very Low Sodium Chunk White Albacore Tuna in Water. "One serving of white tuna in water provides 0.22 grams of EPA and DHA omega-3 fatty acids."

A snazzy claim like that can only come from the way-off-Madison-Avenue writers at the Food and Drug Administration.

Few companies use the confusing FDA-approved health claim. (Even the FDA's own studies show that it misleads consumers.)

Instead, most labels don't mention heart disease. Bumble Bee Wild Alaska Sockeye Red Salmon simply says "contains 1.0g Omega-3 fatty acids per serving." Chicken of the Sea Pink Salmon labels say "heart healthy omega-3s." That's a "structure-or-function" claim that requires no approval because it doesn't mention a disease. (Bet you didn't notice.)

The (really) small print on Chicken's back adds that the salmon "contains 245mg of EPA and DHA combined per serving, which is 153% of the 160 mg Daily Value for

a combination of EPA and DHA." (Ignore all Daily Value claims. There are no DVs for EPA, DHA, or ALA, so companies are making up their own.)

Bottom line: Seafood is the best source of omega-3s, but levels (and serving sizes) vary. Bring your reading glasses.

Smart Marketing

Breyers is one of the first companies to add DHA to foods. And it comes from algae, not fish oil, which may appeal to vegetarians.

But calling a yogurt "Smart!" takes chutzpah. "Boost your brain," says the front label. "DHA Omega-3 is an important brain nutrient that supports brain function and development," says the lid. "DHA also supports a healthy heart," it adds.

"Boost your brain"? Does that mean a higher IQ or SAT score? No worries about Alzheimer's? The evidence that DHA can improve memory is still very uncertain. But claims with words like "support," "maintain," or "boost" don't need evidence. Unfortunately, few people—outside of the FDA and food-industry marketers—know that.

Here's the kicker: Breyers' label doesn't say how much DHA is in Smart! Yogurt. Is that because it's so little? A 6-oz. container has just 32 mg of DHA—about as much as you'd get in 3/4 teaspoon of salmon. (And the salmon has 20 mg of EPA to boot.)

Slick Silk

Like Breyers Smart! Yogurt, Silk Soymilk Plus Omega-3 DHA has added algae (algal oil, to be precise). And Silk also makes a no-evidence-needed claim ("Helps support heart, brain & eye health").

But Silk pulls a fast one. On one panel, the carton says "400 mg of beneficial Omega-3," implying that each cup has that much DHA. Only a few dedicated label readers will notice that Silk Plus also has flax oil, which contains ALA, the far-less-useful omegas-3, and fewer may notice the tiny type on a side panel that whispers, "contains 32 mg of DHA per serving."

Horizon Organic Lowfat Milk Plus DHA has the same 32 mg of DHA per cup—less than what's in a bite of salmon. But you'd never know that from the label, which discloses no DHA numbers at all ("because we're not required to," the company told us). Hello, FDA. Anyone home?

Eggsaggeration

Omega-3 claims are all over the egg case, from brands like Land O Lakes to Best, Gold Circle Farms, Full Spectrum Farms, Giving Nature, Safeway, and more. Clearly, producers are trying to counter the egg's reputation as a heart threat by giving their hens DHA-rich feed.

But omega-3s don't compensate for the 210 mg of cholesterol in each large egg yolk. (That doesn't mean you can't eat eggs. Just stick to no more than four yolks a week, as the American Heart Association recommends.)

And some omega claims are misleading. Land O Lakes Omega 3 Eggs, for example, contain "350 mg of omega-3 fatty acids per serving," according to the label. Yet our independent laboratory analysis found only 150 mg of DHA plus EPA in each egg. The remaining 200 mg was less-beneficial ALA.

At least some companies are more honest. Eggland's Best promises 100 mg of omega-3 on its label. Our lab test found 130 mg of DHA plus EPA.

Our favorite trick: Full Spectrum Farms boasts that its eggs have 30 mg of omega-3s. Yet an egg from a hen dining on ordinary feed has 20 mg of DHA plus EPA.

Bring out the ALA?

"Naturally rich in Omega 3 ALA," says the label of Hellmann's Mayonnaise. "Contains 650 mg ALA per serving; 50% of the Daily Value of ALA (1,300 mg)." Likewise Kraft Real Mayonnaise is a "natural source of 690 mg ALA Omega-3."

Since When Did Mayo Have ALA?

It always has. Mayonnaise is largely soybean oil, which packs 925 milligrams of ALA per tablespoon. (Canola oil has 1,300 mg, while flaxseed oil has 7,250 mg.) Hellmann's Light Mayonnaise has 260 mg of ALA per tablespoon because it has more water than oil.

The question is: do you want more ALA? Like other unsaturated fats, it helps lower blood cholesterol. But experts disagree over whether it reduces the risk of heart disease. And some studies have found that men who eat an average of 1,500 mg a day of ALA have twice the risk of advanced prostate cancer of men who average 700 mg.

Bottom line: If you want the (potential) benefits of omega-3s, go for DHA and EPA. And until experts clarify the possible link with prostate cancer, men shouldn't go out of their way to get more ALA.

Women needn't worry about getting too much. And it's tough to get too little ALA, what with all the soybean and canola oil in the food supply.

Slippery Spread

Smart Balance is Peanut Butter to Omega Oatmeal, Omega Cooking Oil, and Omega Plus Light Mayonnaise, the brand is a regular omega-3 mart.

But only one Smart Balance item gets some of its omega-3s from a source other than the ALA in flax, canola, soybean, or other vegetable oils. A serving of Omega Plus Buttery Spread has "560 mg Omega-3's" and "contains natural plant sterols & fish oil," according to the big print on the front label.

Shoppers have to read the fine print on the side—there's no shortage—to find out that each tablespoon has only 160 mg of "Long-Chain Omega-13 (DHA, EPA)" along with 400 mg of "Short-Chain Omega-3 (ALA)."

There's nothing wrong with getting fish oil from a "buttery spread" . . . as long as you know that you're getting a dollop of ALA along with it.

Track the Flax

You'll find omega-3 claims on Quaker Take Heart oatmeal, Kashi TLC granola bars, Barilla Plus spaghetti, and a host of other cereals, pastas, frozen waffles, and other foods.

Some, like Kashi Mediterranean Pizza, make clear what they contain ("260 mg ALA—an Omega-3"). Others, like Kashi GOLEAN Crunch! Honey Almond Flax cereal, simply say "omega-3 500 mg." How do you know if it's ALA or DHA or EPA?

If the food is made with flaxseed or flax oil, odds are you're getting only ALA. Soybean or canola oil may also supply enough ALA to warrant a claim, but flax is a dead giveaway.

In fact, it's safe to assume that any omega-3 claim refers to ALA unless the label promises EPA and DHA (which should show up in the ingredients list as fish or fish oil) or just DHA (which shows up as algal oil).

Wouldn't it be helpful if the FDA required labels with claims to say how much of each omega-3 the food contained? Don't hold your breath.

UNIT 3

Diet and Disease

Unit Selections

17. **Food for Thought: Exploring the Potential of Mindful Eating,** Sharon Palmer
18. **Eating Disorders in Childhood: Prevention and Treatment Supports,** Catherine Cook-Cottone
19. **The Diet-Inflammation Connection,** Sharon Palmer
20. **The Best Diabetes Diet for Optimal Outcomes,** Rita Carey
21. **Diet Does Matter: Nutrition's Role in Cancer Prevention and Treatment,** Marie Spano
22. **Alzheimer's—The Case for Prevention,** Oliver Tickell
23. **Living Longer: Diet,** Donna Jackson Nakazawa

Key Points to Consider

- How can a person who multitasks while eating benefit from mindful eating practices?

- Do you know someone with an eating disorder? If so, what symptoms does he or she exhibit?

- Are there programs at your college/university for students with eating disorders? If so, is the program well publicized?

- How is inflammation linked to chronic diseases such as diabetes and cardiac disease?

- Does your diet follow the principles of an anti-inflammation diet? Explain why or why not.

Student Website

www.mhhe.com/cls

Internet References

American Cancer Society
www.cancer.org
American Heart Association (AHA)
www.americanheart.org
The Food Allergy and Anaphylaxis Network
www.foodallergy.org
Heinz Infant & Toddler Nutrition
www.heinzbaby.com
LaLeche League International
www.lalecheleague.org
National Eating Disorders Association
www.nationaleatingdisorders.org/

In ancient cultures and in many countries of the world today, the practice of "medicine" or healing includes diet, exercise, and the power of the mind to cure disease. Since those times, research that focuses on the connection between diet and disease has unraveled the role of many nutrients in disease prevention or reversal, but frequently results in controversial or contradictory messages. With the increasing interest in health and disease prevention among Americans, media outlets publish scientific findings prematurely and without the physiological context in which the message should be conveyed. Scientific research takes time to answer the questions about health, nutrition, disease, and medicine, whereas consumers want answers to these questions much quicker than scientifically possible. Medical and nutrition research has changed since mapping of the human genome. We have come to better understand the role of genetics in the expression of disease and its role in how we respond to dietary change. In addition, research about diet and disease has enabled us to understand the importance and uniqueness of the individual (age, gender, ethnicity, and genetics) and his or her particular response to dietary interventions.

Research has been uncovering that a certain food or food components may contribute to one cancer but help prevent another, and specific dietary changes may vary among individuals depending on their genotype, their overall health, and many other factors. Individualizing one's diet to prevent disease and promote health is a new concept that we will see developing in the near future. One of the articles in this unit describes in detail why a Western diet, obesity, and physical inactivity all contribute to a higher risk for cancer, and discusses the importance of lifestyle changes on cancer gene expression. This is a promising picture, especially for people with a family history of cancer, if lifestyle changes are made.

Scientific research has shown that phytochemicals (such as flavonoids, carotenoids, saponins, indoles, and others in foods—especially fruits and vegetables) have the potential to prevent disease, thereby increasing both the quality of life and life expectancy. Research has also shown that inflammation is a risk factor in cardiovascular disease, obesity, diabetes, and a number of other chronic diseases. A lifestyle change plan to decrease inflammation has been developed and is presented in one of the readings in this unit.

As the population is getting older and obesity is on the rise, degenerative diseases that decrease the quality and quantity of life are on the rise. Animal studies have shown that restricting calories prevents disease and prolongs life. Scientists searching for ways to decrease degenerative disease incidence and increase longevity have discovered that restricting or wisely selecting our caloric intake will reduce free radical production and thus lower our risk. Alzheimer's, another disease of aging, is also on the rise. Nutrition research offers many cost-effective, scientifically proven ways for its prevention. A diet high in monounsaturated fats, long-chain omega-3s, and antioxidants is just one of a few suggestions offered by another article in this unit.

Approximately 15 percent of children in the United States between the ages of 6–19 are obese, and 30 percent are overweight. Because of this, childhood obesity has gained much needed attention in the media and health arenas. Another

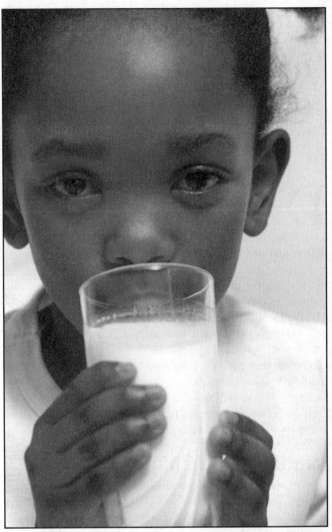

© Greatstock Photographic Library

concern with this population is with the increased incidence of eating disorders (ED) among school-aged children. Although the highest incidences of ED are seen on college campuses, we are seeing increasing incidence of ED among children. The latest estimates of eating disorders among Americans is 36 million who suffer from anorexia, bulimia, or binge eating. The article published by Catherine Cook-Cattone addresses the types of ED, treatment recommendations, and school-based prevention practices of this growing problem. One very promising treatment used by many ED counselors is mindful eating coaching. Mindful eating is a new concept that has proven beneficial in eating disorders treatment, lowering cardiac disease risk, and weight loss in the overweight/obese. The busy lifestyle of Americans has changed our perception of food. We have desensitized ourselves of the normal homeostatic regulation of hunger cues and have a detached view of food. The article by Sharon Palmer introduces the concept of mindful eating and gives tips on how to slow down, appreciate, and change your view of food.

Food for Thought: Exploring the Potential of Mindful Eating

SHARON PALMER

Do you eat when you're not hungry? Do you find yourself wolfing down food without even remembering it? If you're like most people, the answer is yes. In today's world, people barely notice the act of eating, as they feed on demand from fast food drive-thrus, vending machines, and snack food cartons. The net result is that we've become increasingly out of touch with our body's sense of hunger and fullness, as well as the pleasures of eating. In a 2008 General Mills online hunger and eating survey that included 1,049 men and women aged 18 and over, only 6% indicated that they almost always notice physical hunger such as a growling stomach before they eat. When subjects were asked how often they multi-task (driving, walking, working, watching television, shopping online, etc.) while eating, a scant 3% reported never. Only 34% of participants indicated that they decide a meal or snack is over when they feel full.

Mindless Munching

It seems as if our society has refined the art of mindless eating as it grows ever busier and less connected to food and food preparation. "Mindless eating is when people are not paying attention when they are eating. They look down at their empty plate or bag of cookies and ask 'where did it go?' People are eating on the run without tasting food; without an awareness that they are putting it into their mouths. By buying prepared foods, people are putting less personal preparation into it. Even when you make a sandwich, there is a level of awareness and appreciation for the food," says Nancy Ostreicher, M.S., health educator for the University of New Mexico Center for Life Mindful Eating and Living (MEAL) program, a mindfulness-based stress reduction program that incorporates eating exercises. What's the downside to a mindless eating habit? Experts believe that it may be contributing to our nation's obesity problem, which increases the risk for chronic disease.

A New Focus on Food

There is growing support for a new concept that is centered upon mindful eating. Mindful eating draws upon the recognized practice of mindfulness-based stress reduction, which helps people focus on the present moment rather than continuing habitual and unsatisfying behaviors. Mindfulness-based stress reduction has been shown to improve pain, anxiety, and depression. Building upon this strategy, mindful eating practices promote a satisfying relationship with food and eating on a deep emotional level and encourage a better sense of well-being.

"Mindful eating has to do with paying attention to your own personal experience with food. There is a physical awareness of the food; the taste, smell, texture, and how it feels traveling to your belly. There are all of the mental thoughts, including memories about food being pleasurable or displeasurable. Then you can expand that awareness to observations like who grew the food, how it was packaged, where it comes from, and who prepared it," explains Ostreicher.

Evidence supports the benefits of mindful eating in both mental and physical health. Researchers from the University of New Mexico recruited 25 participants for a mindfulness-based stress reduction course that included eating exercises. There was an observed decline in binge eating, as well as anxiety and depressive symptoms. This study was co-authored by Brian Shelley, MD, founder of the University of New Mexico Mindfulness-Based Stress Reduction Program.

On April 14, 2008, Shelley presented findings from a recent study on the effects of mindful eating at the 5th Annual Nutrition and Health Conference: State of the Science & Clinical Applications in Phoenix, Arizona, which was sponsored by the University of Arizona College of Medicine. When study subjects were provided with a MEAL curriculum that included mindfulness-based stress reduction and eating principles, there was an observed decrease in weight, improvements in markers of cardiovascular disease risk, and improvements in measures of mindfulness and binge eating. This study was followed up with a randomized control trial with a group of 20 mindfulness treatment subjects and a group of 20 support group control subjects. The overall weight loss between the groups was similar, but the effect size was slightly larger in the mindfulness group, and was accompanied with greater changes in waist-to-hip ratio and cardiovascular disease risk markers. At the 12-month mark, mindfulness participants maintained and continued to lose weight. Shelley believes that MEAL might be a viable option for treating obesity.

Practicing Mindful Eating

Mindful eating seems like a logical approach to managing your weight. The question is: Are you a mindful eater? Put yourself to the test. According to The Center for Mindful Eating, a mindful eater:

- Acknowledges that there is no right or wrong way to eat, but there are varying degrees of awareness surrounding the experience of food.
- Accepts that his/her eating experiences are unique.
- Is an individual who, by choice, directs his/her awareness to all aspects of food and eating on a moment-by-moment basis.
- Is an individual who looks at the immediate choices and direct experiences associated with food and eating, not to the distant health outcome of that choice.
- Is aware of and reflects on the effects caused by unmindful eating.
- Experiences insight about how he/she can act to achieve specific health goals as he/she becomes more attuned to the direct experience of eating and feelings of health.
- Becomes aware of the interconnection of earth, living beings, and cultural practices and the impact of his/her food choices on those systems.

Thinking Food Through, Step by Step

If you'd like to be more mindful in your eating approach, here are a few handy tips from mindful eating instructor Nancy Ostreicher when you sit down to your next meal:

1. Imagine that this is the first time you've ever seen this food.
2. Take one piece of the food and notice your impression of the food before you put it in your mouth: color, smell, texture, and how it feels in your hand.

3. Bring it to your nose and lips. Notice your feelings, thoughts, memories, expectations, and anticipation before you put it into your mouth.
4. Put it in your mouth. Without biting or swallowing it, notice the initial taste, texture, sensations, and activity inside your mouth.
5. Biting the food and chewing slowly, notice these same sensations and transformations of the food in your mouth.
6. Swallowing the food, notice the feeling of the food traveling to your stomach.
7. Think about what is going on in your mouth, throat, and stomach after swallowing.
8. Eat the second piece of food with awareness. Was your experience different than the first?
9. Consider how this experience with this food was different from how you usually eat this food. Think about your experience of feeling finished, satisfied or wanting more. What insights have you learned from this experience?

Mindful Eating at Your Fingertips

Looking for help on becoming a more mindful eater? Check out these resources:

- University of New Mexico Center for Life developed a Mindful Eating and Living (MEAL) six week training program to help guide participants through the practice of mindful eating (http://hsc.unm.edu/som/cfl/mindfulnessprog.shtml).
- The Center for Mindful Eating offers a wealth of information on mindful eating techniques, as well as links to articles, books, handouts, and workshops on mindful eating (www.tcme.org).

Eating Disorders in Childhood
Prevention and Treatment Supports

CATHERINE COOK-COTTONE

Sarah is a sensitive child who thrives on praise. She works hard to succeed, believing that success is what truly defines a person. Her efforts are often taken for granted, however. Sarah's high-achieving, impeccably dressed parents expect achievement. They regularly attend teacher conferences. They offer continuous support of Sarah's academics and sports. Like any family, they have problems at home, but this family is exceptionally private. Thus, Sarah knows not to discuss the problems with anyone. For Sarah, failure is not an option—not in school, and not on the playing field. She believes that success depends on being what others need you to be. School, her parents, and the media have all influenced how she determines success.

On the surface, Sarah is the type of student that teachers love. She is always smiling, her homework is done perfectly, and she is an active team member across the board. However, it is what is happening inside, beneath the surface, that places Sarah at high risk for developing an eating disorder. Eating disorders (EDs) are chronic clinical mental disorders that are disruptive to the psychological and social development of children and adolescents (Hoek & van Hoeken, 2003). They can be difficult to prevent and treat and are considered among the most chronic and medically lethal of mental disorders (American Psychiatric Association [APA], 2000; Keel & Herzog, 2004). Research suggests that the incidence and prevalence of eating disorders are increasing and that the age of onset may be decreasing (e.g., Rastam, Gillberg, van Hoeken, & Hoek, 2004). Luckily for Sarah and others like her, school can provide a safe and protective environment in which to heal from an ED.

> **Research suggests that the incidence and prevalence of eating disorders are increasing and that the age of onset may be decreasing.**

The keys to preventing and successfully treating EDs are the efficient integration of mental health and school practices in effective prevention programs, timely and efficient risk identification, and support of treatment (Cook-Cottone & Phelps, 2006). However, few education publications offer information and guidance as to *how* early childhood educators can be part of prevention and intervention of EDs (Haines, Neumark-Sztainer, & Thiel, 2007). To help educators support prevention and treatment of EDs, this article provides: 1) a detailed description of symptoms and risk factors associated with EDs; 2) an overview of ED definitions, prevalence rates, and treatment protocol; and 3) a review of school-based prevention practices, with explicit recommendations for childhood educators.

Eating Disorder Risk

It is important for school professionals to have a solid understanding of the risks and causes of EDs (Yager & O'Dea, 2005). The risks are complex, and the pathway to ED behavior is determined by a combination of factors. Although this pathway appears to vary from patient to patient, a combination of biological, psychological, and environmental factors affect each student's risk.

Risk Factors

The two strongest predictors of eating-disordered behaviors are body dissatisfaction and dieting (Cook-Cottone & Phelps, 2006; Mintz, Borchers, Bledman, & Franko, 2008). Gender is a strong risk factor, with only a small proportion of documented clinical cases being male (APA, 2000). Other individual risk factors include: genetic predisposition, early pubertal onset, emotional sensitivity, perfectionism, emotional-regulation difficulties, and disordered development of self-concept (Mintz et al., 2008). A history of physical and sexual abuse also is believed to increase risk (Wonderlich et al., 2001). Family factors include low levels of parental attunement and poor communication (Wonderlich et al., 2001). Participating in activities that emphasize appearance and weight adds to the risk (Patel, Greydanus, Pratt, & Phillips, 2003); such activities include boxing, wrestling, dancing, crew, and gymnastics (Patel et al., 2003). Adding to the risk, today's children and adolescents are eating more calorie-dense foods that are void of nutritional value (i.e., junk food) and spending more time on sedentary activities (e.g., involving hand-held technologies, computer applications, and television) (Haines et al., 2007). Thus, those already at risk for an ED face a consequent risk for weight gain, which, when combined with cultural pressures that idealize thinness, fuels greater anxiety.

Examples of factors that undermine self-image are the media, a cultural focus on dieting, and weight-related teasing. Media influence is considered a particularly important and, some suggest, causal factor leading to ED (e.g., Becker, Burwell, Gilman, Herzog, & Hamburg, 2002). Specifically, chronic exposure to unrealistic media images influences how children think and feel about their bodies (Becker et al., 2002; Haines et al., 2007). The cultural focus on dieting has created unprecedented exposure to diet commercials, diet talk, and dieting behavior (Haines et al., 2007). Finally, researchers have recently started to explore the rate and impact of weight-related teasing among children (Haines et al., 2007).

Pathway to Disorder

For some children and adolescents, the risk factors combine and the pathway toward disorder begins. The trajectory toward illness often involves the onset of body dissatisfaction, accompanied by restrictive dieting behaviors (Mintz et al., 2008). School personnel should note that restrictive dieting is no longer limited to adolescents and adults; it is now found in children as young as 8 years old (Thomas, Ricciardelli, & Williams, 2000). As the disorder evolves, a subset of these children and adolescents continue their food restriction to the pathological levels that characterize anorexia nervosa. Another subset of children and adolescents struggles with adherence to the restrictive diet and begin a binge and purge cycle in an attempt to maintain their weight (as seen in bulimia nervosa). Some of the behavioral signs of eating disorder onset include: excessively exercising; losing weight; eating only certain foods; obsessing over food, body, weight, or dieting; adopting odd eating rituals; lying or making excuses about eating; hiding weight loss with loose clothing; refusing to eat in front of others; frequenting the bathroom after meals; and exhibiting moodiness and withdrawal (Cook-Cottone & Scime, 2006).

Eating Disorder Prevalence, Definition, and Treatment

The Diagnostic and Statistical Manual of Mental Disorders, Fourth Edition, Text Revision (DSM-IV-TR, APA, 2000) currently lists anorexia nervosa (AN) and bulimia nervosa (BN) as the two main manifestations of eating disorder. For both AN and BN, symptoms can interfere with learning, relationships, and family functioning (Hoek & van Hoeken, 2003).

Anorexia Nervosa

According to the APA (2000) and Rastam and colleagues (2004), the average prevalence rate for AN is 0.3% for young women and is approximately 0.03% for males. These rates represent an increase in AN over the past 50 years (Rastam et al., 2004). In a study of AN survivors, less than 50% had recovered, 33% had improved but were not considered recovered, and 20% remained chronically ill (Steinhausen, 2002). AN is associated

with one of the highest risks for premature death among all the psychiatric disorders, with over 5% of those diagnosed dying of the disease or a related complication (Keel & Herzog, 2004). Those diagnosed with AN perceive the size or shape of their bodies in a distorted way and are deeply afraid of gaining weight (APA, 2000). They pursue and/or maintain excessive thinness (i.e., less than 85% of expected weight for age and height) through a reduction in food intake (i.e., food restriction) (APA, 2000; Cook-Cottone & Phelps, 2006).

It is important for school personnel to note that younger children may not experience loss of weight; instead, they may fail to make expected weight gains as they increase in age and height (Cook-Cottone & Phelps, 2006). For girls, low weight is often accompanied by hormonal changes and loss of menstruation. Patients may appear younger than their chronological age (Herzog & Eddy, 2007). Weight loss is achieved through food restriction and purging (e.g., self-induced vomiting and misuse of laxatives or diuretics), as well as excessive exercise (Cook-Cottone & Phelps, 2006). Individuals with AN can appear to be hyperactive. In this case, however, the activity is related to the pursuit of thinness rather than to the neurological tendency to be active that is often seen in attention deficit hyperactivity disorder (ADHD) (Herzog & Eddy, 2007).

Bulimia Nervosa

The prevalence rate for BN is estimated at 1% in young women and 0.1% for young men (Rastam et al., 2004). Outcomes have been relatively promising, with evidence of up to 75% of those diagnosed not meeting criteria at 5 years (Ben-Tovim, 2003). For those diagnosed with BN, approximately 0.3% die of BN or related complications. Those with BN overemphasize body shape and weight in their overall self-evaluation (APA, 2000). They are often within average weight ranges, with a subset falling into overweight and obese categories (Herzog & Eddy, 2007). The symptoms in BN are quite intense and time-consuming. Specifically, individuals with BN manifest frequent, recurrent episodes of binge eating and use inappropriate compensatory behaviors to prevent weight gain (e.g., self-induced vomiting; misuse of laxatives, diuretics, enemas; fasting; or "obligatory" exercise) (Cook-Cottone & Phelps, 2006). Symptoms often occur when the individual is emotionally overwhelmed, and those with BN use the binge-purge cycle to cope (Cook-Cottone, Beck, & Kane, 2008).

Treatment

Children and adolescents with clinical level EDs require comprehensive and multifaceted care (American Academy of Pediatrics [AAP], 2003). Treatment may be done on either an inpatient or outpatient basis, depending on the level of symptomatology and the patient's health status (Cook-Cottone, 2006).

The Treatment Team

Current best practice in treatment recommends a multidisciplinary team that specializes in the treatment of ED to attend to: health status and medication issues, nutrition and meal planning, and psychosocial treatment (American Psychiatric Association

Work Group on Eating Disorders [APAWGED], 2000; Yager & O'Dea, 2005). Outpatient medical treatment typically involves attention to the patient's holistic wellness and the monitoring and treatment of physiological status (e.g., electrolyte levels, weight, vital signs, medications). A nutritionist often works with the patient to develop a nutrition plan to address restriction, to address chaotic eating patterns that can trigger bingeing and purging cycles, and to prevent hunger (American Dietetic Association [ADA], 2001). Psychosocial issues are typically addressed by a licensed mental health professional with training in the treatment of eating disorders. Treatment of AN often includes both individual and family therapy (APAWGED, 2000). Treatment for BN often includes cognitive behavioral as well as individual psychotherapy modalities, augmented with group therapy and support groups (Wilson, Grilo, & Vitousek, 2007).

Teachers and Treatment

The role of the teacher can take many different forms. For example, teachers and other school personnel can provide valuable support by providing coursework and guidance for hospitalized students (Yager & O'Dea, 2005). In addition, it is often very difficult for these students to eat on their own, because they perceive eating to be very scary. Teachers can suggest snack breaks and offer to be a meal buddy for kids struggling to eat. Physical education teachers can provide alternative activities for students who cannot partake in physically demanding tasks (exceptionally low-weight patients likely have medical restrictions). Treatment often involves frequent medical appointments (up to five a week), and so school personnel must work to be understanding and supportive. Children and adolescents in treatment often worry that teachers are angry about their absences, thus leading to additional distress that could distract them from recovery as well as increasing their resistance to necessary treatment sessions. An effective and supportive home-treatment-school bridge is critical for continued academic growth and healing.

Key School-based Prevention and Support Practices

Prevention and intervention at the elementary school level is critical (Haines et al., 2007). For many years, prevention efforts focused on later middle school and high school students, because it was thought that eating disordered beliefs and behaviors were rare among younger children (Thelen, Powell, Lawrence, & Kulnert, 1992). It is now known that ED risk and associated behaviors may emerge as early as 4th grade (Thelen et al., 1992). Accordingly, prevention programs are considered most effective in the lower elementary years, before crystallization of the preoccupation with body shape and weight within the assessment of self (Cook-Cottone, 2006). Childhood educators can play an important role in both the prevention of EDs and support for those struggling with the clinical disorder (Yager & O'Dea, 2005). Effective prevention in the schools includes implementing universal and targeted prevention practices (Cook-Cottone & Scime, 2006). Specifically, universal prevention efforts target the whole school population through application of strategies known to reduce risk and prevent disorder (Mintz et al., 2008). Targeted prevention efforts entail the provision of focused supplemental interventions involving frequent, small-group sessions that target key risk factors (Mintz et al., 2008).

Universal Prevention

Universal prevention efforts focus on healthy development and the prevention of eating disordered attitudes and behaviors (i.e., before symptoms begin) (Scime & Cook-Cottone, 2008). Universal prevention efforts involve creating and maintaining a prevention-oriented school atmosphere. The four core areas of prevention practices are: encouraging body acceptance decreasing appearance-related teasing, addressing nutrition and physical activity, and increasing coping skills.

Practices That Address Body Acceptance

Effective prevention efforts aimed at body acceptance include media literacy, media policy, and self-concept work. Media literacy refers to the ability to critically evaluate media messages. Activities help students deconstruct the media's overly simplified presentation of beauty and self-evaluation and explore the role of media in product sales and promotion (Cook-Cottone, 2006). Specific content may include a critical analysis of the thin female ideal and the excessively lean and hyper-muscular male ideal (e.g., by asking students if these images are normal and healthy). Demonstrations of image editing techniques can be very effective. Several online resources address image editing, including the award-winning *Evolution* film by Dove Soap (see www.campaignforreal-beauty.ca/flat2.asp?id=7134). In-depth work explores marketing motivations and consumer effects, including the practice of companies linking themselves with positive community service to enhance their image (such as Dove). Students also can explore gender-role stereotyping and its effects on them (e.g., How do we feel about patterns of girls passively looking pretty and boys being engaged in active, traditionally male behaviors?). To address media exposure, childhood educators can create and enforce policies that limit in-school advertising (e.g., Cook-Cottone & Scime, 2006). For example, some schools allow the inclusion of advertising content within the curriculum in the context of media and information literacy (e.g., considering the source and author's purpose, and critically analyzing the message).

Self-concept work typically emphasizes the multifaceted aspects of the self and deemphasizes appearance-based self-evaluation. This is done in many ways. For example, messages that promote acceptance for all body types and sizes can be integrated into all diversity messages (Haines et al., 2007). Also, teachers can highlight achievement and interest-based self-evaluation by modeling this in class through biographical studies in both social studies and writing curricular content (Haines et al., 2007). Finally, coaches and physical education teachers can reinforce effort and personal improvement behaviors that go beyond weight and peer comparisons (e.g., Yager & O'Dea, 2005).

Practices That Address Appearance-related Teasing

Childhood educators can prevent and respond to weight-related teasing. First, prevention efforts should include adoption of zero-tolerance policies related to appearance-based teasing (Cook-Cottone & Scime, 2006). For some schools, this means adding explicit behavioral guidelines for teasing behaviors and associated consequences (Haines et al., 2007). Further, teachers can conduct role-plays and highlight books in class that focus on understanding and preventing teasing (Haines et al., 2007). Such efforts also should include content designed to help children learn ways to respond to teasing and find supportive adults. Accordingly, support should be offered for students who are victims of teasing to address resultant negative emotional impact and feelings of isolation (Haines et al., 2007).

Practices That Address Nutrition and Physical Activity

There are several ways to provide opportunities for enhanced nutrition and physical activity. Initially, student motivation can be addressed through inclusion of basic nutrition information and the explanations of long-term effects of dietary intake and exercise (Haines et al., 2007). Such health information can be embedded in science, health, and physical education curricula (Cook-Cottone & Scime, 2006). Next, students should be given the opportunity to make healthy choices. School lunch plans should be evaluated to ensure inclusion of healthful options (Haines et al., 2007). To enhance exposure, snack time can include taste-testing of nutritious options (Haines et al., 2007). Notably, effective schools offer many opportunities for positive physical and expressive experiences (e.g., soccer, yoga classes, track, swimming, art, and music) (Cook-Cottone & Scime, 2006). Also, it is critical for school faculty and staff to model healthy attitudes towards eating and exercise (e.g., eating and exercising with a goal of health rather than a goal of weight loss) (Cook-Cottone & Scime, 2006). This approach includes the elimination of diet discussions in the presence of children.

Practices That Increase Coping Skills

Coping skills and stress management may have positive risk-reduction effects (Steiner-Adair et al., 2002). Coping skills often involve instruction in problem solving and use a cognitive behavioral approach. That is, the children are taught how to break down their challenges (e.g., interpersonal struggles and stressors) into manageable pieces—1) the event or challenge, 2) associated feelings, 3) associated beliefs and thoughts, 4) what the child might plan to say or do in response to the event, and 5) analysis of the associated consequences (Heffner & Eifert, 2004). The final analysis includes: validation of the child's experience, thoughts, and feelings; a review of whether or not the child's needs were met; and consideration of the safety level and respect for the self and others inherent in behavioral choices (Cook-Cottone, 2006). Skills can be practiced in role-plays, reviews of characters in literature, and explorations of individual experiences (Cook-Cottone, 2006). Stress management practice can vary from audiotaped examples (Gharderi, Martensson, & Schwan, 2005) to active

practice, and can include breathing and relaxation through yoga classes (e.g., Scime & Cook-Cottone, 2008). Such instruction can be embedded in daily school routines (e.g., stress relief breaks), as well as provided in discrete afterschool programs.

Targeted Prevention

Targeted prevention efforts focus on the identification and correction of eating disordered attitudes and behaviors in the very early stages (Cook-Cottone & Phelps, 2006). Keeping groups small and single-gender may be the most effective strategy (Haines et al., 2007). The current trend in prevention is to use an interactive, experiential approach that embraces wellness and increasing coping skills (Cook-Cottone & Phelps, 2006). Active learning is believed to increase content acquisition, and the positive psychology model may reduce symptom learning (Haines et al., 2007). Group curriculum often includes such topics as: self-care (e.g., instruction in relaxation techniques), self-concept work, life skills (e.g., assertiveness training), coping skills (e.g., instruction in emotional regulation), and media literacy (Scime & Cook-Cottone, 2008).

Recent innovations in prevention practices have provided compelling outcomes in the areas of dissonance-based prevention, the integration of body-focused relaxation techniques, and technology-based interventions. First, dissonance-based interventions have been empirically supported for use in ED prevention for populations at all levels of risk (Mintz et al., 2008). The theoretical underpinning of dissonance-based prevention is that it is stressful for individuals to hold competing beliefs (such as, beauty comes from within and only those who fit the media image are beautiful). Therefore, individuals will work to resolve cognitive conflict. Dissonance-based group curriculum involves exploration of the following topics: 1) the origin and perpetuation of the thin ideal, 2) the negative consequences of the thin ideal, 3) media image review, 4) "fatism," 5) self-objectification, and 6) feminist perspectives of the history of thinness and the oppression of women (Mitchell, Mazzeo, Rausch, & Cooke, 2007). Second, emerging evidence points to the therapeutic utility of yoga (Scime & Cook-Cottone, 2008). Third, researchers have documented the utility of using interactive, video-based prevention programs to deliver prevention content (Franko et al., 2005; Mintz et al., 2008). More development is needed to provide these types of video tools at the elementary school level.

Referral and School-based Treatment Support

Children and adolescents who demonstrate behavioral indicators or symptoms of eating disorders should be referred to an eating disorder specialist for further assessment and possible treatment (Yager & O'Dea, 2005). Treatment of clinical level EDs typically is facilitated through referral to out-of-school specialists (Cook-Cottone & Scime, 2006). In order to facilitate a timely referral process, every school should have a resource person handle eating disorder concerns (Yager & O'Dea, 2005). The responsibilities associated with this role include: being knowledgeable about how to approach individuals who are at risk for an eating disorder, organizing inservices and booster sessions, communicating with parents, and making referrals to an appropriate professional source (Yager & O'Dea, 2005).

School-support practices require flexibility and empathy on the part of childhood educators and can considerably aid treatment and back-to-school transitions (Manley, Rickson, & Standeven, 2000). In cases of an extended inpatient hospitalization, academic consultation also may be necessary. If hospitalization or day treatment is required, re-entry to school will be an important transition (Manley et al., 2000). Possible academic accommodations can include: reduced workload, alternative assignments for some physical education requirements, extended time for assignments and tests, peer tutoring for missed coursework, copies of class notes, and access to quiet study locations (Cook-Cottone & Scime, 2006). It will be important to allow alternative assignments for class activities that may be triggers for those with eating disorders, such as weighing-in, co-education swimming classes, or counting calories in nutrition class. In addition, inschool counseling and support can nicely augment out-of-school efforts.

Summary and Implications

Eating disorders, considered among the most chronic and medically lethal of mental disorders, are disruptive to children's development and difficult to prevent and treat. They often strike students who are overlooked because they are compliant. Sarah can be helped now, before she begins to struggle, and it is the childhood educator who can make the difference. For those who already struggle with ED, childhood educators can help make school a supportive, safe, and accommodating place in which to recover.

References

1. American Academy of Pediatrics [AAP]. (2003). Policy statement: Identifying and treating eating disorders. *Pediatrics, 111,* 204–211.
2. American Dietetic Association [ADA]. (2001). Position of the American Dietetic Association: Nutrition intervention in the treatment of anorexia nervosa, bulimia nervosa, and eating disorders not otherwise specified. *Journal of the American Dietetic Association, 101,* 810–819.
3. American Psychiatric Association [APA]. (2000). *The diagnostic and statistical manual of mental disorders, 4th edition, text revision (DSM-IV-TR).* Washington, DC: Author.
4. American Psychiatric Association Work Group on Eating Disorders [APAWGED]. (2000). Practice guideline for the treatment of patients with eating disorders (revision). *American Journal of Psychiatry, 157,* 1–39.
5. Becker, A. E., Burwell, R. A., Gilman, S. E., Herzog, D. B., & Hamburg, P. (2002). Eating behaviors and attitudes following prolonged exposure to television among ethnic Fijian adolescent girls. *British Journal of Psychiatry, 180,* 509–514.
6. Ben-Tovim, D. I. (2003). Eating disorders: Outcome, prevention and treatment of eating disorders. *Current Opinion in Psychiatry, 16,* 65–69.
7. Cook-Cottone, C. (2006). The attuned representation model for the primary prevention of eating disorders: An overview for childhood educators. *Psychology in the Schools, 43,* 1–8.
8. Cook-Cottone, C. P., Beck, M., & Kane, L. (2008). Manualized-group treatment of eating disorders: Attunement in mind, body, and relationship (AMBR). *The Journal for Specialists in Group Work, 33,* 61–83.
9. Cook-Cottone, C. P., & Phelps, L. (2006). Adolescent eating disorders. In G. G. Bear & K. M. Minke (Eds.), *Children's needs III* (pp. 977–988). Bethesda, MD: National Association of School Psychologists.
10. Cook-Cottone, C. P., & Scime, M. (2006). The prevention and treatment of eating disorders: An overview for school psychologists. *The Communiqué, 34,* 38–40.
11. Dove © (2008). *Campaign for real beauty: Evolution project.* Retrieved April 30, 2008, from www.campaignforrealbeauty.ca/flat2.asp?id=7134
12. Franko, D. L., Mintz, L. B., Villapiano, M., Green, T. C., Mainelli, D., Folensbee, L., Butler, S. F., Davidson, M. M., Hamilton, E., & Budman, S., H. (2005). Food, mood and attitude: Reducing the risk for eating disorders in college women. *Health Psychology, 24,* 567–578.
13. Gharderi, A., Martensson, M., & Schwan, H. (2005). "Everybody's different": A primary prevention program among fifth grade school children. *Eating Disorders, 13,* 245–259.
14. Haines, J., Neumark-Sztainer, D., & Thiel, L. (2007). Addressing weight-related issues in an elementary school: What do students, parents, and school staff recommend? *Eating Disorders, 15,* 2–21.
15. Heffner, M., & Eifert, G. (2004). *The anorexia workbook: How to accept yourself, heal your suffering, and reclaim your life.* Oakland, CA: New Harbinger Press.
16. Herzog, D. B., & Eddy, K. T. (2007). Diagnosis, epidemiology, and clinical course. *Clinical Manual of Eating Disorders,* 1–26.
17. Hoek, H. W., & van Hoeken, D. (2003). Review of the prevalence and incidence of eating disorders. *International Journal of Eating Disorders, 24,* 383–396.
18. Keel, P. K., & Herzog, D. B. (2004). Long-term outcome, course of illness and mortality in anorexia nervosa, bulimia nervosa, and binge eating disorder. In T. D. Brewerton (Ed.), *Clinical handbook of eating disorders: An integrated approach* (pp. 97–116). New York: Marcel Dekker.
19. Manley, R. S., Rickson, H., & Standeven, B. (2000). Children and adolescents with eating disorders: Strategies for teachers and school counselors. *Intervention in School & Clinic, 35,* 228–231.
20. Mintz, L., Borchers, E., Bledman, R., & Franko, D. (2008). Preventing eating and weight-related disorders: Towards an integrated best practices approach. In R. Brown & S. Lent (Eds), *Handbook of counseling psychology* (4th ed., pp. 570–587). Hoboken, NJ: Wiley.
21. Mitchell, K., Mazzeo, S. E., Rausch, S. M., & Cooke, K. L. (2007). Innovative interventions for disordered eating: Evaluating dissonance-based and yoga interventions. *International Journal of Eating Disorders, 40,* 120–128.
22. Patel, D. P., Greydanus, D. E., Pratt, H. D., & Phillips, E. L. (2003). Eating disorders in adolescent athletes. *Journal of Adolescent Research, 18,* 280–296.
23. Rastam, M., Gillberg., C., van Hoeken, D., & Hoek, H. W. (2004). Epidemiology of eating disorders: A developmental overview. In T. D. Brewerton (Ed.), *Clinical handbook of eating disorders: An integrated approach* (pp. 71–96). New York: Marcel Dekker.
24. Scime, M., & Cook-Cottone, C. P. (2008). Primary prevention of eating disorders: A constructivist integration of mind and body strategies. *International Journal of Eating Disorders, 41,* 134–142.
25. Steiner-Adair, C., Sjostrom, L., Franko, D., Pai, S., Tucker, R., Becker, A., & Herzog, D. B. (2002). Primary prevention of risk factors for eating disorders in adolescent

girls: Learning from practice. *International Journal of Eating Disorders, 32,* 401–411.

26. Steinhausen, C. (2002). The outcome of anorexia nervosa in the 20th century. *The American Journal of Psychiatry, 159,* 1284–1293.

27. Thelen, M. H., Powell, A. L., Lawrence, C., & Kuhnert, M. E. (1992). Eating and body image concerns among children. *Journal of Clinical Child Psychology, 21,* 41–46.

28. Thomas, K., Ricciardelli, L. A., & Williams, R. J. (2000). Gender traits and self-concept as indicators of problem eating and body dissatisfaction among children. *Sex Roles, 43,* 441–458.

29. Wilson, G. T., Grilo, C. M., & Vitousek, K. M. (2007). Psychological treatment of eating disorders. *American Psychologist, 62,* 199–216.

30. Wonderlich, S., Crosby, R., Mitchell, J., Thompson, K., Redlin, J., Demuth, G., et al. (2001). Pathways mediating sexual abuse and eating disturbance in children. *International Journal of Eating Disorders, 29,* 270–279.

31. Yager, Z., & O'Dea, J. A. (2005). The role of teachers and other educators in the prevention of eating disorders and child obesity: What are the issues? *Eating Disorders, 13,* 261–278.

CATHERINE COOK-COTTONE is Associate Professor, Licensed Psychologist, Certified School Psychologist, Department of Counseling, School & Educational Psychology, University at Buffalo, The State University of New York.

The Diet-Inflammation Connection

The emerging science on how diet contributes to inflammation, thus influencing chronic disease, is big news—especially for dietitians.

SHARON PALMER, RD

You know something's big if Oprah covers it. Yes, the anti-inflammation diet was recent fodder for *O, The Oprah Magazine,* so you know it's being discussed. Some even speculate that the anti-inflammation diet will be the next diet craze, which may explain why scores of books have been written on the subject. A recent Amazon.com query uncovered 671 books using the search terms "inflammation and diet." There's even *The Complete Idiot's Guide to the Anti-Inflammation Diet.*

"I think that anti-inflammation is sort of the new buzz word or phrase these days, so I do get a lot of questions about what it means," says Lynn Goldstein, MS, RD, CDN, HHC, a dietitian and holistic health counselor in New York.

Andrew Weil, MD, director of the Program in Integrative Medicine of the College of Medicine at the University of Arizona, put the anti-inflammatory diet on the map thanks to his popular books, including *Healthy Aging: Your Lifelong Guide to Physical and Spiritual Well-Being,* and Web site, www.drweil.com, where people can sign up for his Healthy Aging Anti-Inflammatory Diet.

"People ask about the anti-inflammatory diet. Dr. Andrew Weil is really getting out there influencing people," says Jessica Siegel, MPH, RD, a California Dietetic Association spokesperson who believes that a healthy, educated, affluent consumer base is attuned to the issue.

Weil, who spoke at the Nutrition and Health: State of the Science and Clinical Applications Conference in San Diego earlier this year, says, "All age-related diseases, including cancer, have their roots in inflammation. Vascular disease begins as an inflammatory process, and Alzheimer's disease results from inflammation of the brain. You can go through life in a proinflammatory state or an anti-inflammatory state. Food choices can either up-regulate inflammation or down-regulate inflammation."

Understanding Inflammation's Repercussions

Interest in inflammation is flourishing. "Anything in the inflammation area in the research world is of large interest, especially in the areas of pain relief," says Cheryl Reifer, PhD, RD, LD, director of Sprim USA, an independent research-driven company focused on health.

"There's enough evidence to support that unhealthy characteristics are associated with increased inflammatory markers to warrant targeted approaches to reduce inflammation," says Cynthia Thomson, PhD, RD, an assistant professor in the University of Arizona's department of nutritional sciences. Thomson says a few years ago, scientists didn't know whether increased inflammation was linked to the risk of chronic diseases, but several studies have shown how diseases such as diabetes and obesity are associated with increased inflammatory markers. "In diabetes and cancer, there are more and more studies suggesting that modulation of inflammatory end points may reduce disease risk," Thomson says.

Inflammation is the first organized reaction to an injurious challenge to the body, whether it's a bacterial infection or oxidized low-density lipoprotein cholesterol. During this process, blood leukocytes migrate to specific tissues, and leukocytes are activated to guide a series of biochemical and cellular events. Researchers are discovering that inflammation is emerging as a root of many chronic diseases. Cardiovascular disease, the primary diet-related disease of our time, has an underlying connection to inflammation, as atherosclerosis is in part due to the accumulation of lipids and inflammatory factors within the vessel wall.

Inflammation is also a significant component of obesity, metabolic syndrome, type 2 diabetes, osteoporosis, periodontal disease, rheumatoid arthritis, neurological degenerative disorders, and inflammatory bowel disorders. Both epidemiological studies and intervention trials support a link between the role of diet and the reduction in the risk of many chronic diseases, and it appears that creating a proinflammatory milieu may be one way that unhealthy diets are linked with metabolic and cardiovascular diseases.

The role that inflammation and oxidative stress may play in brain aging is of particular interest. Inflammatory markers, as well as cellular and molecular oxidative damage, increase during normal brain aging, which is accompanied by the decline in cognitive and motor performance in older populations, even in the absence of neurodegenerative diseases. Epidemiological studies have suggested that diets rich in antioxidant and anti-inflammatory compounds, such as those found in fruits and vegetables, may lower the risk of developing age-related neuro-degenerative diseases such as Parkinson's and Alzheimer's. Additional research suggests that the polyphenolic compounds found in fruits may produce their beneficial effects through signal transduction and neuronal communication.[1-3]

Inflammation normally protects against infection, but when it is ongoing for many years due to infection or hormonal stimulation, it can lead to excess oxidation and cancer, according to David Heber, MD, PhD, FACP, FACN, a professor of medicine and public health and director at the UCLA Center for Human Nutrition, who also spoke at the conference. In rapidly expanding abdominal fat cells and many cancer cells, the inflammation system is turned on all the time, thus leading to the excess production of cytokines (peptide hormones secreted by inflammatory cells) and stromal/adipocyte cells that mediate the inflammatory response. Cytokines are signals that can promote atherosclerosis and tumor growth.

Connecting the Dots: Lifestyle and Inflammation

"Through changes in the diet, you can demonstrate improvements in even low-grade chronic inflammation in people associated with chronic disease as they age," says Thomson. A number of recent studies are looking at various aspects of healthful eating and how they can reduce markers of increased inflammation.

According to a 2007 review in the *Asian Pacific Journal of Cancer Prevention,* C-reactive protein is one of the acute-phase proteins in inflammation; thus, high-sensitivity C-reactive protein (hs-CRP) serum concentrations have intrigued researchers. Studies have linked high concentrations of hs-CRP and obesity, as well as smoking. Moderate alcohol consumption and high physical activity have been associated with low levels of hs-CRP. Many prospective studies have also found an increased risk of type 2 diabetes associated with high concentrations of hs-CRP, independent

---

Dr. Weil's Eating Plan to Avoid Inflammation

Andrew Weil's, MD, anti-inflammatory regime is a no-nonsense approach to eating on which most dietitians would happily place their stamp of approval. "It really comes down to the same things I would tell anyone for a healthy diet," says Lynn Goldstein, MS, RD, CDN, HHC, a dietitian and holistic health counselor in New York, of anti-inflammatory diet strategies.

According to Weil, the basic principles of anti-inflammatory eating include the following:

- Eat a variety of foods.
- Emphasize fresh foods that have better nutritional quality.
- Avoid processed foods of all kinds.
- Eat an abundance of fruits and vegetables.
- Consume an appropriate number of calories to maintain optimal weight and metabolic needs.
- Choose less refined carbohydrates with an emphasis on low glycemic index/glycemic load carbohydrates.
- Focus on whole grains that are truly "whole," rather than pulverized and reformulated (eg, flours and processed breakfast cereals).
- Avoid high fructose corn syrup.
- Decrease consumption of animal proteins, except fish.
- Increase intake of omega-3 fatty acids.
- Take advantage of whole soy foods.
- Support organic agriculture to avoid exposure to multiple agents.
- Drink tea instead of coffee.
- Enjoy red wine if alcohol is consumed.
- Consume small amounts of dark chocolate with a minimum of 70% cocoa.
- Flavor foods with antioxidant spices such as ginger and turmeric.
- Increase fiber intake through fruits, vegetables, beans, and whole grains.
- Choose healthy fats by avoiding trans fats and saturated fats, limiting polyunsaturated fats to maintain a better omega-6/omega-3 ratio, and emphasizing extra virgin olive oil, nuts, and avocados.
- Drink more water.
- Consider a multivitamin with mineral supplement for insurance.

---

of obesity and other cardiovascular risk factors, but the findings are inconsistent. Numerous studies have discovered that high concentrations of hs-CRP are associated with increased risks of colorectal and other cancers, but these findings are also inconsistent. High intakes of carotenoids and vitamin C, but not vitamin E, seem to decrease the level of circulating hs-CRP. In addition, high consumption of vegetables and fruits is associated with lower levels of circulating hs-CRP.[4]

Certain dietary strategies may be associated with a lower generation of inflammation, according to a state-of-the-art paper published in a 2006 issue of the *Journal of the American College of Cardiology*. Dietary patterns high in refined starches, sugar, and saturated and trans fatty acids; low in natural antioxidants and fiber from fruits, vegetables, and whole grains; and poor in omega-3 fatty acids may cause an activation of the innate immune system through an excessive production of proinflammatory cytokines associated with a reduced production of anti-inflammatory cytokines. The report also notes that the whole diet approach seems particularly promising in reducing inflammation associated with the metabolic syndrome. Choices such as healthy sources of carbohydrate, fat, and protein, regular physical activity, and avoidance of smoking are critical to fighting the war against chronic disease. The bottom line is that the Western way of eating warms up inflammation, and changing the diet can cool it down.

The results of a 10-week dietary intervention study involving 17 healthy subjects that was published in 2007 in the *European Journal of Clinical Nutrition* found a decreased omega-6/omega-3 polyunsaturated fatty acid ratio resulted in multiple potentially favorable effects on the metabolic and inflammatory profiles. And data from the Iowa Women's Health Study pointed to a reduction in inflammatory mortality associated with habitual whole grain intake that was larger than what was previously reported for coronary heart disease and diabetes. Because various phytochemicals are found in whole grains that may directly or indirectly inhibit oxidative stress and because oxidative stress is an inevitable consequence of inflammation, the researchers concluded that oxidative stress reduction by constituents of whole grain is a likely mechanism for the protective effect.[5]

The ATTICA epidemiological study, which included 625 men and 712 women with abdominal obesity from the Attica area in Greece, discovered that among the subjects studied, low-grade systemic inflammation may be associated with an unfavorable lifestyle, including physical inactivity and unhealthy dietary habits, as well as increased blood pressure levels and low high-density lipoprotein cholesterol.

Send in the Clowns

Even though the field of anti-inflammatory nutrition appears promising, consumers must brace themselves for questionable anti-inflammation science. Unfortunately, when the public is drawn to new diet science, so are the vultures. The anti-inflammatory diet has already attracted less-than-credible advocates to its flock. Today, it's easy to find hundreds of dietary supplements marketed as reducing inflammation, as well as diets promising to "reduce toxicity and inflammation in order to lose 10 pounds in seven days and reduce your pain." Thomson notes that when new science comes out, "Quacks jump on board and sell supplements."

This scenario adds to consumer confusion. "Most people have no idea what an anti-inflammatory diet is. The most they usually know is in regards to omega-3 fatty acids because they have been advertised as having anti-inflammatory properties all over the place," says Goldstein. Reifer agrees, noting that while people are more familiar with antioxidants and omega-3 fatty acids, they are not as familiar with diet and inflammation.

An Anti-Inflammation Diet in Practice

The big question is whether there's enough science to support dietary recommendations specifically aimed at reducing inflammation. Many leading health organizations have yet to jump on the diet-inflammation bandwagon. Thomson reports that for many organizations, it may be too soon to establish guidelines on inflammation and nutrition. "The problem with the science now is that we haven't yet determined the most appropriate study design or inflammatory biomarkers to test dietary effects and build a consensus," says Thomson. She urges dietitians to develop their own evidence base for new science. "You need to define your own data and knowledge base; nobody should be your gatekeeper."

The plain truth is that an anti-inflammatory diet makes sense. "For example, if you're telling people to eat less fat and to increase omega-3 fatty acids and vitamin D in order to alleviate inflammatory symptoms, there is little risk of harm. The likelihood of good is real," says Thomson. Goldstein paints a picture of an inflammation-reducing diet to her clients as one that reduces sugar, refined carbohydrates, saturated fats, and red meat with an increase in fruits and vegetables, whole grains, legumes, nuts, seeds, lean proteins, healthy fats such as olive oil, natural healthy spices and seasonings such as turmeric and garlic instead of salt, and lots of water. It's a portrait of a healthy diet straight out of the rule book.

"I work anti-inflammation into my recommendations," says Siegel. "A healthy diet is anti-inflammatory, good for blood sugar control, heart disease, and cancer prevention." Siegel reports that while she doesn't always use the term anti-inflammation, dietary recommendations such as omega-6/omega-3 fatty acid balance, minimally processed foods, and more fresh fruits and plant foods are all part of her recommendations that cross over into anti-inflammation and wellness.

By focusing on wellness and treating inflammation, dietitians can experience more opportunities to get away from disease management and focus on prevention, according to Reifer. It's something that can help the entire field of dietetics. Thomson adds, "Anti-inflammatory dietary counseling should expand our opportunities for diet intervention. People are likely to welcome information on how foods have a role in decreasing the inflammatory response." Given the burgeoning field of anti-inflammation before us, it looks like it's time to jump in with both feet.

References

1. DeBusk RM, Fogarty CP, Ordoras JM, et al. Nutritional genomics in practice: Where do we begin? *J Am Diet Assoc.* 2005;105(4):589–598.

2. Esposito K, Giugliano D. Diet and inflammation: A link to metabolic and cardiovascular diseases. *Eur Heart J.* 2006;27(1):13–14.

3. Lau FC, Shukitt-Hale B, Joseph JA. Nutritional intervention in brain aging: Reducing the effects of inflammation and oxidative stress. *Subcell Biochem.* 2007;42:299–318.

4. Nanri A, Moore MA, Kono S. Impact of C-reactive protein on disease risk and its relation to dietary factors. *Asian Pac J Cancer Prev.* 2007;8(2):167–177.

5. Jacobs DR Jr, Andersen LF, Blomhoff R. Whole-grain consumption is associated with a reduced risk of noncardiovascular, noncancer death attributed to inflammatory diseases in the Iowa Women's Health Study. *Am J Clin Nutr.* 2007;85(6):1606–1614.

SHARON PALMER, RD, is a contributing editor at *Today's Dietitian* and a freelance food and nutrition writer in southern California.

The Best Diabetes Diet for Optimal Outcomes

Researchers have explored whether certain combinations of macronutrients more effectively manage the disease, but does a perfect eating plan exist?

RITA E. CAREY, MS, RD, CDE

To say that dietary prescriptions for diabetes have varied over the last hundred years is an understatement. From the very-low-carbohydrate diets initiated before insulin was discovered and used therapeutically to the high-carbohydrate, high-fiber vegan diets endorsed today by some medical researchers, recommendations for optimal macronutrient intake for both type 1 and type 2 diabetes have covered nearly every conceivable option. Good scientific studies have identified a number of specific components in foods that may improve clinical diabetes outcomes and others that likely accelerate the pathogenesis of the disease. Yet, the optimal diet profile—the best balance of carbohydrate, protein, and fat—remains a topic of serious debate.

The following review will touch on the primary therapeutic diet patterns for diabetes considered today and some of the data that either support or refute their effectiveness in reducing hyperglycemia, promoting long-term weight loss, and reducing the risk of cardiovascular disease, the most common cause of death for individuals with diabetes.

Not One, but a Variety

The 2008 American Diabetes Association (ADA) position statement, as reported in *Diabetes Care,* notes that "although numerous studies have attempted to identify the optimal mix of macronutrients for the diabetic diet, it is unlikely that one such combination of macronutrients exists." Rather, the ADA indicates, the best mix of carbohydrate, fat, and protein varies depending on an individual's circumstances, caloric needs for weight control, and specific metabolic status (eg, lipid profile).

In other words, the ADA recognizes that a number of healthy diet patterns may be effective for maintaining good glycemic control and reducing the risk of comorbidities. The position statement also notes the important considerations of cultural and personal preferences, stages of change, and physical and social pleasures of eating in its dietary recommendations. Indeed, one of the goals of medical nutrition therapy for individuals with diabetes that's listed in the position statement is "to maintain the pleasure of eating by only limiting food choices when indicated by scientific evidence."

The ADA recognizes that a number of healthy diet patterns may be effective for maintaining good glycemic control and reducing the risk of comorbidities.

With the previous considerations in mind, the ADA does make some specific nutrition recommendations for weight loss, glycemic control, and the prevention of diabetic complications (see sidebar). Low-fat, calorie-restricted diets are traditionally recommended for weight loss. However, the ADA notes that low-carbohydrate diets (less than 130 g carbohydrate/day) may be effective for weight loss in the short term (ie, less than one year). Whether such diets sustain weight loss and support optimal lipid profiles over the long term remains to be determined. Evidence suggests that after one year, the difference in maintained weight loss between low-carbohydrate or low-fat diet patterns is insignificant.[1] In addition, a meta-analysis published in the *Archives of Internal Medicine* in 2006 found that some individuals had elevated LDL levels when following a low-carbohydrate diet.

Long-term effects of low-carbohydrate/high-protein diets on kidney function are also undetermined. Because very-low-carbohydrate diets can eliminate important nutrient- and energy-dense foods, the ADA maintains that the long-term benefits and metabolic effects of low-carbohydrate diets remain unclear.

Benefits of High-Fiber, Vegetarian Diets

The ADA position statement makes no mention of the effectiveness of high-fiber vegetarian or vegan diets for supporting good glycemic control or the overall health of individuals with diabetes. The ADA does, however, note that foods that make up the base of vegetarian and vegan diets (eg, grains, fruits, vegetables, legumes) offer considerable health benefits to people with diabetes, as does the reduction of saturated fat from animal products. The ADA recommends fiber intake of about 14 g/1,000 kcal/day, although data suggest that higher intake of fiber (about 50 g/day) improves glycemic control in people with type 1 and 2 diabetes, as well as lipid profiles in those with type 2.[2]

A study by Barnard et al published this year in *The American Journal of Clinical Nutrition* compared the effects of a low-fat vegan diet (less than 5% saturated fat, 10% total fat, 15% protein, and 75% carbohydrate) and a conventional diabetes diet following 2003 ADA guidelines (less than 7% saturated fat, 15% to 20% protein, 60% to 70% carbohydrate and monounsaturated fat, and less than 200 mg/day cholesterol) on glycemic control, weight loss, and plasma lipid levels. Individuals following the vegan diet ate an average of 22 g fiber/1,000 kcal/day, while those adhering to ADA guidelines consumed approximately 14 g/1,000 kcal/day. The actual trial lasted 52 weeks, but researchers followed the participants for 22 weeks afterward to assess long-term effectiveness of and adherence to the diets.

At the end of the extended observation period, researchers found that both diets were associated with modest sustained weight loss (–4.4 kg in the vegan group vs. –3 kg in the conventional group), as well as comparable reductions in hemoglobin A1c. However, more individuals in the vegan group were able to reduce medications. After controlling for these medication changes, significantly greater reductions were seen in A1c and total and LDL cholesterol concentrations in the vegan group.

A particularly interesting outcome was the greater reduction of triglycerides in the vegan group compared with the conventional group (−33.9 + 12.7 vs. −7.8 + 28.9). These results contrast with previous studies finding elevated triglycerides in high-carbohydrate diets.[3,4] Barnard et al argue that the participants in previous studies were not encouraged to consume most of their carbohydrates from high-fiber, low-glycemic index foods. Refined, carbohydrate-dense foods that are low in fiber are more likely to raise triglyceride levels. Weight loss was also cited as having an effect on lipid levels in this study, as was the ability of participants to self-regulate their caloric intake on either diet.

A Mediterranean Approach

Another macronutrient pattern considered for diabetes is the high-monounsaturated fatty acid (MUFA) or Mediterranean-style diet. The ADA recommends a diet that provides 60% to 70% of calories from a mix of carbohydrate and monounsaturated fat.

ADA Recommendations

- Either low-carbohydrate or low-fat, calorie-restricted diets may be effective strategies for weight loss in the short term.
- Monitor renal function, lipid profiles, and protein intake (in patients with nephropathy) and adjust hypoglycemic therapy as necessary for those following a low-carbohydrate diet.
- Monitoring carbohydrate is a key strategy for achieving glycemic control.
- Patients with diabetes should consume an assortment of fiber-containing foods and attain the USDA dietary fiber recommendation (14 g/1,000 kcal).
- There is not enough consistent, sufficient evidence to prove that low-glycemic load diets reduce diabetes risk. For diabetes management, the use of the glycemic load/index may provide an added, though modest, benefit over that observed when only total carbohydrate is considered.
- Limit saturated fat to less than 7% of total calories and minimize trans fat intake.
- For good health, include carbohydrate from fruits, vegetables, whole grains, legumes, and low-fat milk in the diet.

—Adapted from the American Diabetes Association. Nutrition Recommendations and Interventions for Diabetes. *Diabetes care.* 2008:31(Suppl 1):S61–S78.

Gerhard et al attempted to determine the optimal energy distribution from MUFA and carbohydrate in the diabetic diet in a study published in *The American Journal of Clinical Nutrition* in 2004. This study was very small (only 11 subjects) but yielded interesting results.

Researchers found that a low-fat (20% of calories from fat) vs. a high-MUFA diet (40% of calories from total fat, 26% MUFA) resulted in more weight loss and improved triglyceride levels. Glycemic control did not differ significantly between the two groups. The low-fat diet was higher in fiber and contained foods with a lower caloric density than those in the high-MUFA diet. Subjects in this study were also allowed to self-regulate their intake. The authors suggest that when individuals are allowed to regulate their intake according to satiety, a low-fat, high-fiber, high-volume diet may have advantages for weight loss (but not necessarily glycemic control) over a high-MUFA diet.

A more recent study published this year in *Diabetes Care* found no significant difference in outcomes (weight, lipid levels, and glycemic control) between two groups consuming either a high-MUFA or high-carbohydrate diet over one year. Both groups had modest weight reductions over 52 weeks (approximately 4 kg) along with improved lipid, blood pressure, A1c, and fasting glucose levels. No detail was offered regarding the fiber content or glycemic index of the carbohydrate-dense foods that participants consumed. The authors of this study concluded that both low-fat and high-MUFA diets provide clinical benefits to individuals with type 2 diabetes.

Some researchers have expressed concern over the effects of a high-fat diet on pancreatic beta-cell health and insulin resistance. However, most of the deleterious effects of a high-fat diet seem to be attributable to saturated fatty acids, not MUFAs. A study published in *Diabetes* in 2003 concluded that the fatty acids in monounsaturated oils mitigate the negative effects of saturated palmitic acid on beta-cell death. In addition, circulating saturated fatty acids appear to cause pronounced insulin resistance, whereas MUFA apparently does not.[5]

Low Carb and Beyond

The ADA position statement names low-carbohydrate diets as a viable alternative for weight loss in the short term. Low-carbohydrate diets have been defined as providing anywhere from 50 to 150 g carbohydrate/day.[6] Weight loss is believed to occur not when individuals replace carbohydrate with fat or protein but when deficits in appetite cause a drastic reduction in caloric intake from high-carbohydrate foods. Still, questions about the sustainability of the diet and long-term effects on lipid profiles, glycemic control, cardiovascular disease, and kidney function remain.

Some scientists are now considering diet/genome interactions to explain differences between individual glycemic responses to food. Apparently, a number of genetic factors may influence how an individual reacts physiologically to his or her dietary pattern. For example, a gene implicated in diet/genome interactions is Rad.[7] In experiments with mice, Rad overexpression caused mice eating a high-fat diet to become more insulin resistant and glucose intolerant than normal mice eating the same diet. Rad overexpression has been identified in humans, and this finding suggests that a high-fat diet may have a more profound impact on glucose homeostasis in some individuals.[7] Genetic studies may eventually provide a way to fine-tune individual diets for optimal glycemic control and improved clinical diabetes outcomes.

Best Advice

So what is the optimal macronutrient balance in a diet for someone with diabetes? It appears that low-fat, high-fiber diets may be more effective than low-carbohydrate diets over the long term for sustaining weight loss and improving clinical diabetes outcomes (eg, lipid profile, glycemia). This may also be true of low-fat vs. high-MUFA diets.

The bottom line is that no one can truly say which diet is best. One of the biggest barriers to determining the ultimate diet profile for individuals with diabetes is likely the lack of consistency in study design and size. Not all studies encourage the intake of unrefined, carbohydrate-dense foods that are high in fiber or rate low on the glycemic index scale.

Cohort sizes are often very small. Observation time can range from three to 72 months or more. Most studies also rely on the diet recall of free-living subjects to determine compliance with dietary prescriptions or establish intake patterns. Feeding subjects a controlled diet in a controlled environment would yield more accurate results, but this is usually not feasible or affordable in a study lasting several months or years.

Considering the circumstances and metabolic profile of each individual before suggesting a dietary pattern for diabetes is likely still the best practice.

Notes

1. Gardner CD, Kiazand A, Alhassan S, et al. Comparison of the Atkins, Zone, Ornish and LEARN diets for change in weight and related risk factors among overweight premenopausal women: The A to Z weight loss study: A randomized trial. *JAMA*. 2007;297(9):969–977.
2. Franz MJ, Bantle JP, Beebe CA, et al. Evidence-based nutrition principles and recommendations for the treatment and prevention of diabetes and related complications. *Diabetes Care*. 2003;26 (Suppl 1):S51–S61.
3. Barnard ND, Scialli AR, Turner-McGrievy G, Lanou AJ, Glass J. The effects of a low-fat, plant-based dietary intervention on body weight, metabolism, and insulin sensitivity. *Am J Med*. 2005;118(9):991–997.
4. Nordmann AJ, Nordmann A, Briel M, et al. Effects of low-carbohydrate vs low-fat diets on weight loss and cardiovascular risk factors: A meta-analysis of randomized controlled trials. *Arch Intern Med*. 2006;166(3):285–293.
5. Chavez JA, Summers SA. Characterizing the effects of saturated fatty acids on insulin signaling and ceramide and diacylglycerol accumulation in 3T3-L1 adipocytes and C2C12 myotubes. *Arch Biochem Biophys*. 2003;419(2):101–109.
6. Westman EC, Feinman RD, Mavropoulos JC, et al. Low-carbohydrate nutrition and metabolism. *Am J Clin Nutr*. 2007;86(2):276–284.
7. Dedoussis GV, Kaliora AC, Panagiotakos DB. Genes, diet and type 2 diabetes mellitus: A review. *Rev Diabet Stud*. 2007;4(1):13–24.

RITA E. CAREY, MS, RD, CDE, is a clinical dietitian and diabetes educator at Yavapai Regional Medical Center and the Pendleton Wellness Center in Prescott, Ariz.

Diet Does Matter

Nutrition's Role in Cancer Prevention and Treatment

MARIE SPANO

"Study: Fiber doesn't cut colon cancer risk," said MSNBC (December 2005). "Cereal fiber may reduce the risk of colon cancer," said *Natural Products Insider* (September 2006). "Study shows a low-fat diet may not reduce breast cancer risk," according to Yale New Haven Hospital's Web site (June 2006). "Reducing Total Fat Intake May Have Small Effect on Risk of Breast Cancer, No Effect on Risk of Colorectal Cancer, Heart Disease, or Stroke," said a National Institutes of Health news release (February 2006).

What part does diet really play in preventing disease and how important is maintaining proper nutrition throughout the healing process?

The picture that the media portray is very confusing. Does nutrition really matter when it comes to cancer prevention? Can it prolong one's life once cancer is diagnosed? Will the typical medical treatments of chemotherapy and radiation be more comfortable if a sound diet is adopted? We can answer these questions by turning to both clinical and epidemiological research.

The American Cancer Society estimates that 1,399,790 men and women will be diagnosed with and 564,830 men and women will die of all cancers in 2006.[1]

The most common type of cancer, representing more than one half of all cancers diagnosed in the United States, is nonmelanoma skin cancer (basal cell and squamous cell), with more than 1 million new cases expected in the United States in 2006. (For more information on incidence and mortality, see Table 1.)

According to the annual report on cancer trends spanning 1975 to 2003, cancer incidence rates for men have been stable from 1995 to 2003 while rates for women increased from 1979 to 2003. Additionally, the risk of death from cancer is on the decline. This decline was greater for men than women and is attributed to reductions in tobacco exposure, earlier detection through screening (thanks in part to awareness efforts), and more effective treatments.[2]

Table 1   Cancer Incidence Rates and Death

Cancer Type	Estimated New Cases	Estimated Deaths
Bladder	61,420	13,060
Breast (female/male)	212,920/1,720	40,970/460
Colon and rectal (combined)	148,610	55,170
Endometrial	41,200	7,350
Kidney (renal cell)	31,890	10,530
Leukemia (all)	35,070	22,280
Lung (including bronchus)	174,470	162,460
Melanoma	62,190	7,910
Non-Hodgkin's lymphoma	58,870	18,840
Pancreatic	33,730	32,300
Prostate	234,460	27,350
Skin (nonmelanoma)	>1,000,000	Not available
Thyroid	30,180	1,500

For more statistics:
American Cancer Society: Cancer Facts and Figures 2006. Atlanta: American Cancer Society, 2006. Available at: http://www.cancer.org/docroot/stt/stt_0.asp

Source: *The National Cancer Institute*, http://www.cancer.gov/cancertopics/commoncancers.

The past few decades have spurred an explosion in our understanding of cancer's risk factors and treatment. Though many people still view nutrition and diet primarily as a means to gain or lose weight, dietitians know there are a multitude of connections between what we eat and cancer risk. And new developments are rapidly unfolding.

Nutrition and Cancer Prevention

To understand nutrition's role in cancer prevention as well as the dietary components that may contribute to cancer, we must take epidemiological, in vivo, and in vitro research into account. The statistic that frequently emerges is that diet accounts for approximately 30% of cancer in industrialized countries and 20% in developing countries. Dietary components that may help prevent cancer and those that may contribute to its progression are outlined in Table 2. The mechanisms behind two specific dietary components, alcohol and fruits and vegetables, will be discussed here.

Alcohol

When most people think of cancer and alcohol, liver cancer is typically the first that comes to mind. However, alcohol consumption is also associated with an increased risk of cancers of the mouth, esophagus, pharynx, larynx, and possibly colorectal cancer in men and women, and breast cancer in women.[3] And it doesn't take much—just one drink per day for women and two for men, according to the *Cancer Trends Progress Report.* (One drink equals 12 ounces of regular beer, 5 ounces of wine, or 1.5 ounces of 80-proof liquor.) Risk increases with greater consumption, and the earlier that heavy consumption starts, the greater the risk. Additionally, combining alcohol and tobacco— a bar favorite—creates a synergistic risk, increasing the chances of cancer of the mouth, throat, and esophagus.

Why is ethanol carcinogenic? During metabolism, ethanol generates acetaldehyde (AA) and induces cytochrome P4502E1, which stimulates free radical production. AA binds to DNA and proteins, destructs folate, and leads to secondary hyperproliferation. What is the combined link behind alcohol plus smoking and cancer? Smoking also increases AA production. Lastly, alcohol also increases estradiols—a potential link between alcohol consumption and increased risk of breast cancer.[4]

Aside from liver cancer, alcohol has a very strong relationship with the most common cancer in women: breast cancer. In the Prostate, Lung, Colorectal, and Ovarian Cancer Screening Trial, researchers examined the relationship between dietary folate, alcohol, and postmenopausal breast cancer in a cohort of women. They used food frequency questionnaires and questions on supplemental vitamin and mineral use (from the age of 25) from 25,400 women aged 55 to 74 (at the beginning of the trial) and followed these women between 1993 and 2001.

Why look at the two of these dietary components together? Alcohol has been associated with an increased risk of breast cancer, possibly due to alcohol's interference with estrogen pathways and subsequent effect on hormonal levels.[5–7] However, high consumption of alcohol is known to lower folate status, thereby providing another possible mechanism by which alcohol may increase breast cancer risk.[7,8]

In this particular study, 691 women developed breast cancer during the observed period. Alcohol consumption was positively related to breast cancer risk and this risk was greater in women with lower total folate intake. However, a high folate intake did not decrease risk and in fact, a high supplemental folic acid intake was related to increased risk.[9] Other studies have supported these results—that adequate folic acid intake (up to 350 micrograms per day) may attenuate breast cancer risk associated with high alcohol consumption—but there is no association between greater consumption of folic acid (above 350 micrograms per day) and breast cancer incidence.[10]

Folate's role in DNA methylation may be the important factor in one specific type of breast cancer: aberrant methylation of the estrogen receptor (ER) gene. Folate deficiency may be partially responsible in ER gene-negative breast tumors where drinking approximately 1.5 servings of alcohol per day necessitates the need for adequate folate consumption.[11] Even one drink per day could be harmful, according to researchers of a controlled feeding study in healthy postmenopausal women. Consumption of just one drink per day led to increases (7.5%) in estrone sulfate, a breakdown product of estrogen.[12]

Fruits and Vegetables

The link between fruit and vegetable consumption and a decreased risk of several chronic diseases is old news. Populations with high levels of produce intake have a decreased risk of diabetes, heart disease, hypertension, several types of cancer, and possibly overweight and obesity. Cancerwise, consuming the recommended 2 cups of fruit and 2.5 cups of vegetables per day may lower your risk of developing mouth, throat, colorectal, pharynx, esophagus, stomach, lung, and prostate cancers.[13–15]

While some compounds within specific fruits and vegetables have been identified, scientists are still working on the possibility of utilizing these components as targeted cancer treatments. A few of those identified and researched that can interfere with several cell-signaling pathways include resveratrol (red grapes, peanuts, berries), lycopene (tomatoes), genistein (soybeans), capsaicin (red chilies), ursolic acid (apples, pears, prunes), catechins (green tea), beta-carotene (carrots), curcumin (turmeric), diallyl sulfide (allium), S-allyl cysteine (allium), allicin (garlic), diosgenin (fenugreek), 6-gingerol (ginger), ellagic acid (pomegranates), silymarin (milk thistle), anethol (anise, camphor, and fennel), eugenol (cloves), indole-3-carbinol (cruciferous vegetables), limonene (citrus fruits), and dietary fiber.[16]

Because we have yet to uncover many additional components within the myriad fruits and vegetables that exist, government agencies have always recommended consuming a variety of fruits and vegetables to expose oneself to as many different cancer-fighting compounds as possible.

Visit www.5aday.gov for more specific recommendations based on age.

Impact of Nutrition at the Gene Level

The epidemiological data surrounding various diseases and cancer continue to grow. For example, obesity increases one's risk for colon, postmenopausal breast, uterine, esophageal, and renal cell cancers. Additionally, overweight and obesity may increase the risk of death from many cancers—up to 14% of cancer deaths in men and 20% in women.[3] The relationships between these diseases and cancer have led to an increased awareness of how a person's diet and lifestyle can impact both the onset and progression of these diseases.

An area of research that has begun to further explore the inner workings of obesity and cancer risk is taking place at the gene level. Identification of the obesity gene, related receptors (eg, leptin, ghrelin, insulin), nuclear transcription regulators (eg, nuclear factor family, peroxisome proliferator-activated receptor family), and substrate regulation (eg, glucose, insulin), to name a few, have paved the way for this research. Although

Table 2 Nutrition and Cancer: What Is the Relationship?

Dietary Component	May Decrease the Risk of:	May Increase the Risk of:
Aflatoxin		Liver cancer
Alcohol		In both men and women: oral, esophagus, pharynx, larynx, and possibly colorectal cancers
		Women: breast cancer in women; death from breast cancer
Fiber/whole grains	Colon and gastric cancers	
**Heterocyclic amines/polycyclic aromatic hydrocarbons		Prostate, stomach, colorectal, pancreatic, and breast cancers
Overweight/obesity		Postmenopausal breast, uterine, esophageal, and renal cell cancers; colon and breast cancer recurrence
Saturated fat		Risk of advanced prostate cancer, breast cancer
Soy	Prostate, breast, and colorectal cancers	
Beta-carotene supplementation	Dying from prostate cancer; esophageal cancer	Lung and prostate cancers in male smokers
Vitamin C supplementation (above the Recommended Daily Allowance)	Breast cancer recurrence; esophageal, prostate, and skin cancers	
Vitamin D	Prostate, breast, colon, and skin cancers	

**Heterocyclic amines (HCAs) are formed when muscle meats such as beef, pork, fowl, and fish are cooked at high temperatures. Cooking temperature, time, and method of cooking all affect their formation in meat. Frying, broiling, and barbecuing are associated with the highest amounts of HCAs.

Resources: The American Cancer Society: The Cancer Atlas. Available at: http://www.cancer.org/docroot/AA/content/AA_2_5_9x_Cancer_Atlas.asp
National Cancer Institute. Nutrition in Cancer Care. Available at: http://www.cancer.gov/cancertopics/pdq/supportivecare/nutrition/Patient/page6

genetics is an important component, it accounts for only a portion of the factors that must be considered when determining what foods are responsible for disease development and ensuing increased cancer risk.

People's overall phenotype, including their overall health status, is achieved and maintained by the sum of metabolic activities that function under different circumstances within the life cycle and all the complex interactions among their genotype, metabolic phenotype, diet, lifestyle, and the environment. The metabolic regulation that occurs—from genes to metabolites—dictates biochemical functions, as well as the nutritional and dietary needs of each individual.

As a result, genetic disposition and metabolic needs are important in determining each individual's optimal diet. Fortunately, advances in molecular biology research technology has enabled researchers to measure and analyze many of the underlying sequences, transcripts, and translational products that result from these interactions. Much research is being done in these areas to start identifying the components within certain foods and their cellular targets.

The exciting aspect of this research is its ability to link certain nutrients in food that for years have been suggested to be good for your health. These dietary agents have been shown to impact numerous levels of cell function, many of which relate to cancer development (metastasis factors), obesity (insulin receptor substrate, leptin receptors), apoptosis, various cell signaling pathways, etc. As research progresses, the relationship between these nutrients and various genetic factors will continually develop, further clarifying the role that various foods play in the development of diseases such as cancer, and also lead to the development of personalized nutritional regimens that can help prevent these diseases altogether.

Nutrition Recommendations for Cancer Prevention

- Consume alcohol in moderation; if breast cancer runs in your family, minimize alcohol intake as much as possible.
- Maintain a healthy weight: avoid overweight and obesity.
- Minimize exposure to aflatoxin.
- Consume various fruits and vegetables each day. Aim for 2 cups of fruit and 2.5 cups of vegetables daily.
- Keep total fat intake between 20% and 35% of calories, with most fats coming from sources of polyunsaturated and monounsaturated fatty acids, such as fish, nuts, and vegetable oils.

Proper nutrition during cancer treatment is vital—and a challenge. A sound diet at this time can help a patient feel healthier and better tolerate treatment.

- Maintain a diet of less than 10% of calories from saturated fatty acids.
- Keep trans fatty acid consumption as low as possible.
- Avoid tobacco.
- Eat only moderate amounts of salt-preserved foods.

Nutrition during Cancer Treatment

Proper nutrition during cancer treatment is vital—and a challenge. A sound diet at this time can help a patient feel healthier and better tolerate treatment. This can be a challenge because chemotherapy and radiation may cause several nutrition-related side effects, most notably difficulty eating due to anorexia, cachexia, nausea, vomiting, diarrhea, constipation, mouth sores, trouble swallowing, and pain. In addition, chemotherapy can alter the taste and smell of many foods, making them unappealing. At a time when patients need all the strength they can get, malnutrition may result as a side effect of treatment, making the individual feel tired and weak, and thereby making handling the therapy or even higher doses of some treatments, healing, and fighting infection that much harder.

Over time, almost all patients develop a loss of appetite or desire to eat (anorexia). Cachexia is another common development. This wasting syndrome causes weakness and loss of both fat and muscle. How do anorexia and cachexia differ? While they often occur hand in hand, cachexia can also occur in people who are eating plenty of calories but cannot absorb a good portion of the nutrients they consume.

For more specific dietary advice for relieving nutrition-related side effects of cancer and cancer treatment, visit www.cancer.gov/cancertopics/pdq/supportivecare/nutrition/Patient/page5.

Though there is still much to learn about nutrition's role in both cancer prevention and progression, it is clear that diet affects a variety of cancers and nutrition is of utmost importance during treatment. In the future, we can expect developments on the mechanisms behind the preventive action of various dietary components and possibly tailored diets for prevention of many genetically linked cancers. The toughest part for dietitians will always be motivating clients to make behavior changes that may or may not be beneficial, and the potential benefits may not be crystal clear to them.

MARIE SPANO, MS, RD, is an exercise physiologist; vice president of the International Society of Sports Nutrition (ISSN); spokesperson for the Tea Council of the USA and the ISSN; and a freelance writer, consultant, and speaker in the nutrition, fitness, and health industries.

For references, view article on our archive at www.TodaysDietitian.com.

From *Today's Dietitian,* vol. 8, no. 11, November 2006, pp. 39–42. Copyright © 2006 by Great Valley Publishing Co., Inc. Reprinted by permission.

Alzheimer's—The Case for Prevention

Are we losing our minds? And could something as simple and inexpensive as diet and lifestyle prevent it from happening?

Oliver Tickell

Alzheimer's and other dementias are dreadful diseases. They are also expensive. Just how expensive was revealed by the Alzheimer's Society in its *Dementia UK* report in February. The cost to the UK is £ 17 billion a year, or around £ 25,000 a year for each of the 700,000 sufferers of late-onset dementia. The number of sufferers is projected to rise: to 940,110 by 2021, and to 1,735,087 by 2051.

In response to the looming crisis, the Society makes seven sound recommendations. But something essential is missing: prevention. There are many cost-effective, scientifically robust steps that could dramatically reduce the incidence of dementia and enable elderly people to retain their cognitive faculties, especially in the areas of diet, nutrition and lifestyle. Applied systematically, these measures have the potential to transform the entire Alzheimer's risk landscape.

The brain is a fatty organ, and works best when fed the right kinds of oil and fat. It responds especially badly to the industrial trans fats found principally in hydrogenated oil. A 2003 study in the *Archives of Neurology,* which surveyed 815 people over 65, found that the 20 percent with the highest trans fat consumption were four times more likely to develop Alzheimer's than the 20 percent with the lowest trans fat consumption.

The same study found that the 20 percent with the lowest consumption of polyunsaturated vegetable oils were five times likelier to develop Alzheimer's than the 20 percent with the highest consumption. Combine these effects, and someone eating a diet high in trans fat and low in polyunsaturated fat is nine times more susceptible to Alzheimer's than someone eating a low trans fat, high polyunsaturated fat diet.

A 1999 study in the journal *Neurology* is one of many to show the benefit of mono-unsaturated oil, especially the oleic acid in olive oil. It suggests that, as people age, their brain chemistry may need more monounsaturated fat to prevent degeneration: 'High MUFA [monounsaturated fatty acid] intake *per se* could suggest preservation of cognitive functions in healthy elderly people. This effect could be related to the role of fatty acids in maintaining the structural integrity of neuronal membranes.'

Omega-3 oils, especially the long-chain EPA and DHA essential fatty acids, are a prerequisite of a healthy brain function and have successfully treated depression, attention deficit hyperactivity disorder (ADHD) and other mental conditions. Evidence published in the *Journal of Neuroscience* in 2005 shows that these oils reduce build-up of the amyloid plaque linked with Alzheimer's in mice, and may also help humans.

This supposition was supported in an October 2006 study in the *Archives of Neurology.* The one-year study of 204 Alzheimer's sufferers showed that the decline of very early-stage patients was significantly slowed by taking Omega-3 supplements. 'It seems that not only is DHA an important structural component of brain cells but DHA and its metabolites seem to exert a preventive effect against development of brain cell death,' commented the authors. 'These positive findings now indicate that early treatment with Omega 3 can help to reduce memory decline in patients experiencing the early symptoms of Alzheimer's.'

The risk of dementia is strongly correlated with higher levels of homocysteine—a rogue amino acid associated with low levels of folic acid and vitamin B12—as noted in the *American Journal of Clinical Nutrition,* February 2007. Treatment with B12 is protective: 'Higher plasma vitamin B12 may reduce the risk of homocysteine-associated dementia or CIND (cognitive impairment without dementia).'

Vitamin D also protects against dementia, as shown in a 2006 study of 80 participants, half with mild Alzheimer's and half without. It concluded: 'Vitamin D deficiency was associated with low mood and with impairment on two of four measures of cognitive performance.'

Protection is also conferred by the polyphenol antioxidants in fruit and vegetables, as shown in a 2006 paper in the *American Journal of Medicine,* based on a study of 1,836 Japanese Americans. Those who drank juice at least thrice weekly were a quarter as likely to contract Alzheimer's as those who drank juice less than once a week: 'Fruit and vegetable juices may play an important role in delaying the onset of Alzheimer's disease, particularly among those who are at high risk of the disease.'

Turmeric, the base spice of every curry, is strongly protective. It is rich in the oily chemical curcumin, which triggers our defence mechanisms against free radicals, a cause of cellular damage and a key part of the ageing process. There's a host of evidence for curcumin's benefits, not just in Alzheimer's but in a broad range of pathologies from Crohn's disease to psoriasis. This is supported by the low incidence of Alzheimer's in India. One 2001 study in *Neurology* of a rural population at Ballabgarh, India, found a 0.3 percent incidence, 'among the lowest ever reported'—and roughly a quarter of that of a reference US population.

The same dietary changes that reduce the risk of Alzheimer's would also strongly benefit cardiovascular health, reducing heart disease and stroke. Mental and cardiovascular health are strongly correlated, as shown by a 21-year study of 1,500 Finns by Miia Kivipelto of the Karolinska Institute, Stockholm. 'Midlife obesity, high total cholesterol level, and high systolic blood pressure were all significant risk factors for dementia', each doubling the risk, 'and they increased the risk additively', so that people with all three risk factors were 6.2 times more likely to succumb to dementia.

Another vital dementia-prevention strategy is to stay lively and mentally active. In June 2003 the *New England Journal of Medicine* published a study of 269 healthy adults between 75 and 85 over a 21-year period, which found that 'reading, playing board games, playing musical instruments, and dancing were associated with a reduced risk of dementia'—a 75 percent reduced risk, for those who were most mentally active. 'It seems that remaining mentally agile makes the brain more healthy and more likely to resist illness, just as physical exercise can protect the body from disease,' said lead author Dr Joe Verghese. Numerous other studies have confirmed these findings.

Loneliness is another important factor, as a study by Professor Robert Wilson, professor of neuropsychology at Rush University Medical Centre, revealed in February 2007. His study of 823 older people in the Chicago area found that the risk of Alzheimer's 'was more than doubled in lonely persons' compared with those who were not lonely. 'Loneliness was associated with lower level of cognition at baseline and with more rapid cognitive decline during follow-up,' his team also found.

In recent months the Alzheimer's Society has accepted the need to assess the potential benefits of low-cost preventative measures. But the vast majority of its efforts are still aimed at securing drug therapies (many of dubious efficacy and with undesirable side effects) and adequate care for sufferers. Disproportionate medical research funding is also applied to patentable genetic technologies such as the role of inherited genetic predispositions, and the use of genetically modified cell transplants to produce Nerve Growth Factor.

The greatest disgrace is that the growing compendium of medical knowledge has had no policy response from the Government.

But the greatest disgrace is that the growing compendium of medical knowledge about diet, nutrition, lifestyle and dementia has produced no policy response from the Government. It is hard not to question whether it suits the Government to have the elderly population die relatively young. All the measures that would slow or prevent the onset of dementias would also extend life, especially through improved cardiovascular health, and thus increase pension, benefit, housing and other health costs.

But with the cost of Alzheimer's and other dementias projected to rise to alarming levels in the absence of preventative action, a rethink should (sooner or later) be on the way. Meanwhile, all of us can try, in our own lifestyles, to stay out of the dementia danger zone.

OLIVER TICKELL is a writer and campaigner on health and environmental issues. He is the founder of the tfX campaign against trans fats (www.tfx.org.uk) and architect of the Kyotoz proposals for an effective climate protocol (www.kyotoz.org).

Living Longer: Diet

In the search for the fountain of youth, researchers keep coming back to one fact: what you eat has a tremendous impact not only on your health but on your longevity. Here's why every bite you take counts.

DONNA JACKSON NAKAZAWA

It's hard to get through your first cup of morning coffee without reading a headline about food. Eat blueberries! Inhale kale! Such antioxidant-rich foods will clear your arteries and help prevent the buildup of Alzheimer's plaque in your brain. Add in a cup of green tea in the morning and swish down an ounce or two of dark chocolate with a glass of red wine in the evening and you will be nicely tanked up on healthy fuel for the day.

Or will you? Almost every day, it seems, new studies emerge on the antiaging properties of various foods. One day, soy is good; the next, we find out soy's health benefits may have been oversold. To add to the confusion, this year *The Journal of the American Medical Association* (*JAMA*) published a study that found caloric restriction—eating about 25 percent less than normal—could extend your life.

So which headlines should we believe? And why should we believe them? The answers lie in research that shows exactly how various foods work at the cellular level. In particular, antioxidant-rich fruits and vegetables are emerging as powerful medicine in the fight against cellular aging.

Here's how it works. In the normal process of metabolism, cells produce unstable oxygen molecules—called free radicals—that damage cells. Worse still, the older we get, the more free radicals we produce. Recent studies suggest that the havoc free radicals wreak "plays a central role in virtually every age-related disease, including cardiovascular diseases such as stroke and atherosclerosis, Parkinson's disease, Alzheimer's, and type 2 diabetes," says Mark Mattson, Ph.D., chief of the Laboratory of Neurosciences at the National Institute on Aging at the National Institutes of Health.

It sounds pretty grim, but in this battle there are, thankfully, superheroes. Enter the vibrant world of antioxidants—substances that bind with free radicals and inhibit them from damaging cells. They are abundant in the most colorful fruits and vegetables, including spinach, broccoli, spirulina (blue-green algae), red apples, cranberries, blueberries, cherries, and grapes, as well as in chocolate and red wine. When you hear doctors say that eating five helpings of fruits and vegetables a day is good for you, antioxidants are the main reason. In the past five years an impressive body of research has emerged showing how antioxidants may protect the body and brain against the ravages of aging.

Paula Bickford, Ph.D., a researcher at the University of South Florida Center of Excellence for Aging and Brain Repair, is particularly interested in the role of antioxidants in brain health. The brain is a good place to study the benefits of antioxidants, says Bickford, because it has one of the highest percentages of fats of any organ in the body, and it is in our fats that free radicals inflict much of their damage. As we age, "communications between neurons become damaged, kind of like what happened to the Tin Man in *The Wizard of Oz*," she explains. "Oxidative damage caused the Tin Man to grow rusty—until Dorothy came along and oiled him." Similarly, antioxidants help to "regrease the lines of communication" in the cells in our brain, says Bickford.

To measure how the communication between cells was affected when groups of rats ate different diets, Bickford and her colleagues placed electrodes in the brains of 20-month-old rats—the equivalent of 60-year-old humans. She then fed one group of rats a diet supplemented with spirulina, another with apples, and a third with cucumbers, which lack the antioxidant qualities of spirulina and apples. Bickford and her colleagues were surprised by the robustness with which "both the spirulina and apple groups demonstrated improved neuron function in the brain, a suppression of inflammatory substances in the brain, and a decrease in oxidative damage." By contrast, there was no improvement in rats fed a diet containing cucumbers.

Red Wine and Chocolate: The Reality

A glass of red wine and a little dark chocolate and you'll live forever—that's what the media would have us believe. But should we? The answer is not really, though these foods in moderation do have powerful health benefits.

Chocolate contains flavonoids, particularly potent antioxidants that possess "a very good ability to clear free radicals and protect against inflammation, which helps in protecting your heart," says diet and aging researcher Paula Bickford, Ph.D. Indeed, one study found that people who ate 1.6 ounces of dark chocolate a day (about four squares, or 220 calories' worth) for two weeks gained strong antioxidant benefits. Of course, you'd have to cut something else out of your diet—or run two to three miles a day—to justify those extra calories. Instead, Bickford recommends adding a teaspoon of plain cocoa powder (which has fewer calories and no sugar) to chili or other southwestern recipes. Or treat yourself to one square of dark chocolate a day—60 percent or 70 percent cocoa is ideal because it has less sugar and higher levels of flavonoids than chocolate with lower levels of cocoa.

Red wine contains an abundance of the antioxidant resveratrol, which naturally stimulates the sirtuins—genes that help mop up free radicals, stabilize blood glucose levels, and otherwise make our cells healthier. To produce significant life-extending effects, though, you would probably need to drink 5 to 15 glasses of red wine a day. Long before you'd benefit from cellular rejuvenation, you'd be facing liver and other organ damage. That's why few longevity scientists recommend drinking more than one or two glasses of red wine a day. (Studies also have found that drinking a modest amount of red wine has other benefits than those obtained by its resveratrol content.) "Better to get your antioxidants from a range of healthy sources than to overindulge in any one of them," says Bickford. One thing to look for in the future: some wineries are starting to add resveratrol content to their labels. While some wines contain 3 to 4 micromolar of resveratrol (a micromolar is a way to measure the concentration of any compound in a liquid), others may have as much as 46 micromolar. As labeling resveratrol grows more popular, higher amounts, says Bickford, would be something to look for when browsing at your local wine shop.

—D.J.N.

Bickford, who calls the findings "dramatic," reproduced her results in another study, in which rats fed a spinach-rich diet had a reversal in the loss of learning ability that occurs with age.

Most recently, Bickford examined whether eating a diet high in antioxidant-rich spinach and blueberries makes a difference in lab animals suffering from stroke and Parkinson's. "We've seen very positive effects with both of these diseases, as well," she says. "We believe that antioxidants can help people either to delay the onset or to slow the progression of a range of diseases that we tend to get as we age."

Tempting though it may be now to go out and gorge on antioxidant-rich dark chocolate, resist the urge. The hottest discovery in the search to find the fountain of youth through the foods we eat is to—gulp!—eat a lot less of them. A 2006 article in *JAMA* caused a stir by announcing that in both men and women, caloric restriction—as spartan as 890 calories a day—resulted in a decrease in fasting insulin levels and body temperature, two biomarkers of longevity. Why? Because restricting calories also helps to eliminate those nefarious free radicals. Mattson explains: "When you overeat and more energy comes into the cells than you burn off by being active, you are going to have more excess free radicals roaming around." Still, he advises, don't panic over the idea of having to subsist on 890 calories a day. Mattson, who calls such a diet "starvation," believes we can all gain the benefits of healthy eating with a lot less pain.

Richard Miller, MD, PhD, a researcher and professor of pathology at the University of Michigan, agrees. He has spent the last 20 years studying the ways in which dietary and genetic changes can slow the aging process. The research has shown that mice, rats, and monkeys that have undergone severe caloric restriction demonstrate all kinds of mental and physical benefits such as better mental function, less joint disease, and even fewer cases of cataracts. But it's unrealistic to try to replicate that in humans. "To copy what's happening in the lab, a man weighing 200 pounds would have to decrease his caloric intake by 40 percent for life, which would put him at about 120 pounds," Miller explains. "That's just not tenable."

Instead, Mattson and Miller advocate a more moderate approach. According to the Centers for Disease Control and Prevention, the average man in the United States consumes about 2,475 calories a day. That's roughly 500 more, on average, than he really needs. Likewise, the average American woman consumes 1,833 calories, yet probably needs only about 1,600. One way to ratchet down your caloric consumption would be to follow this simple equation: men should aim for about 500 calories at both breakfast and lunch, while women should strive for about 300 at each meal. Both sexes can then shoot for 1,000 calories at dinner.

5 Foods That Can Add Years to Your Life

New research suggests that including a combination of antioxidants on your plate yields a more powerful advantage than eating any one type of antioxidant-rich food alone. Try to make the following foods a part of your daily diet.

1. Spirulina (blue-green algae). Spirulina contains not only the antioxidant phycocyanin but also a bundle of protein, plus omega fatty acids. Once a mainstay food of the Aztecs, spirulina additionally works as an ibuprofen like nonsteroidal anti-inflammatory. Add one teaspoon to one tablespoon of spirulina a day to smoothies or yogurt, or take it in capsule form. Caution: for some people, spirulina can be over-stimulating (kind of like too much coffee), so experiment to find the right balance.

2. Cranberries, blueberries, blackberries. These are jam-packed with antioxidants called anthocyanins and polyphenols, which also have anti-inflammatory qualities. Try to work in a cup of berries a day.

3. Leafy greens (such as kale or spinach). They're full of lutein, another super-antioxidant; it's been proven to protect against macular degeneration of the optic nerves, thus protecting eye-sight. Scientists recommend eating a cup of cooked kale or one to two cups of raw spinach each day.

4. Almonds and walnuts. These nuts are a fantastic source of omega-6 fatty acids, as well as phytosterols (plant sterols) and vitamin E (tocopherols). People who regularly consume nuts tend to have both a lowered risk of Parkinson's and lower cholesterol. Try to eat a quarter cup of these nuts a day whenever you can.

5. Flaxseed. It contains fiber and omega-3 fatty acids that help to clear plaque and bad fats from the cardiovascular system. The fiber also protects against colon cancer. For best results, buy flaxseed ground (or grind it yourself) and throw one teaspoon to one tablespoon a day into everything from meat loaf to muffins.

Finally, don't forget to add these superfoods into a diet rich with lean meat, fish, and whole grains.

—D.J.N.

Bickford, who prefers to think of caloric restriction as caloric selection, underscores the importance of getting as much of your caloric intake as you can not only from antioxidant-rich fruits and vegetables but also from nuts and flaxseed, which are loaded with vitamin E and omega-3 and omega-6 fatty acids. In fact, Bickford takes a page out of her own lab studies and starts her day with an antioxidant smoothie. You can try it at home by blending together one cup of frozen blueberries with half a tablespoon of spirulina (available in any health food store), half a cup of nonfat plain yogurt, one teaspoon of ground flaxseed, one tablespoon of almond butter or a half-handful of almonds, and a dash of soy milk. Consider what's in that blender as a gas tank full of high-antioxidant fuel for the day.

Of course, one can't help but ask: what's the fun of living to 102 if you're subsisting on spirulina shakes? Not to worry. If you splurge on a stack of pancakes with eggs, bacon, and sausage—packing in 2,000 calories before 10 A.M.—you can always take heart in new data about to emerge from Mattson's lab, which show that periodic fasting—skipping a meal here and there—can also help to eliminate free radicals quite beautifully. "From an evolutionary standpoint we just aren't used to constant access to food," he explains. "Our bodies are used to going days without eating anything. Yet all of a sudden, we are taking in calories all day long."

In other words, we have gone from thousands of years of intermittently restricting our calories and eating a high-antioxidant diet to, in the past century, constantly eating a low-antioxidant diet. And that means more free radicals and more disease. So indulge in the pancakes or the cheese steak, but not both. Then skip a couple of meals and make your next one an all-out antioxidant feast. It may be counter to the don't-skip-meals philosophy our mothers all taught us; yet as it turns out, Mother Nature just might know better.

DONNA JACKSON NAKAZAWA is a health writer whose next book, a medical mystery about *What's Behind Rising Rates of Autoimmune Disease,* will be published by Touchstone/Simon & Schuster in 2007.

UNIT 4

Obesity and Weight Control

Unit Selections

24. **Why We Overeat,** David Kessler
25. **Still Hungry?,** Janet Raloff
26. **The Health Diet Face-Off,** Christie Aschwanden
27. **Will Your Child Be Fat?: How to Prevent Obesity—for Babies on Up,** Jessica Snyder Sachs
28. **Are We Setting the Stage for Obesity and Poor Oral Health?,** Terri Lisagor
29. **Cancer: How Extra Pounds Boost Your Risk,** Bonnie Liebman
30. **The World Is Fat,** Barry M. Popkin

Key Points to Consider

- Discuss some of the causes behind a person becoming obese.

- What are the primary factors that have contributed to the obesity epidemic in the world?

- What are some of the reasons that people with high BMI and waist circumference have increased risk for cancer?

- How are you going to ensure that the website you use to manage your weight is credible and reliable?

Student Website
www.mhhe.com/cls

Internet References

American Society of Exercise Physiologists (ASEP)
www.asep.org
Calorie Control Council
www.caloriecontrol.org
Shape Up America!
www.shapeup.org

Overweight and obesity have become epidemic in the United States during the last century and are rising at a dangerous rate worldwide. Approximately 5 million adults are overweight or obese according to the new standards set by the U.S. government using a body mass index (BMI) range of 30 to 39.9. Reports suggest that by the year 2050, half of the U.S. population will be considered obese. This problem is prevalent in both genders and all ages, races, and ethnic groups. Twenty-five percent of U.S. children and adolescents are overweight or at risk, which emphasizes the need for prevention, as obese children become obese adults. The catastrophic health consequences of obesity are heart disease, diabetes, gallbladder disease, osteoarthritis, and some cancers. The cost for treating this degenerative disease in the United States is approximately $100 billion per year. Even though professionals have tried to prevent and combat obesity with behavior modification, a healthy diet, and exercise, it seems that these traditional ways have not proven effective. Fast-food eateries are the mainstay because they offer quick, inexpensive foods. Supersizing has become the norm because it's cheaper to order a biggie combo than smaller items individually. Americans are so accustomed to our fast food nation that many people become infuriated when asked to pull up and wait an extra minute for a 2,400 calorie meal. The problem is exacerbated by the food industry's historical plight to earn profit and market share by providing U.S. consumers with the fatty, sugary, and salty foods that we demand. Considering all of these challenges, we should not be surprised that obesity has become an epidemic. Food companies spend millions of dollars in advertising foods loaded with simple sugars, fat, and salt. Their aggressive advertising, coupled with food accessibility and large portion size, has created the current obesity pandemic. Other obstacles to maintaining a healthy diet are low accessibility and high cost of eating a healthy diet. These challenges are being addressed by programs such as urban community gardens and gleaning programs discussed further in Unit 1 and Unit 7.

More recently, scientists have reported that fat is a dynamically active endocrine organ that releases hormones and inflammatory proteins that may predispose a person to chronic diseases including heart disease. In addition, research has discovered the role of the "hunger hormone" and how individual differences affect our ability to lose weight. A positive association was recently found between obesity, especially central obesity, and different types of cancer. Thus, there is a great need for a multifaceted public health approach that would involve mobilization of private and public sectors and focus on building better coping skills and increasing activity. The role of fiber in protecting against overweight and obesity has been repeatedly documented. However, not all fibers are equally effective; isolated or functional fibers may not aid in weight maintenance like naturally occurring, unrefined fibers. Understanding how to choose foods with the most beneficial types of fiber is explained in one of the readings.

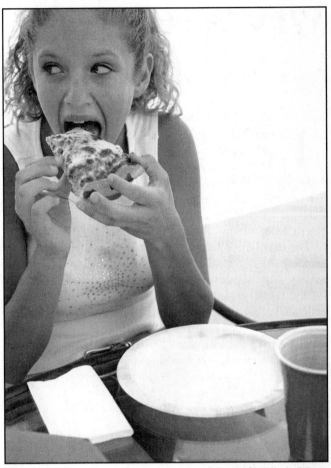

© BananaStock/JupiterImages

Globalization is causing the rest of the world and especially third world countries to mimic the unhealthy Western diet that contributes to obesity. So obesity is now a global epidemic. Sweetened beverages and the sedentary Western way of life that has been adopted by many developing countries are some of the major contributors of this epidemic. Intervention should be the top priority of policy makers. At the public sector, inclusion of health officials, researchers, educators, legislators, transportation experts, urban planners, and businesses that would cooperate in formulating ways to combat obesity is crucial. A sound public health policy would require that weight-loss therapies have long-term maintenance and relapse-prevention measures built into them. Healthy people 2010 is the U.S. government's prevention agenda designed to ensure high quality of life and reduce health risks. One of the 28 areas it focuses on is overweight and obesity. Its main objectives are to reduce the proportion of overweight and obese children, teens and adults to 15% and to increase the proportion of adults who are at a healthy weight.

Why We Overeat

DAVID A. KESSLER AND BONNIE LIEBMAN

"In 1960, when weight was relatively stable in America, women ages 20 to 29 averaged about 128 pounds," writes David Kessler in *The End of Overeating*. "By 2000, the average weight of women in that age group had reached 157." Among women 40 to 49, the trend was similar. "The average weight had jumped from 140 pounds in 1960 to 169 in 2000."

Two out of three American adults are now either overweight or obese. One in six children aged 2 to 19 is obese. Excess weight increases the risk of diabetes, heart disease, cancer (of the breast, colon, esophagus, kidney, and uterus), stroke, gallbladder disease, arthritis, and more.

Americans spend billions on weight-loss schemes, yet most diets fail over the long term. "That is because we have not understood why eating certain foods only makes us want to eat more of them," says Kessler. "No one has recognized what's really happening."

Here's how the food industry leads us to overeat . . . and how to fight back.

Q: *Why did you write* The End of Overeating?

A: There was a fundamental mystery that I wanted to understand. Why is it so hard for so many of us to resist eating even if we're not hungry? Why does that chocolate chip cookie have so much power over me? Why do we engage in behavior we don't want to engage in?

I started listening to people say, "I eat when I'm hungry, I eat when I'm not hungry, I eat when I'm happy, I eat when I'm sad." And I'd ask, "Do you understand why?" And they'd say "No."

Q: *Do people blame themselves?*

A: Yes. The result is a lot of misinformation and myths or people feeling bad about themselves or just throwing in the towel and saying, "There's nothing I can do."

I wanted to help people understand why it's so hard to resist food. And for the first time, we now have the science to say to people, "It's not your fault, and there are things you can do to control it."

Q: *What does the science say?*

A: First, we know what drives overeating. We published a paper called "Deconstructing the Vanilla Milkshake." We asked: Is it sugar or fat or the flavor that drives intake?

Chocolate Chip Cookie Molten Cake. Cake (fat, sugar), chocolate filling (fat, sugar), ice cream (fat, sugar), chocolate shell (fat, sugar).

Cheese Dip. Heavy cream (fat), cheese (fat), tortilla chips (fat, salt).

Southwestern Eggrolls. Fried tortilla (fat), chicken (salt), cheese (fat), ranch dressing (fat, salt).

Bacon Cheeseburger. Ground beef (fat), bacon (fat, salt), cheese (fat), sauce (fat, salt).

Buffalo Chicken Wings. Fried wings (fat), hot sauce (salt), butter (fat), dressing (fat, salt).

Cheese Fries. Fried potatoes (fat), beef chili (fat, salt), cheese (fat), dressing (fat, salt).

Java Chip Frappuccino. Coffee mix (sugar), whipped cream (fat, sugar), chocolate chips (fat, sugar), chocolate drizzle (sugar).

We gave rats a series of solutions containing combinations of sugar, corn oil, and vanilla, and found that sugar was the prime driver. But when you add fat to sugar, you increase the drive synergistically.

Q: *The rats pressed a lever more times to get it?*

A: Yes. If you combine sugar and fat, animals will work harder to get it. They'll want it more. If you give sugar alone, you'll get some dopamine spike, but if you put sugar and fat together, you stimulate more brain activation. And we know that humans prefer sugar mixed with cream more than the same amount of sugar mixed with skim milk.

Q: *How is dopamine—a neurotransmitter that conveys messages from one nerve cell to another—part of overeating?*

A: Dopamine focuses your attention. As human beings, we are wired to focus on the most important stimuli in our environment. If a bear walked into your office right now, your dopamine would spike. If your child is sick today, that's what you're thinking about. That's what captures your attention.

For some, alcohol can be a salient stimulus. Or illegal drugs, gambling, sex, smoking. But for many of us, it's food.

Of all the cues in this room right now, of all the things I could be thinking about, those little chocolate chip cookies over there are capturing my attention. Why? Because of my past experience, chocolate chip cookies will activate my brain.

Q: *Before you take the first bite?*

A: Yes. I'm not tasting them. It's not genuine hunger, but the anticipation, that makes us eat long after our calorie needs are satisfied.

Q: *And the sight of the cookies is the cue?*

A: Yes, but I could also be cued by the location, the time of day, or just getting in my car because it anticipates the consumption.

I could be walking down Powell Street in San Francisco and I start thinking about chocolate-covered pretzels because six months earlier I went into a store on Powell Street that had chocolate-covered pretzels. I didn't even remember that, but the street itself was a cue. And we're such effective learners.

The street cue stimulates brain activation. It causes arousal. And then it becomes part of working memory. You're thinking about it. You want it.

Food or Drug?

Q: *Do some foods keep the brain activated more than others?*

A: Yes. We've known that dopamine would spike—and stay elevated—in response to drugs like cocaine or amphetamines. But with food, we thought you would get a little dopamine elevation and then we would habituate—that is, the food would lose its capacity to activate our brains.

But if you combine sugar and fat, that brain activation doesn't always habituate. And as you make food more multisensory, some people don't get habituation. Their dopamine stays elevated.

Q: *What do you mean by multisensory?*

A: I mean that the food is more complex. For example, ice cream combines sugar and fat and cold. But if you add Heath bars, Reese's Peanut Butter Cups, crumbled cookies, and hot fudge, that adds more texture and aroma and temperature. The more multisensory you make food, the more reinforcing it becomes. The more people come back for more.

Q: *So it gets harder to resist over time?*

A: For some people, yes. I was talking to an individual who works in publishing. Big guy. The hardest thing for him to do every day, he says, is to get past the newsstand on the way to the train because the newsstand sells KitKat candy bars. For each of us, it's something different. But at its core, fat, sugar, and salt are highly salient stimuli.

Q: *How does salt make us want to eat more?*

A: A food industry executive told me that the industry creates dishes to hit what he called the three points of the compass. Sugar, fat, and salt are what make food compelling and indulgent. The most palatable foods have two or three

of them. [See boxes.] They lead to a roller coaster in the mouth—the total orosensory experience. We get captured.

Q: *What's the roller coaster?*

A: It's the cycle of cue-activation-arousal-release. We get cued—by sights, sounds, smells, time of day, location. The brain circuits get activated. There's arousal. And then you either distract yourself with something that's more important or you consume it and there's a release.

Q: *So eating is a thrill ride?*

A: Yes. If I gave you a pack of sugar and said, "Go have a good time," you'd look at me and say, "What are you talking about?"

Now I add to that sugar some fat, I add texture, color, temperature, mouthfeel, the outward appearance, the smell, and I put it on every corner, make it available 24/7.

Then I add the emotional gloss of advertising. I say you can eat it with your friends. Have a good time. I make it into a food carnival, and what do you expect to happen?

Q: *It's hard to resist.*

A: Right. Let me give you another example. Nicotine alone is a moderate reinforcing substance in animals. I add to that nicotine the smoke, the cellophane crinkling of the pack, the color of the pack, the image of the cowboy, the sexiness, the glamour that the industry created 50 years ago, the emotional gloss of advertising.

And what did I do? I took a moderately reinforcing substance and made it into an addictive product. So sugar alone is not enough.

Q: *Is everyone equally vulnerable to these foods?*

A: No. You can ask people if they have these three characteristics:

One: Do you lose control in the face of highly palatable foods? Is it very hard to resist them?

Two: Do you feel a lack of satiation—a lack of feeling full—when you're eating?

Three: Do you have a preoccupation? Do you think about foods in between meals? Or as you're eating something, are you thinking about what you'll be eating next?

When you ask these questions, some people have no idea what you're talking about. But about 50 percent of obese, 30 percent of overweight, and 20 percent of healthy-weight individuals score very high on those three characteristics.

Q: *Are these normal people?*

A: Yes. We're not talking about eating disorders. This is in the normal spectrum. There's no psychopathology. So when you add them up, it's some 70 million Americans who have this constellation of characteristics. It's not a disease. It's a syndrome that I call conditioned hyper-eating.

Q: *Is there evidence of what's going on in their brains?*

A: Yes. If you expose these people to the cues—a picture of chocolate, say—and you scan their brains, you see elevated activation in a part of the brain called the amygdala.

Q: *What does the amygdala do?*

A: That's where we process and store memories of emotions. When individuals who aren't conditioned hypereaters start to consume chocolate, for example, the activation shuts off. But in conditioned hypereaters, the activation remains elevated and it doesn't stop until they stop consuming the chocolate.

So the reason some foods are so hard for conditioned hypereaters to resist is that the reward circuits of the brain are in overdrive, and they're overriding the body's homeostatic mechanisms.

Q: *Those mechanisms should have made them stop eating?*

A: Yes. If you look at children at the age of two or three, they compensate. If you give them more calories in one meal, they'll eat less later in the day. But if they get exposed to sugar, fat, and salt all day for a few years, they lose the ability to compensate. By age four or five, they're eating all the time.

Q: *So eating these foods changes your brain?*

A: Yes. Every time you get cued and consume the stimulus, you strengthen the neural circuits, so the next time you're more likely to do it again. Strengthening those circuits is what we define as learning, even though it's not the kind of conscious learning we think about.

Q: *Does that explain why it's tough to keep weight off?*

A: Yes. Why don't diets work? Sure, I can deprive someone by cutting their calories for 30, 60, or 90 days. And they'll lose weight.

But, first of all, deprivation increases the reward value of food unless you substitute something you want more. And after you lose the weight, the old circuitry is still there.

Unless you've replaced it with new circuitry—new learning—if you're put back in your old environment, you continue to get bombarded by the old cues, so of course you'll gain the weight back.

Q: *Because the old circuitry remains?*

A: Yes. And if I become stressed, fatigued, hungry, if I'm trying to catch a plane and there's nothing else around, I will still grab those chocolate-covered pretzels. For most of us, the trick is to learn new circuitry. (See "Food Rehab," box)

The Food Industry

Q: *How does the food industry take advantage of conditioned hypereating?*

A: They understand that sugar, fat, and salt drive consumption. They've layered and loaded it into foods. They understand the combinations that will drive intake by giving you the greatest neural activation.

Industry also knows the bliss points—how much sugar, fat, and salt is just enough and not too much. And they understand the outputs—that people keep coming back for more.

Food Rehab

Here's some of the advice David Kessler gives in *The End of Overeating* (Rodale, $25.95) to help you resist the pull of unhealthy foods.

1. **Replace chaos with structure.** Determine ahead of time what you'll eat for meals and snacks. Block out everything else.
2. **Practice just-right eating.** Figure out how much food you need. (Odds are, it's less than you think.) Put it on your plate and don't go back for more.
3. **Pick foods that will satisfy, not stimulate, you.** What satisfies you is personal, but try foods that occur in nature, like whole grains, beans, non-starchy vegetables, and fruit, combined with lean protein and a small amount of fat.
4. **Rehearse.** Anticipate your moves like an elite athlete before a competition. For example, tell yourself, "If I encounter chocolate-covered pretzels, I'll keep walking."
5. **Seize control.** Stay alert to emotional stressors or other stimuli that trigger automatic behavior. Recognize emotions (like sadness, fatigue, or anxiety) that might lead you to overeat.
6. **Stop that thought.** Change the channel. Turn off the image of the trigger food before you start to debate whether to eat it.
7. **Think negative.** Pair the unhealthy food with a stream of (unappealing) images. "That's the flip side of what advertising agencies do when they link an Olympic athlete to a pair of sneakers or an attractive woman to a new piece of technology," says Kessler.

They haven't necessarily understood the black box in between—the neuroscience. Industry would say that it's just giving consumers what they want. But what they're giving consumers is food that excessively activates the brains of millions.

Q: *So we get a fatty, salty food like french fries smothered in cheese and bacon, which adds even more fat and salt?*

A: Right. They've optimized those ingredients to maximize the drive for food. We used to eat for nutrition—to satisfy ourselves. Now we eat for stimulation.

We're getting cued. We get that arousal. That attention. That release. The food isn't satisfying us. It's taking us on a roller coaster ride.

Q: *It's food as entertainment?*

A: Yes. If you go at 5 P.M. to a food court like the one at Washington D.C.'s Union Station, it's a food carnival. You optimize sugar, fat, and salt to drive consumption and add the emotional gloss, which amplifies the reinforcing value.

You'll want it. You'll love it. You'll have a good time. They make it into a carnival. Who doesn't want to get on the rides?

Q: *How can people fight back?*

A: How do you cool down the stimulus? The same way we did it with tobacco. We used to look at tobacco as something we wanted, something that would make us feel better, that would make us cool, sexy.

The real success was that we changed how people viewed the stimulus. We changed from seeing tobacco as glamour to perceiving it as a deadly, disgusting product.

When you're dealing with a reinforcing stimulus, that's important. If you view it as something that you want, something that's going to comfort you, you'll approach it. If you view it as something you don't want, that's your enemy, you're going to avoid it. So social norms and attitudes do affect us and affect brain impulses.

Q: *Did it help to tell teens that the tobacco industry was trying to hook them?*

A: Yes. And if our behavior is becoming conditioned and driven, that has immense policy implications. Then you start seeing advertising not just as information protected under the First Amendment, but as a cue that stimulates and drives consumption.

Once our kids become conditioned and their behavior is driven by sugar, fat, and salt, then that vending machine in the hallway and that fast food restaurant are cues.

Q: *Don't we want the food industry to make good-tasting food?*

A: Yes. We need foods that are rewarding. Food has to be pleasurable. But we've taken highly reinforcing substances and made them more reinforcing. And we've taken down the barriers by putting fat, sugar, and salt on every corner, making it socially acceptable and available 24/7.

Q: *What policies could help people?*

A: First, restaurants should list calories on the menu. We also need well-funded campaigns to let people know that big food—food that's layered and loaded with fat, salt, and sugar—is unhealthy. And we need to rethink advertising for highly palatable foods.

Q: *How?*

A: Advertising is not just neutral information. It's a cue that amplifies the reward value of highly stimulating foods. It affects how the brain responds. Once you understand that, then I think that's a legitimate reason to limit advertising of foods that have excess fat, sugar, and salt. And we need to go to the next step on food labeling.

Q: *Beyond Nutrition Facts?*

A: Yes. I was recently in the cafeteria at Google's headquarters. It was striking. They have red, yellow, or green in front of each lunch item. Green means have as much as you want. Yellow means have a moderate amount. Red means taste it but be careful how much you eat. It had a real effect on me.

We need something like that on the front of food packages. It's not just about individual ingredients any more.

Also, the industry needs to set responsible portion sizes. The reality is that we're going to finish the package because once our brains are activated, it's virtually impossible to stop.

Q: *How have people responded to the book?*

A: It takes courage for people who weigh 300 pounds to come to these book events. But to see them shake their heads and say, "Finally, someone is explaining to me why I do this," that's why I wrote the book.

DAVID A. KESSLER was commissioner of the U.S. Food and Drug Administration from 1990 to 1997, during which the agency overhauled and redesigned the Nutrition Facts labels that are on most foods. His first book, *A Question of Intent: A Great American Battle with a Deadly Industry,* describes the FDA's attempt to regulate cigarettes as nicotine-delivery devices. In 2000, the Supreme Court ruled that the FDA did not have the power to regulate tobacco. In June, Congress passed legislation to give the FDA that authority. Kessler spoke to *Nutrition Action*'s Bonnie Liebman by phone from San Francisco.

From *Nutrition Action HealthLetter*, July/August 2009. Copyright © 2009 by Center for Science in the Public Interest. Reprinted by permission.

Still Hungry?

Fattening revelations—and new mysteries—about the hunger hormone.

JANET RALOFF

Too busy to cook, you drop by the neighborhood café and treat yourself to fried chicken with a side of macaroni and cheese. You wash it all down with a bottle of apple juice—to balance the high-fat entrees with something healthy. Although you've put away far more calories than usual, you still don't feel really full, so you select a slice of chocolate torte from the dessert case.

Recent studies have begun pointing to a wide variety of factors, including body weight, food choices, and lack of sleep, by which we can unwittingly alter not only when we experience hunger but also what items appear appetizing and how much food it takes to trigger a feeling that we've had enough.

Our bodies rely on a host of involuntary cues to regulate food consumption. In 1999, researchers discovered a hormone that contributes to strong feelings of hunger. Throughout the day, its concentration in our bodies rises and falls. Although we're not aware of these ups and downs, they drive our behavior, either moving us toward the table or letting us get on with the rest of our lives.

Cycles of this powerful hormone—dubbed ghrelin, after a Hindu word for "growth"—reflect a complex interplay of chemical signals that scientists are now beginning to untangle. In the last 2 years, research has also begun pointing to an array of diet and lifestyle factors that modify the body's production of ghrelin and other eating-related signals.

Such findings are not just curiosities. As the complex picture of ghrelin and its allies has been getting clearer, the medical community has begun considering new drugs, lifestyle changes, and other interventions to counter people's penchant for overeating. On the table are billions of dollars and the health of millions of people.

Gut Reactions

Although many endocrinologists glibly refer to ghrelin as the "hunger hormone," it's got plenty of accomplices when it comes to making people eat—and stop eating—notes Aart Jan van der Lely of Erasmus University in Rotterdam, the Netherlands. Some 2 dozen chemical agents—many of them hormones—stimulate food intake, and a similar number suppress appetite, he says. But only a few of these substances appear to hold feature roles in dinner theater, while the rest serve as understudies or the chorus.

According to recent studies, ghrelin stars as a trigger of appetite (*SN: 2/16/02, p. 107*). The featured players in appetite suppression include insulin, which is made in the pancreas, and leptin, which fat cells manufacture. These two hormones turn down the dial on ghrelin production. Another appetite suppressor is PYY, a gut hormone that also appears to curb ghrelin manufacture.

All these hormones travel through the body, carrying their eat or don't-eat messages. They also trigger nerve signals running from the gut to the brain and are influenced, in turn, by messages returning from the brain.

As in a great theater production, there's depth in the cast of appetite regulators. When top-billed performers, such as ghrelin, are no-shows, the body turns to understudies to figure out when to eat and, somewhat less effectively, when to stop.

For instance, David E. Cummings of the University of Washington in Seattle and his coworkers reported in the October 2004 *Endocrinology* that the spike in insulin secretion that occurs after eating usually correlates with a dip in ghrelin production. The researchers found that when they killed rats' insulin-producing cells to model uncontrolled diabetes, food intake still suppressed ghrelin concentrations in the blood, but only about half as effectively as when insulin was present. One or more understudies must take a portion of ghrelin's role, the team concludes.

This study also showed that lack of insulin increased a rodent's sensitivity to ghrelin's call to eat. When Cummings and his coworkers infused a small amount of ghrelin into the diabetic rats, the animals more than tripled their food intake compared with that of healthy rats given the same treatment.

Related studies are homing in on other factors that perturb the normal checks and balances on ghrelin—changes that might keep the hunger bell ringing long after people would otherwise feel full. People may overeat not just when there's a problem with the ghrelin signal but also when something goes amiss in other parts of the control system.

With this new conceptual framework, scientists are looking for means to confront what many have characterized as a worldwide epidemic of obesity (*http://www.sciencesnews.org/articles/20020803/food.asp*).

All Calories Aren't Alike

Although most health guides recommend that we eat less fat, people have a hard time complying. The late Walter Mertz, when he was head of the Department of Agriculture's Human Nutrition Research Center in Beltsville, Md., used to sympathize: "The trouble with fat is that it tastes so good."

Cummings' new research points to a related problem: Calorie for calorie, fat is less effective than other nutrients at suppressing ghrelin's hunger call. During one recent study, his team on different days infused into rats' gastrointestinal tracts equal-calorie quantities of pure sugar, protein, or fat. In the February *Endocrinology,* the group reports that sugar and protein each prompted a rapid, 70-percent drop in the concentration of ghrelin circulating in the rodents' blood. When rats instead received fat, ghrelin concentrations fell far more slowly and by only about 50 percent.

"We've now found the same thing with humans," Cummings told *Science News.*

These results are consistent with earlier work by his team. For example, the researchers observed in 2003 that prebreakfast, or background, ghrelin concentrations rise as most people lose weight—as if the body is attempting to regain the pounds. However, when people trimmed their waistlines over several months via a low-fat diet, their prebreakfast ghrelin levels remained unchanged.

This "leads us to hypothesize," Cummings says, "that one of the mechanisms behind weight gain typically associated with high-fat diets is that they don't suppress the hunger hormone as well [as low-fat fare does]."

When it comes to sugars, different types can have different effects on ghrelin. For example, Peter J. Havel of the University of California, Davis and his coworkers gave 12 women standardized meals served with custom-prepared drinks sweetened with either of the two table sugar components: glucose, the sugar that cells use for energy, or fructose, the primary sugar in fruits and many soft drinks.

The meals silenced participants' ghrelin signals only about half as much on the days when the accompanying drinks had been sweetened with fructose compared with the days of glucose drinks, Havel's group reported in the June 2004 *Journal of Clinical Endocrinology & Metabolism (JCE&M).*

Even more interesting is what happened after each day of test drinks, when the women were permitted to eat anything from a buffet. The six women who had reported being careful about their food choices before the study chose fattier fare on the day after imbibing fructose drinks than they did on the day after drinking glucose-sweetened beverages. Moreover, these diners described themselves as being hungrier before meals on the day after getting fructose-sweetened drinks.

The sugar consumed the previous day didn't influence food choice or appetite of the other six women, Havel's team observed.

Though preliminary, these data suggest that even though fewer calories of fructose than calories of other sugars are required to sweeten a food, a high-fructose diet might boost calorie consumption in some people by fostering overeating, Havel notes.

Weighty Problems

One might expect that people with the highest background ghrelin concentrations in their blood would be the hungriest, eat the most, and end up fattest. It's just the opposite. This observation suggests that many people's bodies are misreading or ignoring hunger and satiety signals.

Obese individuals tend to have the lowest background ghrelin production, as if their bodies are encouraging them to fast (*SN: 7/6/02, p. 14*). Meanwhile, unhealthily lean people, such as those with anorexia nervosa, can have sky-high background ghrelin concentrations.

> ## "No wonder these poor people can't lose weight."
>
> —Stephen Bloom, Hammersmith Hospital

Ian M. Chapman of the University of Adelaide in Australia is examining elderly individuals who are healthy except for their poor appetites and inordinately lean physiques. People with this "anorexia of aging" tend to produce twice as much ghrelin as do well-nourished seniors yet claim that they're never hungry, he says.

A similarly perplexing trend appears among 30 non-diabetic but overweight adults whom Arline D. Salbe has studied at a National Institutes of Health center in Phoenix. After being on a weight-maintenance diet for 3 days, the recruits got to eat all they wanted, whenever they wanted, for another 3 days. Each volunteer stayed in a hotel-like hospital suite, and dieticians recorded every calorie consumed.

In the June 2004 *JCE&M,* Salbe's group reported that the higher a volunteer's prebreakfast concentration of ghrelin, the less he or she tended to eat.

Endocrinologist Stephen Bloom of Hammersmith Hospital in London isn't surprised.

Research by Cummings' group last year showed that in normal-weight volunteers, the more calories in a meal, the more it suppressed ghrelin production. But Bloom and his coworkers have found that hunger and satiety signals don't function well in heavy people.

Bloom's team fed 20 normal-weight and 20 heavy adults milkshake-like meals packed with anywhere from 250 to 3,000 calories. In the February *JCE&M,* the London researchers reported that ghrelin concentrations fell with increasing calories only among the normal-weight men and women. In the obese volunteers, the hormone showed the same drop after all meals, regardless of their milkshake's calorie content. The decline was similar to that in normal-weight people eating a meal with 1,000 calories.

In earlier work, Bloom's team had shown that after a meal the satiety-signaling gut hormone PYY rose less in obese volunteers than in people with normal weight (*http://www.sciencenews.org/articles/20030906/food.asp*).

"So now, you've got a double whammy," Bloom told *Science News.* Compared with other people, the obese remain hungry longer and don't feel full as quickly. "No wonder these poor people can't lose weight," he adds.

Hungry for Sleep

Since the mid-1960s, the rate of obesity in the United States has nearly tripled to one in three adults. Over the same period, U.S. citizens have deducted, on average, about 2 hours from their nightly slumber. Is there a connection?

Endocrinologist Eve Van Cauter strongly suspects that there is. She points to seven studies that have linked body weight to how long people sleep.

In her lab at the University of Chicago, Van Cauter has also been showing that blood concentrations of hunger and satiety hormones—as well as food preferences—depend on how well-rested people are. For instance, in the November 2004 *JCE&M,* her research team reported that prebreakfast concentrations of the satiety hormone leptin were roughly 20 percent lower in 11 healthy men who had slept only 4 hours a night for nearly a week than when they had slept 9 hours nightly.

In the December 2004 *Annals of Internal Medicine,* the researchers reported similar leptin differences in 12 healthy men after just 2 nights of each sleep regimen. Moreover, daytime concentrations of ghrelin climbed 28 percent during the sleep-deprived cycle.

After the second night of sleep deprivation, the recruits' appetites and food intake increased by 24 percent, compared with those after a good night's sleep. Moreover, when sleep deprived, the volunteers chose to consume a larger proportion of their food as high-calorie, carbohydrate-rich items, such as crackers and sweets. Those foods represented 33 to 45 percent more of the caloric intake than they did when the participants were well rested.

Van Cauter has also found that sleep loss increases the activity of the vagus nerve, the trunk line for signals between the gut and the brain. During stress, the brain signals the gut to alter its release of appetite-controlling hormones, which might be the mechanism by which sleep loss changes eating behavior. People are the only animals to voluntarily ignore their sleep needs, according to Van Cauter. They stay up to play, work, socialize, or watch television. However, she adds, "We're overstepping the boundaries of our biology because we are not wired for sleep deprivation."

Hunger Therapy

Despite the complexity of appetite control, several large pharmaceutical companies have started developing ghrelin-blocking agents intended to blunt hunger in overweight individuals. Researchers are currently testing these substances on lab animals. From his own work, Cummings notes, ghrelin blockers "look pretty promising."

Currently, Bloom is probing dietary maneuvers to suppress ghrelin peaks and to increase the body's natural production of some of the understudy appetite-quenching hormones. He found that when he injected PYY into people, it suppressed appetite by 30 percent.

With sleep deprivation, "we're overstepping the boundaries of our biology."

—Eve Van Cauter, University of Chicago

The stomach hormone called oxyntomodulin also reduces ghrelin concentration and appetite in people. Indeed, "if we give a fair amount of oxyntomodulin to animals, they don't eat at all," Bloom notes.

In its search for appetite suppressors, van der Lely's team is focusing strictly on ghrelin, which comes in two forms. The type generally described as active is bound to a fatty acid and is called the acylated form. Although the unacylated form "used to be called inactive," van der Lely says, his team has found evidence that it has its own role in eating behavior.

In the February *JCE&M,* van der Lely and an international group of researchers report that unacylated ghrelin acts as a spoiler to the acylated form. "We have observed that if you experimentally co-administer both [ghrelins]—one in the left arm, and the other in the right arm of people—the unacylated ghrelin can completely abolish all of the effects of the other ghrelin on metabolism," he says. The finding suggests yet another means to silence the call to eat.

Ghrelin is emerging as a hunger hormone with multiple personalities.

The Health Diet Face-Off

In a groundbreaking study, we put 1,000 women on 4 popular diets, then tracked them for 6 months. Now, the results: Here's what works best.

CHRISTIE ASCHWANDEN

When it comes to diets, everyone has an opinion. Proponents offer fantastic testimonials. Critics dismiss them as unhealthy, short-term gimmicks. And both claim experts' support. But when we sat down to investigate the hard data on particular plans, we were shocked at how little actually existed.

How well do diets perform in real life? Can anyone stick to them more than a few weeks? How much weight do dieters drop? In short, which plan actually works, and works best? No one had ever done the studies that could tell us for sure, so we came up with an ambitious, unprecedented plan: We joined forces with nutrition guru David Katz, MD, MPH, director of the Yale-Griffin Prevention Research Center in Derby, Connecticut, to design a scientific comparison of four popular diets. We developed a study rigorous enough for a medical journal, one far beyond what magazines usually offer.

Our Diet Face-Off also differs in critical ways from typical studies. For instance, as we began our research, we learned that two other teams had diet trials under way. No question, those analyses are important. But the scientists didn't test diets under real-life conditions; their volunteers met with nutritionists and got other support.

We didn't want to know how well a diet works when a researcher holds your hand. We wanted to know if real women can expect to lose weight on a plan when they're pinched for time, under stress, and feeding a hungry family. So we picked four popular diets (see "The Contenders," above right) that represent distinctly different weight-loss approaches, and randomly assigned 1,000 reader volunteers to them. Now, 6 months later, here's what we found.

The Contenders
Weight Watchers Online

The portion-control program has been popular for decades. We chose the online, do-it-yourself version (at www.weightwatchers.com) because it was cheaper than the regular program and easier to fit into a busy schedule.

Dr. Atkins' New Diet Revolution

This plan spawned the low-carb craze. Even though Atkins Nutritionals Inc. recently filed for bankruptcy, the book has had a seemingly permanent place on best-seller lists.

Eat More, Weigh Less

Developed by renowned physician Dean Ornish, this low-fat program is the only diet proven to reverse heart disease.

The Way to Eat

Katz's Mediterranean-style eating plan focuses on changing unhealthy eating habits. Though he was testing his own diet, we protected against any bias by coding the data: He didn't know which group was which until after his team had tallied the results.

And the Winner Is . . .
Weight Watchers Online

Throw out that box of low-carb pasta: You *can* lose weight without giving up whole categories of food or chewing through cardboard cuisine. In our groundbreaking study, Weight Watchers Online (WWO), with its "no food is off-limits" approach, led the pack with a mean weight loss of slightly more than 11 pounds. We hereby declare it the winner.

But weight loss isn't the only reason to give the nod to WWO. In fact, women on Atkins and The Way to Eat lost nearly as much; the numbers were so close that our team of experts ruled the outcome a three-way tie. But unless a diet morphs from a desperate measure into a lifelong way of eating, the pounds will inevitably return. So we also examined the factors that matter most over the long haul.

"We addressed questions that other studies don't: How difficult was it? Can you make this diet permanent? Did it fit with your family's lifestyle?" Katz says. "When you address these issues, you see a clear dividing line."

WWO bested the others when it came to satisfaction with the diet; its livability; and, most important, our volunteers' confidence that they'd be able to continue the diet long-term. Women on The Way to Eat (another plan without stern carb or fat limits) also reported much more satisfaction and confidence than Atkins and Ornish dieters.

What else did we learn? We asked Katz and other top researchers in the weight-control field to review our findings. Here are the lessons they pulled from our results.

What We Learned
1 Dieting Is Hard—Really Hard

No one needs a study to know that losing weight is tough, but the numbers told a sobering story. No matter what the diet, most people could not stick to it for even 6 months. Within 3 months, 71 percent of our initial participants had dropped out; by 6 months, only 16 percent remained. No diet proved superior to the others in the dropout rates.

"People have trouble losing weight, and that's the message here," says Robert H. Eckel, MD, an obesity expert at the University of Colorado at Denver and Health Sciences Center. That's not a happy finding, but it's worth focusing on for just a minute because other studies have painted a different, perhaps overly optimistic, picture.

In January, for instance, Michael Dansinger, MD, at Tufts–New England Medical Center in Boston, published his comparison of four diets (including Ornish, Atkins, and WWO) and found an attrition rate of 42 percent. But participants in the Dansinger study met with a nutritionist several times for support and individualized advice. Researchers also sometimes give participants an extra nudge to keep going by paying them for their time. "*Health* just told people to get the book," says Christopher Gardner, PhD, a Stanford University nutrition researcher

who has his own four-diet-comparison study under way. "That's real life, and it shows that the average person on the street is going to have a low likelihood of following one of these for even 6 months." To which we add: Don't feel bad if you haven't succeeded so far, but do try again because . . .

2 Some Diets Are Easier to Sustain

When you look at the volunteers who stayed in the study at the 6-month mark, there were clear differences. An astounding 90 percent of those still in the Atkins group had quit their diet; so had 85 percent of the Ornish dieters. But 36 percent of the women on WWO and 33 percent of those on The Way to Eat were still trucking.

These results run counter to some widely held notions. The buzz on Atkins has always been: Damn the nutritionists (who of course, have always raised concerns about the plan's healthfulness)—it's the only approach that doesn't leave a dieter starving or dealing with unmanageable cravings. But despite that reputation, at 6 months Atkins left 59 percent of our volunteers fighting frequent food cravings. Ornish fared only slightly better, with 54 percent reporting snack attacks. Meanwhile, a slim 29 percent of the WWO group and 35 percent of The Way to Eat folks were plagued by cravings. Perhaps that's why people in the Atkins group didn't show stick-to-it-iveness. "Atkins was fast out of the blocks," Katz says, "but it was overtaken by Weight Watchers by 6 months."

3 The More Restrictive the Diet, the Grumpier the Dieter

Even though Atkins allows dieters to eat foods typically forbidden on diets, they pay for that leniency by having to severely limit carbohydrates. And the Ornish plan stringently restricts fats. WWO and The Way to Eat focus instead on steering dieters to healthier foods with fewer calories per serving, rather than placing whole categories off-limits. That seemed to make things easier for dieters at home. A whopping 97 percent of WWO dieters and 89 percent of The Way to Eat participants called the food they were eating at least "somewhat pleasing"; just 67 percent of the Ornish group and 51 percent of the Atkins group said the same.

Family dinners proved especially challenging for those on restrictive programs. A full 92 percent of those assigned to the Atkins plan and 78 percent of those following Ornish said the diets did not address their family's needs. Many women on these plans commented in interviews that they had to do double prep work, making themselves separate meals because their families weren't willing to eat the allowed foods. Few on the other diets experienced this problem, though: Only 21 percent of The Way to Eat folks and 27 percent of the WWO group reported conflicts with their family's eating habits.

When it came to overall satisfaction, the plans with the most varied food choices came out ahead. At 6 months, 64 percent of WWO dieters told us they were "very" or "extremely" satisfied with the program; 42 percent on The Way to Eat said the same. Only 20 percent of Atkins dieters and 18 percent of the Ornish group were as positive. "Clearly, people were not as happy with the restrictive diets," Katz says. It's not that people can't lose weight on Atkins or Ornish diets, he says, but people seem to have a more difficult time sticking to their strict rules.

4 Every Diet Can Work

Despite the overall numbers, our study also proved that each diet worked for some people. At least one person from each group managed to shed 30 or more pounds. "No diet works, and every diet works," Katz says.

While the more-restrictive diets had lower satisfaction on average, "that doesn't mean that they're unsatisfactory for everyone," Dansinger says. For instance, while many participants told us they hated the Atkins diet, our biggest "loser" was Melanie Wagner, who shed 70 pounds on Atkins and declared the program a perfect fit for her.

Success requires finding a diet you can stick to, but none seems to fit everyone's temperament. For this reason, our study may paint a bleaker picture than is warranted. We randomly assigned our volunteers to their diets (ignoring some shouts of protest) to ensure the groups were similar at the start. If we'd allowed people to pick their own diets, we wouldn't know how well the plans worked for the average person—only how they performed for those most inclined to try them. But we received dozens of e-mails from people who refused to even try the diet we assigned. Katz believes we would have seen fewer dropouts had we allowed each volunteer to choose her own diet.

5 It Has to Be Easy Enough to Become Automatic

When we spoke with our successful dieters, we heard the same mantra again and again: "It's not a diet, it's the way I eat now." James Hill, PhD, a weight-loss expert at the University of Colorado Health Sciences Center, emphasized that aspect of our results. He and Rena Wing, PhD, at Brown Medical School in Providence, Rhode Island, have collected information from more than 4,500 people who have lost at least 30 pounds and kept it off a year or more. Their National Weight Control Registry shows that people who shed weight and keep it off share a common mind-set. " 'It's not a diet, it's a way of living my life'— that's what we like to hear," Hill says.

But it was harder for people on the most restrictive eating plans to turn the diets from short-term endeavors to lifelong habits. Only 28 percent of Atkins people and 40 percent of the Ornish group said the diets fit their lifestyles, while 79 percent of WWO dieters and 66 percent of Way-to-Eaters called the plans compatible with theirs.

Many of our dieters, such as Joyce Rodriguez (read her story and accounts from other volunteers in "From the Trenches,"), told us they made the switch from diet to lifestyle with the support of a spouse, friend, or other loved one. "To be successful, you need not just a book but a strong support system around you," Gardner says.

From the Trenches

Here's a closer look at women's real-life experiences with the 4 diets we tested—both pro and con.

Weight Watchers Online

WWO's Flex Plan uses a point system to teach portion control and steer dieters toward low-calorie, high-fiber foods. And its Core Plan allows dieters to select from an extensive "core group" of healthy, nutritious foods without tracking points. Our volunteers were free to choose between the plans.

"It Worked"

Wendy Tackett, 32 Education researcher; Battle Creek, Michigan; 5 feet, 2 inches; Pounds lost: 35

Wendy lost a hefty amount of weight and dropped two dress sizes via WWO. She likes that the plan doesn't put any foods off-limits. "You can find something to eat in any setting," she says. "And you can go out with friends without bringing your own meal."

While WWO provides dieters with an online diary that automatically tracks and calculates points, Wendy opted instead to track her daily points with a charm bracelet. "When I get down to the Mickey Mouse, I know I'm done eating for the day," she says.

The program helped her realize that her generous portions were adding pounds, so she and her husband, who joined her on the diet, bought new, smaller cereal bowls to painlessly reduce their serving sizes. They also took Schlotzsky's Deli off their menu after discovering that a seemingly healthy turkey club sandwich her husband regularly ate burned close to a day's worth of points. In place of such high-calorie fare, she started buying more fresh fruits and vegetables. "I used to think they were too expensive, but now I realize I'm worth it," she says. Since dropping the weight, Wendy feels more energetic. "This is a diet I can live with," she says.

Karen Miller-Kovach, MS, RD, chief science officer for Weight Watchers International, says Wendy's experience reflects Weight Watchers' mission. "We're not a diet; we're a comprehensive lifestyle program," she says. "We may not be the fastest kid on the block, but we're OK with that."

"It Didn't Work"

Robyn Baumbach-Veenker, 33 Graphic designer; Portland, Oregon; 5 feet, 6 inches

Robyn lost a pound or two in the couple of weeks she tried WWO, but she says that recording points at every meal was a hassle, and she tired of trying to figure out whether the chicken on her plate was a 4- or 6-point serving. She wanted to eat without having to grab a book or log on to the computer to calculate points. "It was making me obsess over my food too much," she says. "It felt more stressful than helpful."

Robyn has since adopted the Body for Life diet (a plan we didn't test in our study), which tells her what's allowed at each meal—one small serving each of fruit, vegetable, protein, and carbs. She says that fits her lifestyle much better.

Atkin's New Diet Revolution

Not just a diet but a phenomenon, the Atkins plan started the low-carb craze. The diet tightly regulates carbohydrates but is freer when it comes to the consumption of proteins and fats. Dieters can re-introduce whole grains after the 2-week "induction phase," though carbs are never unregulated.

"It Worked"

Melanie Wagner, 29 Nanny; Kennewick, Washington; 5 feet, 4 inches; Pounds lost: 70

We hereby anoint Melanie our Diet Face-Off superstar: The 70 pounds she dropped was more than any other participant lost. She would have never predicted that. "I was praying, please don't let me get Atkins—that's the one I'll hate the most," she recalls.

Melanie doesn't care much for vegetables, but giving up pasta and bread was difficult. She never felt like she was starving, though, and she's sure she can keep going with the diet. "I have more self-confidence now. I'm not so afraid to be noticed," she says.

Colette Heimowitz, MS, vice president of education and research at Atkins Nutritionals Inc., says Atkins dieters are most successful when, like Melanie, they follow the 2-week induction by adding low-glycemic fruits, vegetables, and whole grains.

"It Didn't Work"

Heather Batalis, 32 Stay-at-home mother of 2-year-old daughter; Warsaw, Indiana; 5 feet, 2 inches

Heather lost about 8 pounds during the 17 days she stayed on Atkins. The weight came off quickly, but she hated cooking separate meals for her husband and daughter. And she felt exhausted: An avid runner, Heather normally runs four or five times a week. While on the diet, though, she couldn't run more than 15 minutes without feeling tired. Her friends and husband questioned the diet's wholesomeness, which made it tough to stay motivated. "We eat a lot of fruits and vegetables at home, and this diet didn't seem very healthy," Heather says. As soon as she went off the diet she gained the weight back, but she feels like her old self again. She is now trying to watch what she eats and ramp up her running.

Eat More, Weigh Less

Physician Dean Ornish's Eat More, Weigh Less program focuses on health. Numerous studies have provided evidence that his vegetarian diet, which limits fat to 10 percent of calories, can actually reverse heart disease. (The average American diet gets more than 30 percent of calories from fat.)

"It Worked"

Katherine Blake-Parker, 47 Library media specialist; Guilford, Connecticut; 5 feet, 5 inches; Pounds lost: 18

Katherine was pleased to draw the Ornish diet. She was recovering from kidney failure, and because excess protein can strain the organ, this diet seemed like a good fit. Of the 18 pounds she initially lost on the diet, she's kept 15 off.

She had been a vegetarian in the '70s and didn't mind going meat-free, but her kids were another story. "I have three athletic teenagers, and it was hard to integrate what I was eating with what they were eating" Katherine says. "I could slip the tofu and soy powders into things, but it wasn't a big hit."

Her family eventually reached equilibrium: She's a bit more permissive with the diet, and they're more accommodating. Katherine intends to continue the diet long-term, though she does stretch the rules here and there. Finding the fat limitation too restrictive, she's added nuts, avocados, and other plant-based fats. "You're supposed to totally avoid alcohol, but I'm not going to deny myself a glass of Merlot once in a while," Katherine says.

Many of our dieters complained about the Ornish diet's no-meat rule. But "what we've found over and over again is that if people make these changes, their quality of life goes up," says Dean Ornish, MD, president of the Preventive Medicine Research Institute in Sausalito, California. "Their cholesterol goes down as much as with drugs, and their blood pressure goes down. What good is it to lose weight if it's not healthy for you?"

"It Didn't Work"

Susan K. Sulfaro, 43 Product-development vice president for a consulting firm; Brighton, Michigan; 5 feet, 7 inches

Before starting, Susan had lost 55 pounds with a medically supervised program and exercise. But she knew her eating habits were standing between her and the nearly 59 pounds she still wanted to drop. When she drew the Ornish plan, she went out and bought an array of fat-free salad dressings and condiments, but "they all tasted awful."

When Susan learned that Ornish gives permission to eat prepared food if it has less than 2 grams of fat per serving, she drove 45 minutes to a Whole Foods Market. "I went through the entire frozen-foods section and couldn't find anything that had less than 2 grams of fat," she says. After a month, she'd lost only a pound and felt so cranky she gave up. She switched to WWO, which is working for her.

The Way to Eat

The Way to Eat plan doesn't tell you what to eat; instead, it outlines strategies for making healthy choices, and promotes habits and food preferences that will help with lifelong weight control. The book steers you to a Mediterranean-style eating program that conforms to current dietary guidelines.

"It Worked"

Joyce Rodriguez, 45 General manager of a wholesale yarn distributor; Cornish, Maine; 5 feet, 3 inches; Pounds lost: 13

When Joyce read The Way to Eat, she was disappointed to find no magic trick to melt the pounds away. "It was like auditioning for Extreme Makeover and being given the runner-up prize of dumbbells and a falafel sandwich," she says.

Her disappointment didn't last. "In the beginning, there was too much thinking," Joyce says. Then she realized that was the point. "I've always been looking for the magic pill when what I really needed was to make better choices." Soon she'd switched from white rice to brown. She tried the protein-rich grain quinoa for the first time, and packed extra fruit and vegetables into her family's meals. Her teenage son still likes his Pop-Tarts, she says, but he also eats the whole grains she puts in front of him. Her husband has lost weight right along with her. "I can mountain-bike 12 or 15 miles now, when I was struggling with just a mile before," she says.

Joyce has dropped 13 pounds and several dress sizes, but it didn't happen quickly. "I was happy with losing only 5 pounds in the first 8 weeks—I actually got the part about having unrealistic expectations before," she says. Joyce calls this plan not a diet but a new way of eating.

Her story reflects the kind of results Katz hopes for. He says the relative success of WWO and The Way to Eat suggests that learning to make good choices works better than restricting options.

"It Didn't Work"

Gail Martino, 44 Assistant director of admissions at a private school; Doylestown, Pennsylvania; 5 feet, 7 inches

Gail read The Way to Eat, but thought it was awful. "Too much theory," she says. With a busy job, and a husband and two young kids to cook for, she was looking for a diet that told her exactly what to do; she didn't have time to make the decisions on her own, or to do the food prep required by The Way to Eat plan. She also wanted more guidance, and concedes that she was looking for a magic formula—one she didn't find in The Way to Eat program. She has since joined Weight Watchers instead. "It's a lifestyle approach, like The Way to Eat, but it has more structure," she says. Gail likes Weight Watchers because she can still have her favorite foods.

By the Numbers

Our volunteers answered hundreds of questions when they started, after 3 months on their diet, and again after 6 months. Here's a look at what they said.

Did You Stick with It?

Percentage of those remaining who stuck with the diet

WWO(*)	36%
The Way to Eat	33%
Ornish	15%
Atkins	10%

*Weight Watchers Online

How Strictly Did You Follow the Diet?

Percentage who kept to the diet most or all of the time

WWO	61%
The Way to Eat	39%
Ornish	23%
Atkins	17%

How Many Pounds Did You Lose?

Mean weight loss (in pounds) for those who stuck it out

WWO	11.2
Atkins	9.8
The Way to Eat	6.1
Ornish	5.0

Did You Like the Diet?

Well, what percentage of volunteers did?

WWO	64%
The Way to Eat	42%
Atkins	20%
Ornish	18%

Did You Battle Food Cravings?

Percentage of those who said yes

Atkins	59%
Ornish	54%
The Way to Eat	35%
WWO	29%

Did You Like Your Food Choices

Percentage who called the food very or extremely pleasing

WWO	69%
The Way to Eat	57%
Atkins	32%
Ornish	23%

Did Your Family Play Along?

Percentage who said the diet fit into their family's lifestyle

The Way to Eat	79%
WWO	73%
Ornish	22%
Atkins	8%

Was the Diet Easy to Follow?

Percentage who said yes

WWO	85%
The Way to Eat	77%
Atkins	53%
Ornish	38%

Did the Diet Fit Your Lifestyle?

Percentage who said yes

WWO	79%
The Way to Eat	66%
Ornish	40%
Atkins	28%

Could You Live with This Diet?

Percentage who were very or extremely confident they could continue it

WWO	50%
The Way to Eat	36%
Ornish	13%
Atkins	12%

Will Your Child Be Fat?
How to Prevent Obesity—for Babies on Up

JESSICA SNYDER SACHS

At 7 months, Zachary Miller was a happy and healthy, but not especially active, baby. "The pediatrician told me, 'The big ones don't like to move'" says Zach's mom, Ellie, of Somerset, New Jersey. "She told me to put him on the floor and on his tummy as often as possible. He hates that. But it does get him to push up on his arms and roll over."

At 20 pounds and 27 inches long, Zach was already overweight. His height was in the 50th percentile for boys his age, but his weight was in the 75th (pediatricians like both numbers to be close together). But does it really make sense to be so concerned about a baby this young?

Yes, say an increasing number of health experts. The more weight a baby gains before age 2, the heavier she's likely to be as an older child and adult, studies show. If one or both parents are overweight, the concern is even greater.

And the eating and activity patterns learned in childhood—for good or ill—tend to persist for a lifetime. Some overweight kids as young as 3 or 4 can already have elevated levels of cholesterol, insulin, or blood pressure.

But many people miss the signs that a child (especially a boy) is too chubby. In one study, only 21 percent of the moms of overweight preschoolers knew it. As more and more kids get heavier—the average child's waist has gone up two sizes in the past 20 years—kids who are overweight increasingly look "normal" to us.

Pediatricians can miss the signs, too, even though the American Academy of Pediatrics (AAP) recommends that they check a child's body mass index (BMI)—a measure of fatness—annually starting at age 2.

So it's up to *you* to be alert to the signs that your child's overweight or gaining too quickly. "Our current lifestyle is putting kids at risk for serious health problems," says pediatrician Sheila Gahagan, M.D., of the University of Michigan's Department of Pediatrics and Center for Human Growth and Development in Ann Arbor, "but we can turn it around." The hard part: Improving their lifestyle usually means changing yours, too.

That means neither obsessive eating nor quick weight-loss plans, which are especially dangerous for children, whose growing bodies require nutrients from a broad variety of foods, including healthful fats. Instead, what's needed is a return to good nutrition centered on family meals, says Naomi Neufeld, M.D., a pediatric endocrinologist and director of KidShape, a family-based pediatric weight-management program in four states.

Here, what you need to know to set your child—from birth through grade school—on a path toward maintaining a healthy weight:

Babies: 0 to 1 Year

Eating well. Nursing reduces the risk of obesity in later childhood and beyond. Not only do compounds in breast milk help regulate appetite and body fat, but breastfed babies also take in only as much as they need, and milk production adjusts accordingly.

For a bottle-fed baby, resist the urge to encourage him to finish that last ounce—whether it's formula or expressed breast milk—after he's signaled he's full. And whether you're nursing or bottle-feeding, don't automatically feed your baby every time he cries, says Dr. Neufeld: "Sometimes all he needs is attention."

Nor should you rush solids. While it's acceptable to start as early as 4 months, it may be best to wait until 6 months—especially if your baby's a little heavy to start with. When you do start, don't invite him into the clean-plate club. "When he turns his head away, the meal's over," says Christine Wood, M.D., the author of *How to Get Kids to Eat Great and Love It!*

Getting active. Infancy is a critical time for new brain-muscle connections, but all you need to provide are soft, safe toys and an unrestricted space, such as a five- by seven-foot rug, where

1,000	Calories that kids ages 1 to 3 need in a day
1,250	Calories that American kids get at this age
1,250	Calories that kids ages 4 to 6 need in a day
1,800	Calories that American kids get at this age

your baby can safely roll over, push and pull up, sit, crawl, and play movement games like patty-cake with you. (But don't force his body into extreme positions, such as feet over head.) "I put Samantha, who's nine months old, where she can watch her older siblings playing," says Anna Toma, of Monmouth Junction, New Jersey. "I can tell by the way her eyes light up and her arms go up in the air that she's going to be right in there running around with them as soon as she can."

Toddlers: 1 to 3 Years

Eating well. Toddlerhood is a time when many parents, without realizing it, set the stage for mindless consumption of empty calories. Even 100 percent juice should be limited to four to six ounces a day for kids ages 1 to 6, according to the AAP; fruit "drinks" and sugary sodas don't belong on toddler menus. The best beverages are low-fat milk—and water.

Try not to start hard-to-quit habits, like snacking on fast food, eating in front of the TV, or pacifying a full but restless (or crying) toddler with convenience snacks when you're in the checkout line or car, or just too busy to play. Instead, find a self-directed activity, book, or other noncaloric distraction.

On the other hand, toddlers need to eat between meals—when they're hungry—and should be offered healthful snacks, such as soft, bite-size pieces of fruits and vegetables, string cheese, or a tube of low-fat yogurt. (Avoid choking hazards such as whole grapes, nuts, and hard chunks of fruits and vegetables.)

Getting active. Once your child is walking, let him act on his natural desire to keep moving. Whenever you can, slow down so he can walk and climb the stairs, and make sure his days include outside play. "When my daughters were two, four, and six, we all loved to go out in the yard, pretend we were the Powerpuff Girls, and chase each other around," says Hannah Storm, coanchor of *The Early Show* on CBS and author of *Go Girl! Raising Healthy, Confident and Successful Girls Through Sports.* (Now that they're a few years older, they all play soccer and T-ball in the yard.)

When it's raining, explore ways to be active indoors—dancing or wrestling on the rug, or climbing on sturdy furniture. Kids under 2 should watch very little TV; those 2 and up, no more than an hour or two a day. And when it's time to shop for daycare or a preschool program, look for a daily schedule that includes both structured games like Duck, Duck, Goose and unstructured run-around time. Experts recommend that toddlers get at least 30 minutes of structured activity and one to several hours of unstructured activity daily.

Preschoolers: 3 to 5

Eating well. Practice portion control. Serve your child one tablespoon per year of age. A typical meal for a 3-year-old might be three tablespoons each of pasta (try whole-wheat), peas, chicken, and fruit. (If your child doesn't want it all, that's fine.)

What about the child who wants only carbs (the infamous "white diet") while leaving everything else on his plate? Saying "veggies first before seconds of pasta" is tempting, but using

---

How to "Sell" Healthy Foods

TV advertising influences what kids as young as 2 want to eat and drink (and bug their parents to buy)—so much so that it may contribute to childhood obesity, finds an Institute of Medicine report. It's a growing threat: Nearly 500 new food products are targeted to kids each year, up from a few dozen a decade ago. What to do:

- **Until age 8,** kids can't understand that the purpose of advertising is to persuade. For little ones, limit exposure, and as they grow, teach them: Point out commercials, Internet "advergames," billboards, sponsored books, and packaging. They'll learn to see them for what they are.
- **Seek out plugs for healthier foods.** Some companies use licensed characters like Arthur and Clifford to promote more nutritious fare.
- **Resist whining.** Little kids don't buy junk; they make us do it. When you shop, let your child pick out his favorite fruit, but let him choose only between the cereals you select.
- **Be a superhero.** Yes, cartoon characters have influence, but so do you. Eat well, and your child will have a good role model.

—Robert Barnett

---

food as a reward can backfire—kids tend to like the reward food even more and the have-to-eat food even less. One solution: Make just enough for one or two toddler-size servings.

Whatever you do, keep offering a variety of healthful choices at every meal. "Tastes mature," says early-childhood educator Harriet Worobey, director of Rutgers University's Nutritional Sciences Preschool, in New Brunswick, New Jersey, which combines early-childhood education with research on childhood nutrition and family development. "Don't stop serving broccoli just because your child rejects it once."

Getting active. Frisbee, hopscotch, bike riding, kickball, dancing—the joy of movement takes dozens of wonderful forms in the preschool years. (Watching a screen isn't one of them.) By age 3, kids need an hour of structured and one to several hours of unstructured play—and shouldn't be sedentary for more than an hour at a time. You don't need to do much to get kids moving at this age: If the weather's nice, just open the door and go outside, or take a nature hike with a plastic bucket, which your child can fill with found "treasures."

Schoolkids: 5 and Up

Eating well. Find fun ways to teach your child about nutrition. Here's what Joy Bauer, a registered dietitian in private practice in New York City, does with her kids: She helps each make a list of the favorite treats that, in quantity, would not be good for their "teeth or insides." She then allows one or two a day, any time they choose. And she keeps the portions within reason by stocking up on small versions, such as "fun-size" candy bars.

If Your Child Is Overweight . . .

To help, the key isn't to count your kid's calories but to change the family's lifestyle:

- **Color-code food.** "Red" for special-occasion, high-calorie foods and drinks (candy, chips, soda); "yellow" for healthy-in-moderation foods (whole-grain bread and pasta, lean meat, low-fat cheese); "green" for anytime foods (fresh fruits, vegetables). Read nutrition labels together.
- **Eat breakfast.** Kids who do so regularly are more likely to control weight.
- **Get moving.** Make time for active family outings, even just playing in the backyard or walking together to nearby playdates.
- **Fight mindless munching.** Post a refrigerator-door list of alternatives to "boredom eating": reading, drawing, coloring, listening to songs, playing favorite games.

Bauer also suggests having kids use sticker charts to log each time they eat fruit, veggies, or other healthful foods. (Go to MealMarkers.com for a $25 kit that takes advantage of reusable vinyl stickers. Another teaching tool, "Food Fun Nutrition Cards," loads lots of facts onto a real playing deck; $10, foodfun4kids.com.)

If you've already let sugar and other empty calories swamp your child's diet, gradually start to dial it back. Bauer recommends cutting sugary cereals, fifty-fifty, with healthful look-alikes.

Getting active. Your child can now share more fully in family outings such as hiking, biking, and skating. The early grade-school years, of course, are also a great time to sample a variety of sports and dance, from team sports like soccer and softball to individual ones like karate and gymnastics, hip-hop and ballet. By this age, kids should get about an hour of moderate to vigorous activity a day, with rest breaks. It doesn't have to be all at once, either—10 or 15 minutes at a time is fine. Now's the time to find creative ways to rein in the mounting temptations of electronic entertainment: TV, DVDs, video games, and Internet sites. "Since my boys were six and nine, they've known that they need to spend a half hour moving for every half hour on the computer or Xbox," says LynnAnn Covell, an exercise physiologist at Green Mountain at Fox Run, a nondiet weight-loss resort in Ludlow, Vermont.

In the older grade-school years, sports and dance can become highly competitive. "That's unfortunate, as it means that less athletically inclined kids tend to drop out," says pediatric exercise physiologist Randy Claytor, PH.D., of Cincinnati Children's Hospital and Medical Center. If that happens to your kid, he suggests, try setting up social situations in which she can play sports with friends "just for fun." Walking or riding bikes to school together can also be an opportunity to chat and bond. (For tips on making it safer in your town, go to the Centers for Disease Control's Walk to School website, Cdc.gov/nccdphp/dnpa/kidswalk. And if you're looking for ways to make your child's school healthier, go to Action for Healthy Kids, a public-private partnership, at actionforhealthykids.org.)

Thanks to his mom's encouragement, at 3 years old, Zachary Miller has become a vigorously active preschooler who loves racing around the backyard with his brothers, Matthew, 7, and Jake, 21 months. At 36 inches and 37 pounds, he's still on the stocky side. But he's developed the kind of habits that favor a lifetime of healthy physical activity. "He's very coordinated, riding his big brother's old training-wheel bike, kicking balls, climbing, and jumping," says his mom. "It's a regular circus around here."

JESSICA SNYDER SACHS is a contributing editor at *Parenting.*

Are We Setting the Stage for Obesity and Poor Oral Health?

America. It's the land of the free and the home of the super-sized soda, where the health of today's children is at risk. The picture may be grim, but there's hope for change through education and collaboration.

TERRI LISAGOR, EdD, MS, RD

"During thousands of years marked by food scarcity, human beings developed efficient mechanisms to store energy as fat. Until recently, we rarely enjoyed the abundance of cheap food that we see today."[1]

And enjoy we do. By some estimates, we experience an average of 5.6 eating episodes (i.e., snacks and meals) per day.[2] That could be translated to as many as 163,000 snacks and meals throughout our lifetime, totaling tons of food. Thus, dietary choices that we make can have a profound effect on overall health, especially for our children. Given the current trends, are we setting the stage for childhood obesity and poor oral health?

Influences on Early Eating Behaviors

Several factors influence what, when, and how often our children and adolescents eat. Today's children glue themselves to the television more than ever before, according to recent research, and many children are watching between 21 and 28 hours of TV per week.[3] This is more than twice what the American Academy of Pediatrics recommends.

Besides the obvious sedentary behavior, while watching television, children are receiving powerful advertising messages about foods. It comes as no surprise that advertisements aimed at youths are generally contrary to what is recommended for healthful eating.[4] Adding to the concern is the fact that among some populations, roughly 38% of children aged 1 to 4 have televisions in their bedrooms.[5] This encourages more TV viewing and less physical activity, while providing an even greater opportunity for advertising messages to influence preschoolers' eating behaviors.

In addition to the influences of television, children are exposed to and often swayed by other children's eating habits. They are exposed to snack machines and opportunities for frequent snacking, an abundance of convenience and fast foods, and super-sized servings. And, unfortunately, foods are frequently used as pacifiers that substitute for a lack of parental attention, time, or an understanding of the need for more nutritious foods.[6] As a result, less nutritious foods are consumed more frequently.

An example of children's changing food habits can be seen in beverage consumption patterns (see Figure 1). Between 1970 and 2000, regular soda consumption climbed from 22 to 49 gallons per person per year. During that same period, milk intake dropped from 31 to 23 gallons per person per year. According to the U.S. Department of Agriculture's (USDA) Continuing Survey of Food Intakes by Individuals (CSFII), 1994 to 1996, 20% of all children aged 1 to 2 consumed soft drinks.[7] The USDA's CSFII also shows that soda consumption exponentially increased through young adulthood (see Figure 1).[8]

Cause for Concern

Why should this be of worry? Because poor eating habits, including excess consumption of sweetened beverages, often lead to increased consumption of sugar and calories, which negatively affects the intake of various essential nutrients. Sweetened beverage intake is also associated with an increased risk of obesity and dental caries.[9–11]

Heavy soft drink consumption has been linked to low intake of magnesium, ascorbic acid, riboflavin, and vitamins A and D, as well as a high intake of calories, fat, and refined carbohydrates.[7] Dietary surveys of teenagers found that in 1996, only one third of boys and girls consumed the number of servings of vegetables recommended by the USDA's Food Guide Pyramid, less than 16% consumed adequate fruit servings, and 29% of boys and 11% of girls consumed the recommended servings of dairy foods.

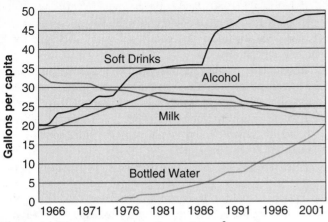

Figure 1 Beverage consumption patterns.[8]
Source: USDA.

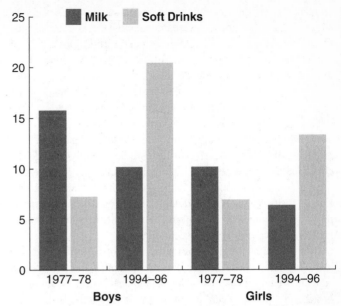

Figure 2 Teens' (ages 12 to 19) comsumption of milk and soft drinks per day.
Source: USDA, NFCS, CSFII.

As shown in Figure 2, 30 years ago, teens drank twice as much milk as soft drinks. By 1996, those numbers reversed, such that young people drank twice as much soda as milk. There is no doubt that youths' dietary inadequacies can increase risk factors for several diseases that manifest in adulthood (e.g., osteoporosis).[12]

From Family-Size to Super-Size

A meta-analysis of research between 1966 and 2005 showed a positive correlation between a greater intake of sugar-sweetened beverages and weight gain in children and adults.[9] In the 1950s, a family-size bottle of soda was 26 ounces. Today, a typical soft drink at fast-food restaurants is 12 to 42 ounces—for one person.

Of course, soda consumption is not the only calorie-dense item that has increased. McDonald's shakes, Dunkin' Donuts Coolattas, Starbucks' Venti lattes, and even canned sweetened iced teas have become super-sized. And as portion sizes have grown, value marketing has skewed Americans' thinking about appropriate portions. According to the American Institute for Cancer Research (AICR), value marketing appeals to the consumer's desire for bargains by offering more (product) for less (money). The result: more calories attendant with less nutrient density.

Super-Sized Consequences

What are some consequences of current eating habits for our nation's youths? Between 1980 and 1994, the mean daily energy intake for children increased by approximately 100 to 300 kilocalories, while energy expenditure decreased (more television, computer usage, and video games and less physical activity), setting the stage for increased risk of obesity and associated diseases.

Based on the National Health and Nutrition Examination Survey (NHANES) II data of 1976 to 1980, only 5% of youths were classified as overweight. By the NHANES III survey, from 1988 to 1994, the number of overweight youths increased to 11%.[13] More current estimates suggest that 25% of children in

the United States are overweight and another 11% are obese.[14] We know that overweight and obese children are at higher risk for cardiovascular disease, type 2 diabetes, asthma, gallbladder disease, and certain cancers.[13,15–18]

As children become more overweight, another health relationship has been observed: Increased obesity rates parallel increased caries rates.[15,19,20] Clearly, a proper diet goes a long way toward reducing the risk for obesity and dental caries, particularly if we once again address types of foods consumed, frequency of exposure, and the amount of food eaten.[21] More than 50 years ago, the classic Vipeholm study demonstrated what other, more current studies have supported: Carbohydrates, including sugars, have a role in caries formation; frequency of sugar consumption and duration of carbohydrate exposure also have a significant impact on dental health.[22,23]

Current health and nutrition behaviors among the nation's youths seem to put them at risk for poor overall health. Childhood is the time for setting the stage for positive health outcomes.

Practical Solutions

What can be done? One answer lies in education, in raising the awareness of all those who influence children's eating behaviors, including the family or main caregivers. It also includes all those who affect the health of children: parents, families, and caregivers; healthcare professionals; food industry and the media; educational authorities and schools; communities; and governmental agencies at all levels. Everyone must step up and set the stage for preventing childhood obesity and dental disease and promoting good overall health.

Parents, families, and main caregivers. It is important for all to understand how subtle messages impact what children learn. Nonverbal cues from primary caregivers, including what and how foods are purchased, prepared, served, and eaten, shape children's habits.[15] Research demonstrates that parents, families, and other main caregivers need to be more aware of their own eating behaviors and attitudes and the impact these may have on their children.[24]

Not surprising is that children's preferences for high-fat, total fat, and sugar, as well as time spent in sedentary activities, have been positively associated with parental behaviors.[25]

Children who eat more family meals together generally eat more healthfully.[26] A National Longitudinal Study of Adolescent Health concluded that parental presence at the evening meal is positively associated with adolescents' higher consumption of fruits, vegetables, and dairy food.[18] Nutrition and health professionals need to educate parents about the role of family mealtimes for healthy adolescent nutrition.

"Parents and caregivers of infants and children often receive little guidance about proper preventive dental and oral health care and dietary measures."[27] It is vital to teach all those involved in a child's primary care about the value of good oral hygiene habits and dietary practices that "emphasize minimum exposure to retentive, fermentable carbohydrates, exposure to fluoridated water, and a varied, balanced diet that should continue throughout childhood."[27]

Parents and caregivers also need guidance with children's use of television, video games, and computers. The American Academy of Pediatrics recommends that parents set limits for their children, but families need to be educated more consistently about why and how this can be accomplished. It is not only that these inactivities encourage sedentary behavior but also that these media can and do deliver unhealthful messages.

In asking again what can be done, another equally important answer lies in collaboration, such as the following:

Healthcare professionals. Pediatric health professionals need to work with one another and parents to form a meaningful alliance resulting in the best possible healthcare for children.[28] As an example of a simple way in which healthcare professionals can collaborate with families, body mass indexes should be routinely checked in children so that counseling and guidance can be provided to the families and/or caregivers.

Pediatricians, pediatric dentists, dietitians, and other healthcare advocates have a duty and an opportunity to be part of our children's healthcare and prevention strategy team. Each brings a unique skill set to the equation and a chance to teach and learn from one another. Through collaboration, this strong alliance can help deliver a consistent message to parents and children: more nutrient-dense foods, less frequency of snacking, proper portion sizes, and adequate oral hygiene.

Food industry and the media. The food industry could be a significant part of a collaborative effort to reduce childhood obesity, promote healthy eating, and prevent poor health outcomes. Think of how powerful their advertising efforts have been at influencing eating behaviors that we find today, and imagine how effective a change in their messaging could be.

Packaged foods and beverages could be more nutritious and nutrient dense; standard serving sizes could return to what they were before the 1980s; and packaging and advertising for the healthier dietary choices could entice the young consumer and replace what we find today with less-healthy packaged foods and beverages.

Restaurants, be they full-service or fast-food, could offer more realistic portion sizes and less super-sized meals; they could offer more nutritious choices and promote these in ways that would appeal to younger audiences. Nutritional information, while available today, could be made more accessible to parents and other caregivers.

Food labeling has been in existence since the early 1970s. From the beginning, the primary purpose of food labels was to be a teaching tool for the consumer. However, food labels need to be clearer and easier for the layperson to understand. Serving sizes of packaged foods also need to be more realistic.

The industry could collaborate with parents, families, schools, and healthcare providers by educating all of those involved with the health and well-being of our children.

School districts and schools. School districts, as well as individual schools, have a unique opportunity to collaborate with families in delivering health-based messages. During the school year, the majority of a child's day is spent in the classroom and elsewhere on campus. Thus, schools present an ideal venue for addressing a child's health.[29] Obviously, the concepts of health should be taught within the classroom, but the application of healthy lifestyles can be demonstrated in many ways: What foods and beverages are served to the students? What items are sold in the machines on campus? What physical activities are provided and promoted? A healthful school environment should be a top priority for the school districts and schools. Through collaborative efforts, the schools could work with families, healthcare workers, and communities to set the standards for good health.

An example of collaboration and education can be found within the California Dietetic Association (CDA). The CDA has formed a childhood obesity task force, partnering with the California School Boards Association. The task force is involved in monitoring and analyzing nutrition-related legislation, increasing overall participation in public policy making, and ensuring that children's health issues remain a priority.

Communities and state and local governments. Communities must rally together to keep children safe and provide opportunities for children to be involved and physically active. Are there places to safely walk, bike, run, or skate? Community coalitions could find creative ways to implement programs especially designed to promote healthy lifestyles and collaborate with state and local governments to garner their support.

Federal government. And finally, at the heart and soul of the charge is the federal government. Obesity prevention and the well-being of our youths must be a national public health priority. As an oversight body, the federal government can develop and promote high standards for health and fitness, enforce guidelines for issues such as advertising to children, be involved in funding prevention research, and convene national conferences aimed at collaborating with and educating those who affect the health of our children.

Summary

Certainly childhood obesity and poor oral health are complex in their etiologies. It therefore behooves us to take a multifaceted approach to finding successful solutions, all of which involve education and collaboration. Childhood must be the time for setting the stage to ensure that children develop healthy eating habits, appropriate levels of physical activity, and good oral hygiene habits that can last a lifetime.

TERRI LISAGOR, EdD, MS, RD, is an assistant professor of nutrition and food science at California State University, Northridge, a registered dietitian in private practice, and a lecturer at the UCLA School of Dentistry.

Cancer: How Extra Pounds Boost Your Risk

BONNIE LIEBMAN

Why worry about XXL size pants? According to a 2006 survey by the American Cancer Society, 83 percent of Americans know that extra flab boosts their odds of a heart attack and 57 percent know that obesity ups their risk of diabetes. Yet only 17 percent know that a growing girth could make them more prone to cancer.

"Five years ago, I would have understood that," says the cancer society's Eugenia Calle. But today, the public's failure to see the connection is even more out of sync with the science.

"I'm just astounded by how much new information is coming out on obesity and cancer," says Calle. "I can barely keep up."

Here's the latest.

Why are researchers seeing a stronger link between obesity and cancer than in the past? "We may not have picked up a link 20 years ago because fewer people were overweight 20 years ago," says Yale's Susan Taylor Mayne.

For example, experts estimate that in the United States, excess weight explains roughly:

- half of all uterine and esophageal cancer,
- a fifth (in women) to a third (in men) of all colorectal cancer,
- a third of all kidney cancer,
- a quarter of all pancreatic cancer, and
- more than a fifth of all postmenopausal breast cancer.[1]

But in Europe, where obesity rates are lower—like ours were 20 years ago—excess weight explains a lower percentage of most cancers.[1]

"The list of cancers related to obesity is growing," says Mayne. "It's alarming."

How much of a spare tire do you need before your risk climbs? It depends. For some cancers, risk starts to rise even before you cross the line that defines "overweight."

"With breast, colon, and endometrial cancer, you can see an increase in risk at the high end of the normal-weight range compared to the low end," says the American Cancer Society's Eugenia Calle. "And then the risk increases in an almost linear fashion from the very lean to the very heavy."

That's partly because the "normal-weight" range is quite large. "Two people of the same height could be 30 to 50 pounds apart and still be normal weight," she explains.

For some cancers, only heavier people appear to be at risk. "For example, it seems like there's no increase in the risk of pancreatic cancer until you get very heavy," says Calle. But that may simply reflect incomplete data.

"Most studies have used Body Mass Index, or BMI, as a measure of obesity, and that's not the best measure for all cancers," she says. "For example, now we're looking at waist circumference and pancreatic cancer and finding a stronger effect."

The lengthening list of cancers linked to obesity, says Mayne, suggests that "it may be a systemic effect."

That's because fat tissue isn't just dormant storage space. It's an active organ, releasing and receiving signals from other organs.

So far, three main theories explain how those signals may help turn healthy cells into tumors.

I. The Insulin Pathway

Insulin is the hormone that allows blood sugar to enter cells, where it is either burned for energy or stored as fat.

But if you have too many overstuffed fat cells, they can become resistant to insulin. It's as though the cells were trying to shut the door that would let in even more sugar.

With insulin losing its punch, the pancreas ramps up its output of the hormone.

"If you have more or bigger fat cells on board, the pancreas is forced to produce more insulin," says Michael Leitzmann, an epidemiologist at the National Cancer Institute.

High insulin levels are especially likely if you have what experts call "central obesity" (see "Waist Not . . ." p. 109).

"These are people who have an apple-shaped body with a big waist instead of the pear-shaped people with big hips," explains Karen Margolis of the University of Minnesota and HealthPartners Research Foundation in Minneapolis.

It's clear that insulin resistance increases the risk of diabetes and heart disease. Now cancer may join those ranks.

"It's likely that the insulin pathway and insulin resistance are important for cancers of the colon, liver, pancreas, and kidney," says Calle.

How? Insulin prompts the body to make insulin-like growth factor 1 (IGF-1). In test tubes, both insulin and IGF-1 make cells proliferate.[1]

"Insulin itself stimulates growth, so it could act directly on cancer cells," says researcher Edward Giovannucci of the Harvard School of Public Health. "And insulin sensitizes the cells to IGF-1."

It's not that overweight people necessarily have more IGF-1. Rather, "insulin decreases IGF-1 binding protein, so there's more free IGF-1 in the blood," he explains.

Here's what researchers know about cancers linked to the insulin pathway.

• **Liver.** "Peripheral fat in the thighs and hips—where a lot of women carry their fat—is not that metabolically active," says Calle.

On the other hand, the "visceral" fat around the waist is constantly sending out signals that promote inflammation or growth elsewhere in the body.

(Inflammation, which is often outwardly invisible, is the immune system's attempt to fight off and repair the damage caused by germs, irritants, or other insults.)

"We're not talking about the subcutaneous layer of fat between the skin and muscles," adds Calle. "We're talking about the fat behind the muscle wall that surrounds the organs." (See "Waist Not . . ." p. 109.)

"People don't realize that once you get beyond a certain level of adiposity, fat starts to infiltrate muscle and organs like the liver."

In the past, excess alcohol accounted for most fatty livers. "But the most common cause of abnormal liver tests in the United States now is non-alcoholic fatty liver disease," says Calle.

A fatty liver starts out benign, but it can lead to cell injury, scarring, and inflammation. "It can progress from fatty liver to hepatitis to cirrhosis to liver cancer," says Calle.

So far, studies suggest that the obese have anywhere from 1½ to 4 times the risk of liver cancer.[1,2] But the disease is still rare in the United States, so it's harder to get a precise risk estimate.

• **Colon.** Colon cancer isn't rare. It kills more non-smokers than any other cancer.

In the National Institutes of Health-AARP Diet and Health Study, which tracked more than 300,000 men and 200,000 women for five years, the heaviest men had twice the risk of colon cancer, while the heaviest women had a 50 percent increase in risk.[3] But that doesn't mean that everyone else is in the clear.

"The risk increases even for people who are mildly over-weight, which isn't reassuring for people who have a couple of extra pounds," explains the National Cancer Institute's Michael Leitzmann.

Why does obesity seem to matter more in men than women? Fat around your waist is the culprit, and men are more likely to gain weight there.

Giovannucci and colleagues found that men with a waist measuring at least 43 inches had a 2½ times greater risk of colon cancer than men with a waist smaller than 35 inches.[4] And a big belly often goes hand in hand with excess insulin.

"In human and animal studies, insulin levels are correlated with risk," says Giovannucci. For example, the higher a rat's insulin level, the more its colon cells proliferate.[5]

"The data linking insulin to risk is stronger for colon than for any other cancer," says Giovannucci.

• **Pancreas.** Pancreatic cancer is deadly. Only one in five patients is alive one year after diagnosis, and only one in 25 survives five years. The only known risk factors are cigarette smoking, diabetes, and obesity.

"In the past six years, a huge number of studies using prospective data have shown a very strong association between obesity and pancreatic cancer," says researcher Dominique Michaud of the Harvard School of Public Health.

In most studies, being obese doubles the risk.[6,7] "For people who are overweight, the link isn't as strong as it is for other cancers," says Michaud. "It shows up more for the obese."

A few studies, like the European Prospective Investigation into Cancer and Nutrition (EPIC), which tracked more than 430,000 men and women for six years, found a stronger link with waist size than with obesity *per se*.[8] But other than EPIC, "there's very little data on waist circumference," Michaud notes.

It's still not clear how excess fat leads to pancreatic tumors. "It's probably a consequence of sustained higher levels of glucose and insulin in the blood," suggests Michaud.

Inflammation may also play a role, she adds, "because people who are obese have higher levels of inflammation."

Again, it's the visceral fat cells deep in the belly that appear to be at fault. "Those fat cells are different," Michaud explains. "They're actively causing trouble."

• **Kidney.** Although kidney cancer accounts for only about 2 percent of cancer deaths, the incidence is rising in the United States and worldwide. Smoking, diabetes, high blood pressure, and obesity all seem to raise the risk, but it's not clear if a large waist matters more than a large number on the bathroom scale.

In many studies, excess fat anywhere in the body raised the risk.[9] But in the Women's Health Initiative, which tracked about 140,000 U.S. women for nearly eight years, those with the largest waists (for a given hip size) had double the risk.[10]

"Central obesity was the strongest risk factor in these women," says the University of Minnesota's Karen Margolis, who co-authored the study.

What's more, U.S. women who had lost or gained over 10 pounds more than 10 times during their lifetime had a 2½ times greater risk of kidney cancer than those with stable weights.

"It appears that weight cycling has a pretty strong relationship with kidney cancer, particularly at the extreme," says Margolis. "But we don't know why."

II. The Estrogen Pathway

If you're overweight but don't carry the extra pounds in your waist, are you off the hook?

No. Fat—whether it's around your hips, thighs, waist, or wherever—produces steroid hormones like estrogen.

"Another main way that obesity can raise the risk of cancer is through the estrogen pathway," says the American Cancer Society's Eugenia Calle.

In premenopausal women, estrogen comes largely from the ovaries. "After the ovaries stop functioning, the primary source of estrogen production is adipose [fat] tissue," Calle explains. "And estrogen is associated with endometrial and breast cancer."

As with IGF-1, obesity depresses levels of binding proteins.

"There's not as much sex-hormone-binding globulin levels in the circulation, so less estrogen is bound" and free estrogen goes up, says Calle. And that increases risk. Some specifics:

• **Breast.** The risk of postmenopausal breast cancer rises by 30 percent in overweight women and 50 percent in obese women.[11] For years, researchers couldn't detect the link because they didn't separate women who take estrogen pills from those who don't.

"Weight is not related to breast cancer in postmenopausal women who take hormones," says Calle. That's because the pills raise estrogen levels—and the risk of cancer—whether the women are skinny or plump.

"The sharp decline in the number of women taking postmenopausal hormones means that weight matters to an increasing segment of the population," she adds.

More than other cancers, postmenopausal breast cancer is related to how much weight you gain as an adult.[12] "That's in part because obesity may lower the risk of breast cancer in pre-menopausal women," says Calle.

Why? Obesity seems to impair their ability to ovulate. "So the woman with the highest risk was normal weight and had regular periods when she was young and became obese when she got older," Calle explains.

In a study of 44,000 postmenopausal women who weren't taking estrogen, those who gained 21 to 40 pounds after age 18 had a 68 percent higher risk of breast cancer that spread beyond the breast than those who gained 20 pounds or less. The risk was nearly double for those who gained 41 to 60 pounds and triple for those who gained more than 60 pounds.[13]

"Excess adiposity is an important contributor to breast cancer risk in postmenopausal women, especially for tumors that are most likely to spread," says Calle.

• **Uterus.** Cancer of the endometrium (the lining of the uterus) is twice as likely in overweight women and 3½ times more likely in obese than in normal-weight women.[1]

"That was the first cancer we recognized as related to obesity," says Calle. And it's clear why excess fat threatens the uterus. "We know that endometrial cancer is associated with estrogen that's unopposed by progestin."

Decades ago, researchers found that women who took estrogen pills had a higher risk of uterine cancer, but the risk disappeared in women who took estrogen combined with progestin.

Recently, researchers have detected a higher risk among women with central obesity. In a study of 223,000 European women, the risk of uterine cancer in those with at least a 35-inch waist was 76 percent higher than in those with a waist smaller than 32 inches.[14]

"Once you get to some level of obesity, you're going to have a certain amount of central adiposity no matter where you carry your weight," says Calle.

III. Local Impact

For some cancers, obesity seems to boost risk because it leads to problems in nearby tissues (rather than by altering circulating hormones). For example:

• **Esophagus.** Two distinct cancers show up in the esophagus. With a five-year survival rate of 16 percent, both are deadly.

But there are differences. The incidence of squamous cell carcinoma (which is common in alcoholics, who are often underweight) is flat or dropping, while rates of adenocarcinoma (which is common in the overweight) are on the upswing.

"The incidence of adenocarcinoma is going up more in men than in women and no one knows why," says Yale's Susan Taylor Mayne. Obesity may have more impact in men, she suggests.

At first, researchers thought that a wider girth led to esophageal cancer because it caused acid from the stomach to flow back into the esophagus, causing inflammation.

"Obesity may be acting to promote cancer in part via acid reflux, but it may also be acting independently," says Mayne.

"In our study, when we controlled for reflux, we still found a strong effect of obesity, so risk is not just driven through reflux."[15]

• **Gallbladder.** The gallbladder is a pear-shaped organ below the liver that collects and stores bile (a fluid made by the liver to digest fat). In about a quarter of all cases, gallbladder cancer is found early (usually when the organ is removed for other reasons), and the five-year survival rate is 80 percent.

But more often, the tumor is discovered too late to be surgically removed. If that happens, only 5 percent of patients live for two years.

While gallbladder cancer is rare, excess weight accounts for more than a third of all cases in the United States. How?

"Obesity is associated with gallbladder stones," explains Calle. "The stones provide a local inflammatory environment," which sets the stage for cancer.

Waist Not . . .

Extra padding *anywhere* seems to boost your risk of cancers of the breast, uterus, esophagus, gallbladder, and prostate. But other cancers—colon, liver, pancreatic, and kidney—are more closely linked to the visceral fat that's underneath your stomach muscles.

Unlike subcutaneous or retroperitoneal fat, which is less active, visceral fat is busy pumping out a slew of hormones—like leptin, adiponectin, and IGF (insulin-like growth factor)—that cause trouble.

"That's why central obesity is related to diabetes, heart disease, and cancer," says Dominique Michaud of the Harvard School of Public Health. "We wouldn't have all those complications if overweight people were just carrying extra weight around."

How do you know how much of your fat is visceral?

You can't tell without a CT-scan, MRI, or other imaging technique. But your waist circumference is a good proxy, because a big belly usually means rich deposits of both visceral and subcutaneous fat.

(When studies measure waist circumference or waist-to-hip ratio, they report on participants' "central obesity" or "abdominal obesity," rather than visceral fat.)

How to measure your waist circumference:

1. Place a tape measure around your bare abdomen just above your hip bone.
2. Be sure that the tape is snug, but does not compress your skin, and is parallel to the floor.
3. Relax, exhale, and measure.

Women with a waist bigger than 35 inches and men with a waist bigger than 40 inches have a higher risk of heart disease and diabetes. But for cancer, the cutoffs are less clear.

The question is: how can you keep fat away from your innards?

On one hand, genes seem to decide whether you end up with an apple or pear shape—with more weight around your middle or around your hips.

Hormones also play a role, since women tend to go up in waist size after menopause. But that doesn't mean you're helpless.

Here's what we know so far:

- **Don't fall for gimmicks.** Despite what you see in ads for weight-loss pills, potions, and gadgets, there is no way to target belly fat when you're losing weight. Sit-ups, crunches, and other exercises can strengthen abdominal muscles, but they don't melt belly fat any more than other fat deposits.

- **Count calories in *and* out.** Cutting calories coming in or boosting calories going out has the same impact. In a six-month study of 35 overweight men and women, there was no difference in visceral fat loss among people who cut calories by 25 percent or who cut calories by 12.5 percent *and* burned 12.5 percent more calories than usual.[1] Both lost about 10 percent of their weight and 27 percent of their visceral fat. Of course, exercise can also help lower the risk of heart disease, diabetes, and cancer, even if you don't lose weight.

- **Cut calorie-dense, nutrient-poor foods.** It's easier to slim down if you fill up on vegetables, fruit, and other foods that aren't calorie-dense. Limit calorie-dense fatty foods (especially if they're high in saturated and trans fats) and carbohydrates (especially sweets, white potatoes, and breads, cereals, rice, and pasta made with refined flour). And don't drink your calories, whether it's alcohol, soda, or juice.

- **Don't just sit there.** The more time you spend on the couch, in the car, or at the computer, the more fat you invite into your abdominal home.

In a study of 175 overweight, sedentary men and women, one group walked 12 miles a week (which took about 3 hours), a second group jogged 12 miles a week (2 hours), a third group jogged 20 miles a week (3 hours), and a fourth group stayed inactive.[2]

After six months, the 20-mile joggers had lost 7 percent of their visceral fat, while the 12-mile walkers and 12-mile joggers—who burned roughly the same calories—had lost no visceral fat. But the real surprise was the control group. In just six months of inactivity, their visceral fat jumped 9 percent. And in a recent rat study, inactivity made rats grow more fat cells.[3]

The bottom line: What matters is how many calories you burn when you exercise—whether it takes you 1 hour, 2 hours, or whatever—not whether it's high intensity (like jogging) or moderate intensity (like walking). But what matters most is that you get off your derriere.

So, for now, eat less and move more—all easier said than done, of course.

Notes

1. *J. Clin. Endocrinol. Metab.* 92: 865, 2007.
2. *J. Appl. Physiol.* 99: 1613, 2005.
3. *J. Appl. Physiol.* 102: 1341, 2007.

Uncertain Pathways

Researchers are still in the dark about how obesity may raise the risk of some cancers. For example:

• **Prostate.** Prostate cancer strikes one out of six men sometime in their lifetime. But only one in 34 dies of the disease.

Researchers saw no consistent link with weight until they separated men with local, less aggressive cancers from those with more aggressive or fatal cancers.[16]

"Obesity is associated only with the more aggressive prostate cancers," says Harvard's Edward Giovannucci. "So it's possible that obesity doesn't cause prostate cancer, but makes prostate cancer more likely to progress."

For example, when researchers followed more than 285,000 men from the National Institutes of Health-AARP Diet and Health Study for five years, the risk of dying of prostate cancer was 25 percent higher in those who were overweight than in those who were normal weight. And the risk was twice as high in the most obese men.[17]

Among the possible explanations: "Obesity may increase the blood supply to the tumor or increased growth factors like insulin could cause it to progress," suggests Giovannucci. "Or it's possible that not all prostate cancers are alike."

In other words, aggressive cancers may have a different cause than those that don't spread.

"It looks like there are at least two distinct types of prostate cancer," explains the National Cancer Institute's Michael Leitzmann.

"We can separate them according to the grade—how abnormal the cancer cells are—and according to the stage—whether they've spread beyond the prostate gland or not."

And obesity may promote only the aggressive (higher grade, higher stage) cancers. In fact, excess fat may protect against localized prostate cancers—those "you'll die with, not from," says Leitzmann.

Why? Higher levels of insulin, free IGF-1, and leptin (a hormone that's secreted by fat cells) are potential culprits.[7] So is testosterone.

"Heavy men have lower testosterone levels," explains Leitzmann. "We know that testosterone leads to the start of prostate cancer."

But testosterone also helps maintain the structure and function of the prostate cells, says Leitzmann. "So the cells are more likely to go awry if testosterone levels are low."

That's speculative, he adds. "But it's possible that high testosterone levels make you more likely to get the disease, but low testosterone levels make the disease worse once you get it."

Notes

1. *Nature Reviews 4*: 579, 2004.
2. *N. Engl. J. Med. 348*: 1625, 2003.
3. *Am. J. Epidemiol. 166*: 36, 2007.
4. *Ann. Intern. Med. 122*: 327, 1995.
5. *Endocrinol. 147*: 1830, 2006.
6. *Cancer Epidemiol. Biomarkers Prev. 14*: 459, 2005.
7. *Gastroenterol. 132*: 2208, 2007.
8. *Cancer Epidemiol. Biomarkers Prev. 15*: 879, 2006.
9. *Int. J. Cancer 118*: 728, 2006.
10. *Am. J. Epidemiol.* DOI: 10.1093/aje/kwm137.
11. *Am. J. Epidemiol. 152*: 514, 2000.
12. *JAMA 296*: 193, 2006.
13. *Cancer 107*: 12, 2006.
14. *Cancer Causes Control 18*: 399, 2007.
15. *J. Natl. Cancer Inst. 95*: 1404, 2003.
16. *Cancer Epidemiol. Biomarkers Prev. 15*: 1977, 2006.
17. *Cancer 109*: 675, 2007.

The World Is Fat

More people in the developing world are now overweight than hungry. How can the poorest countries fight obesity?

BARRY M. POPKIN

Over the past 20 years a dramatic transition has altered the diet and health of hundreds of millions of people across the Third World. For most developing nations, obesity has emerged as a more serious health threat than hunger. In countries such as Mexico, Egypt and South Africa, more than half the adults are either overweight (possessing a body mass index, or BMI, of 25 or higher) or obese (possessing a BMI of 30 or higher). In virtually all of Latin America and much of the Middle East and North Africa, at least one out of four adults is overweight. Although undernutrition and famine remain significant problems in sub-Saharan Africa and South Asia, even desperately poor countries such as Nigeria and Uganda are wrestling with the dilemma of obesity. Worldwide, more than 1.3 billion people are overweight, whereas only about 800 million are underweight—and these statistics are diverging rapidly.

The obesity rates in many developing countries now rival those in the U.S. and other high-income nations. What is more, the shift from undernutrition to overnutrition—often called the nutrition transition—has occurred in less than a generation. When I return to villages that I visited 15 years ago in India, China, Mexico and the Philippines, I see enormous changes: kids guzzle soft drinks and watch television, adults ride mopeds instead of walking and buy their food from supermarkets. In addition to adopting more sedentary lifestyles, people in the developing world are also consuming more caloric sweeteners, vegetable oils and animal-source foods (meat, poultry, fish, eggs and dairy products). The combination of lifestyle and dietary changes has paved the way for a public health catastrophe, with obesity leading to an explosive upsurge in diabetes, heart disease and other illnesses.

To combat this threat, we must look behind the vast social, economic and technological trends that are transforming the Third World. This examination reveals that many governments and industries are contributing to the growth in obesity by flooding developing countries with cheap sweeteners, oils and meat while doing nothing to promote the consumption of fruits and vegetables. Revamping agricultural subsidies and regulating food advertising may help alleviate the damage. But the effort will require new policy research, long-term funding commitments and a hefty amount of political will.

Brazil

Gross domestic product (GDP) per capita	$8,800
Percentage of adults who are overweight	20.0 (1975)
or obese	36.7 (1997)

Note. Supermarkets have proliferated across Brazil and other Latin American nations over the past two decades, leading to a large rise in the consumption of processed foods.

A Problem of the Poor

Mexico is perhaps the most striking example of a developing nation suffering from the obesity epidemic. In 1989 fewer than 10 percent of Mexicans were overweight. In fact, no one in the country even talked about obesity back then; the focus was on poverty and hunger. But national surveys conducted in 2006 found that 71 percent of Mexican women and 66 percent of Mexican men were overweight or obese—figures that approximate those in the U.S. And the health effects are already becoming apparent. Diabetes was almost nonexistent in Mexico 15 years ago, but today almost one seventh of the country's people suffer from type 2 (adult-onset) diabetes, and the disease is spreading quickly.

How could such a radical change have taken place in less than 20 years? Proximity to the U.S. may have exacerbated the problem—many Mexicans are exposed to American culture and media, which could have influenced their dietary or lifestyle choices—but obesity has also burgeoned in countries that have much less contact with the U.S. The migration of people from the countryside to the cities may have also played a role. Studies of more than 157,000 women in 39 developing nations have shown that in nearly all the countries, women in urban areas are more likely to be overweight than women in rural areas. (Researchers have collected more data for women than for men in these studies because their focus was on reproductive health.) But the prevalence of obesity has grown in rural regions, too; for example, in Mexico, Colombia, Turkey, South Africa and Jordan, more than half the rural women are overweight.

Obesity Spreads across the Globe

People who are overweight (possessing a body mass index, or BMI, of 25 or higher) or obese (a BMI of 30 or higher) are now just as common in many developing countries as they are in the U.S., Canada and Europe. In large parts of Latin America, North Africa and the Middle East, the problem has triggered an upsurge in diabetes, heart disease and other illnesses. Obesity rates are also rising quickly in China, India and other Asian nations.

Egypt

GDP per capita	$4,200
Percentage of adults who are overweight or obese	59.1 (1998)

Note. In Egypt the obesity problem is particularly severe for urban women. Poor Egyptians have adopted modern habits that exacerbate obesity, such as television watching.

A better explanation lies in the connection between obesity and poverty. In the developing world, obesity has become predominantly a problem of the poor, just as it is in the U.S. In all countries with a gross domestic product greater than $2,500 per capita—which includes most developing nations outside of sub-Saharan Africa—obesity rates are higher for poor women than for those with higher socioeconomic status. As average incomes in these countries have risen, farm laborers and the urban poor have adopted modern habits associated with obesity, such as watching television and shopping in supermarkets, but still do not have access to education, healthier foods or recreational activities that would help them control their weight.

Compounding the tragedy is the fact that obese people in the Third World may be more likely to develop diabetes or high blood pressure than obese individuals of European descent. Scientists have long hypothesized that Latin American, African and South Asian populations may carry a disproportionate number of "thrifty genes" that evolved to help them survive times of famine by enabling them to store fat more efficiently. Unfortunately, when a person with these genes becomes overweight, body fat tends to accumulate around the heart and liver, increasing the risk of diabetes and cardiovascular problems. In China, where obesity levels are climbing rapidly, nearly one third of the population suffers from high blood pressure. Moreover, I have found in my surveys that only a small fraction of Chinese with hypertension receive treatment for the condition. Whereas Western countries can afford to monitor and provide drugs for diabetic and hypertensive patients, the illnesses go mostly untreated in the developing world, and so health complications appear early on.

A Dietary Disaster

One of the biggest contributors to the obesity epidemic in the Third World is the recent popularity of sweetened beverages. For most of our evolutionary history, the only beverages humans consumed were breast milk after birth and water after weaning. Because water has no calories, the human body did not evolve to reduce food intake to compensate for beverage consumption. As a result, when people drink any beverage except water their total calorie consumption rises, because they usually continue to eat the same amount of food. Although humans have been drinking wine, beer, fruit juice and milk from domesticated animals for thousands of years, the proportion of calories coming from beverages has been relatively small until the past 50 years, when Coca-Cola, Pepsi and other soft drinks began spreading across the globe.

For physicists, a calorie is the amount of heat energy needed to raise the temperature of one gram of water by one degree Celsius. The calorie unit on a food packaging label, though, is equal to 1,000 heat-energy calories, so it is often called a kilocalorie, or kcal for short. Daily energy requirements vary depending on age, weight and activity levels, but most nutritionists recommend a range of 1,800 to 2,200 kcal for women and 2,000 to 2,500 kcal for men. When a person consumes a surplus of 3,500 kcal above his or her requirements, this extra amount will usually produce a weight gain of about 0.45 kilogram (one pound). Researchers estimate that putting sweeteners into beverages added about 137 kcal to the average American's daily diet between 1977 and 2006. Over a year this surplus can cause a weight gain of about 6.4 kilograms (14.2 pounds). In Third World countries, consumption of sweeteners is rapidly catching up to American levels; for example, the average Mexican now consumes more than 350 kcal from beverages every day.

The growing presence of supermarkets in the developing world has greatly increased the availability of both sweetened beverages and processed foods. In country after country, companies such as Wal-Mart, Carrefour and Ahold have opened giant stores offering a wide variety of cheap snacks and soft drinks. In Latin America the proportion of all food expenditures spent in supermarkets jumped from 15 percent in 1990 to 60 percent in 2000 and is still rising briskly. Scientists have not yet quantified the impact of replacing traditional village markets with megastores, but the few studies available suggest that the new way of shopping encourages the consumption of processed foods, particularly products with added sugar.

Another key contributor to obesity is the widespread shift to energy-dense foods that has occurred in many developing nations. The human body regulates appetite based on the volume of food consumed rather than the number of calories in a meal. This adaptation was useful in regions where large seasonal swings in rainfall and temperature affected food production; during the times of plenty, people could load up on calorie-rich meats and vegetable oils, building up their weight to survive subsequent periods of famine. In recent years, however, the consumption of energy-dense vegetable oils—soybean oil, palm oil, corn oil and dozens of variations—has skyrocketed in the developing world. In China, for example, the average daily intake of vegetable oils rose from 14.8 grams per person in 1989 to 35.1 grams per person in 2004, adding an extra 183 kcal to the population's daily diet. Similar increases have taken place in the Middle East, Africa, and parts of South and Southeast Asia. My research has shown that technological advances in the production and processing of oilseeds have made vegetable oil a relatively cheap option for poor families; in China, the poor spend a larger share of their food expenditures on vegetable oil than the rich do.

The third major change in the developing world's diet is the surge in consumption of animal-source foods. Over the past 20 years most of the growth in the world's production of meat, poultry, fish, eggs and milk has come from developing nations. Latin Americans are eating more beef, Chinese are devouring more pork and Indians are consuming more dairy products. In China the consumption of animal-source foods more than tripled in rural areas and almost quadrupled in urban areas between 1989 and 1997. By 2020 developing countries are expected to produce nearly two thirds of the world's meat and half its milk. In addition to raising obesity rates, the intake of all this energy-dense animal-source food threatens to boost the prevalence of heart disease in the Third World by injecting excessive saturated fat into the average diet.

People in the developing world are not only converting to the unhealthy Western diet; they are starting to work, travel and entertain themselves in ways that worsen that diet's effects. When I lived in Asia in the 1970s, only small quantities of electricity reached rural areas, roads were unpaved and farming was the only option for employment. What is more, farming in Asian countries was a backbreaking task: transplanting rice, weeding, hoeing, spreading fertilizer and harvesting were all done by hand. Difficult manual labor was also the norm for people living in the urban slums of Old Delhi in India, where I lived for a year.

The shift from undernutrition to overnutrition has occurred in less than a generation.

Today, however, the various components of modern infrastructure—roads, factories, media access, and so on—are reaching into even the remotest corners of the Third World. Many farmers in Asia and Latin America now use tractors to plow the soil and trucks to carry their produce to market. In China the portion of the population working in jobs with very light activity requirements has grown from 44 percent in 1989 to 66 percent in 2004. In 1989 few Chinese owned a television; today televisions are ubiquitous in the country, with more than half of households owning a color set. Because the shift to a more sedentary lifestyle decreases one's energy requirements, excess calories accumulate faster. In our studies in China, my colleagues and I have shown that all the observed lifestyle changes—increased television use, reduced walking and biking, and less strenuous labor at home and in the workplace—have led to significant gains in weight.

The Big Picture

The overarching trend that is encouraging all these changes in diet and lifestyle is globalization—the freer movement of capital, technology, goods and services across the world. For

Mexico

GDP per capita	$10,700
Percentage of adults who are overweight or obese	61.9 (2000)
	69.3 (2006)

Note. One of the biggest contributors to obesity in Mexico is the consumption of soft drinks. Almost one seventh of the country's people suffer from type 2 (adult-onset) diabetes.

example, the ability of huge retailers to open mega-stores in developing countries has brought all the health effects of modern food processing, both positive and negative, to new populations. Global media companies have enhanced the attraction of television by offering entertaining programs to regions that formerly received only boring government-produced broadcasts. Furthermore, international agencies such as the World Bank have promoted agricultural changes that have encouraged the proliferation of unhealthy diets in the developing world.

It may be difficult to gather support for a fight against obesity, which is still widely viewed as a sign of sloth and gluttony.

The long-held philosophy of agricultural experts is that once a country produces enough grains and tubers, it should massively subsidize its livestock, poultry and fish industries. The result has been a major reduction in the prices of animal-source foods. The wholesale price of beef (in real dollars) on the world market declined from about $530 per 100 kilograms in the early 1970s to about $150 per 100 kilograms in the mid-1990s. The drop in the cost of vegetable oils and animal-source foods, combined with the recent increases in personal incomes in China, India and other developing nations, has led to a consumer revolution. People are rapidly abandoning their traditional low-fat, high-fiber diets and switching to meals of calorie-rich fats, sweeteners and refined carbohydrates.

What can we do to counter such a sweeping and deadly transition? No country in modern times has succeeded in reducing the number of its citizens who are overweight or obese. In fact, the obesity epidemic is accelerating in the U.S. and many other nations. The world is getting fatter, and the annual rates of increase are higher today than they were 15 years ago.

Representatives of the food industry have long insisted that governments should not restrict an individual's dietary choices. Their solution is to teach people how to control their diets and become more physically active. Even most health professionals in the U.S. and abroad focus on the narrow, short-term need to educate children and their parents. But this strategy ignores the vast social, technological and structural changes that are pushing millions of people into debilitating lives of obesity. If left unchecked, the nutrition transition will cause horrendous increases in illness and devastating reductions in life expectancy.

In the developing world, most government and private aid programs still focus on fighting hunger and infectious diseases.

China

GDP per capita	$7,700
Percentage of adults who are overweight or obese	12.9 (1991)
	27.3 (2004)

Note. The booming Chinese economy has increased average incomes, enabling the country's people to boost their intake of calorie-rich foods while shifting to a more sedentary lifestyle.

These efforts can backfire, though; national hunger programs in Mexico and Chile may have increased obesity levels among some recipients of their food aid. For example, the Mexican program called Oportunidades (formerly named PROGRESA) has improved the growth rates of children in the families it has enrolled but has also exacerbated obesity among the urban women receiving its cash payments and food supplements. In response, the managers of the program are now considering halting the distribution of fortified milk to adult women and providing vitamin supplements instead.

It may be difficult for politicians or development officials to gather support for a fight against obesity, which is still widely viewed as a sign of sloth and gluttony rather than as a consequence of global changes. Nevertheless, this new threat demands action. Nongovernmental organizations such as the Bill & Melinda Gates Foundation, which strives to improve public health and reduce poverty around the world, must address the obesity epidemic before it is too late. Unless strong preventive policies are undertaken, the medical costs of illnesses caused by obesity could bring down the economies of China, India and many other developing countries. China already spends more than 6 percent of its gross domestic product on nutrition-related chronic diseases, and this expense is projected to increase steeply over the next 20 years.

Government interventions will also be necessary. We could begin by restructuring the massive agricultural subsidies that encourage the production of meat, poultry and dairy products. Instead of giving billions of dollars to giant agribusinesses growing grain for livestock, the U.S. and other high-income nations could direct some of that money to farmers cultivating fruits and vegetables. This reform could help people in developing countries by adjusting prices on the world market. Making meat more expensive and vegetables cheaper would provide an incentive for healthier food choices. New farm policies should also promote the global consumption of whole grains, which have more fiber, vitamins and minerals than refined carbohydrates.

Revamping subsidies will not be as effective for discouraging the consumption of sweetened foods and beverages, because the cost of sweeteners represents just a small fraction of the price of such products. An alternative might be to tax all caloric sweeteners (including sugar, high-fructose corn syrup and concentrated fruit juice) at a relatively high rate—say, a nickel per gram. In Mexico, which has one of the highest consumption rates of soft drinks in the Third World, I am working with the Ministry of Health to devise taxes on these and other high-calorie beverages. I am also working with the Chinese government on testing

AS THE PRICE OF VEGETABLE OILS HAS DROPPED IN CHINA . . .

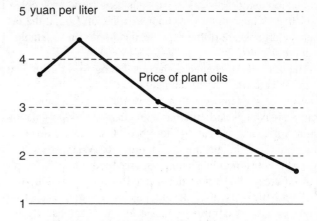

. . . THE COUNTRY'S CONSUMPTION OF THESE CALORIE-RICH FOODS HAS CLIMBED.

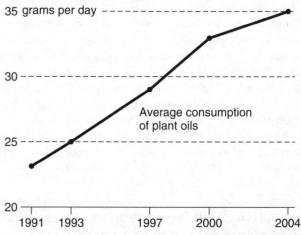

Falling prices for vegetable oils have fostered unhealthy diets in the Third World. In China, a steep drop in the prices of rapeseed, soybean and peanut oils has allowed even the poorest people to increase their intake of these calorie-rich foods.

a tax on vegetable oil in selected provinces. We have found that taxing dietary fat can cut the total calorie intake while increasing protein consumption among the poor in China because they substitute healthier foods for the fats. The impact would be even more positive if the revenues from the tax were spent on encouraging better nutrition.

Researchers and development experts have proposed dozens of similar policies, but they must be designed to meet the specific needs of each country. One particularly intriguing proposal is to ban advertisements for sweetened foods and beverages from children's television or perhaps from all media. At the same time, we cannot forget that many people in developing nations still suffer from hunger. We must design aid programs that can meet the needs of the hungry without increasing obesity in those countries. Conversely, we must ensure that policies designed to fight obesity—such as reducing the consumption of vegetable oils and animal-source foods—do not hurt the undernourished.

Fortunately, some options for fighting overnutrition will be just as helpful for combating undernutrition. For example, the promotion of breastfeeding and the increased intake of fruits and vegetables would alleviate both conditions.

Stemming the tide of obesity in the Third World is a tall order. More policy research is needed to determine the best ways to influence dietary choices in developing countries. Ever since our species arose, we have strived for a tastier diet and a more sedentary way of life. Now we need to reverse those tendencies if we are to create a healthier world.

BARRY M. POPKIN is a professor of nutrition epidemiology at the University of North Carolina at Chapel Hill, where he directs the Interdisciplinary Center for Obesity. His research program includes large nationwide surveys that have tracked changes in diet, activity patterns and body composition in the U.S., China, Russia, the Philippines, Brazil and other countries. He chairs the Nutrition Transition Committee for the International Union for the Nutritional Sciences and has published more than 260 journal articles, as well as many books. In 1998 he was awarded the Society for International Nutrition Research's Kellogg Prize for International Nutrition.

UNIT 5
Health Claims

Unit Selections

31. **Miscommunicating Science,** Sylvia Rowe and Nick Alexander
32. **Shaping up the Dietary Supplement Industry,** Sharon Palmer
33. **Why People Use Vitamin and Mineral Supplements,** Elizabeth Sloan
34. **"Fountain of Youth" Fact and Fantasy,** *Tufts University Health & Nutrition Letter*
35. **Brain Food,** Linda Milo Ohr
36. **Phytosterols: Mother Nature's Cholesterol Fighters,** Jill Weisenberger
37. **The Benefits of Flax,** Consumer Reports on Health

Key Points to Consider

- How can consumers protect themselves from misinformation in the nutrition field?

- Compare the effect(s) of phytosterols versus lipid-lowering medications on heart disease.

- Make a list of the foods that you most commonly eat. Which foods are the health-promoting foods described in Elizabeth Sloan's article on supplements?

- Why do so many Americans take dietary supplements?

Student Website
www.mhhe.com/cls

Internet References

Federal Trade Commission (FTC): Diet, Health & Fitness
www.ftc.gov/bcp/menus/consumer/health.shtm
Food and Drug Administration (FDA)
www.fda.gov/default.htm
National Council against Health Fraud (NCAHF)
www.ncahf.org
QuackWatch
www.quackwatch.com

Technological advances in the twenty-first century have resulted in high-speed communicatin of scientific results and the possibility for miscommunication. Even if the scientific protocol, study, design, data collection, and analysis are impeccable, it is still possible to report the findings in a confusing and biased manner. According to an American Dietetic Association (ADA) survey, 90 percent of consumers polled get their nutrition information from television, magazines, and newspapers. Some Americans are so confused and overwhelmed by the controversies surrounding food and health that they have stopped paying attention to the contradictory claims reported by news media. The media very frequently misinterpret results, simplify them, and take them out of context. In addition, the media is too eager to publish sensational information and not solid science. Another source of confusion is the Internet—about 30 percent of Americans look for information on dietary supplements online.

The dietary supplement business is experiencing a huge transformation. Americans spend approximately $25 billion on alternative treatments. Antioxidant supplements are very popular among Americans, and even though they are available in our diet, many of us choose not to obtain them from food. Consumers, especially baby boomers, are opting for combination or condition-specific supplements. One of the articles in this unit reveals why the baby boomer generation is quickly buying up supplements for specific conditions and why members of generation Y are going for the nutrition and sports-performance type supplements. Additionally, there has been a recent interest in brain health owing the growing incidence of Alzheimer's and cognitive decline in old age. Because of this, there are several new products related to cognitive function on the market. One of the articles provides information on foods, food components, and other products that are thought to improve mental health. The FDA regulates supplements differently than other foods and drugs and has no recall authority over supplements. Thus, initiatives that better protect consumers from charlatans and potentially dangerous products are critical for public health. Recently, the food supplement industry and other organizations, such as the CSPI, are concentrating their efforts on making dietary supplements standardized, safe, and honestly labeled.

Functional foods—foods that may provide a health benefit beyond basic nutrition—constitute one of the fastest growing segments of the food industry, especially among the affluent aforementioned baby boomers. The U.S government has no regulatory category of functional foods at the present time, but has set prerequisites as to what may qualify as a health and structure–function claim. Phytosterols have been documented

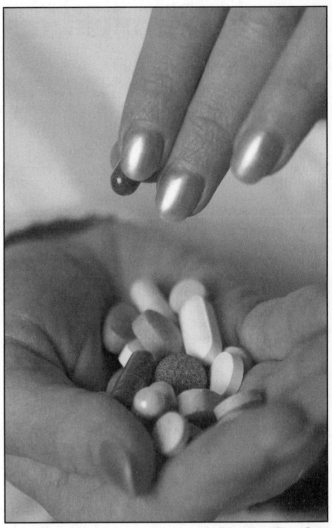

to lower low-density lipoprotein cholesterol and are as effective, safer, and cheaper than medications to lower blood lipids. New food products with added phytosterols are revolutionizing the market and our outlook for disease treatment. Flaxmeal, flaxseeds, and flaxoil are all products derived from flax, which has been reported to lower heart disease risk, reduce inflammation, diabetes, depression, and anxiety among other health benefits. Consumers are increasingly interested in purchasing and using flax for its health-promoting properties.

Miscommunicating Science

This article explores the rapidly evolving nature of communications from the perspective of the food or nutrition scientist who wishes not to miscommunicate; tongue-in-cheek tips are offered to scientists who are not afraid to mislead or misinform the public and hinder public understanding of their work. Analysis is offered of the chief causes of miscommunication and public misunderstanding of science.

SYLVIA ROWE, MA AND NICK ALEXANDER, BA

What follows can be considered a kind of primer on how to tell it wrong—how to take a scientific project, worthy or not worthy, and communicate it so that (1) few people can be expected to understand the project, (2) few people can be expected to care about the project, or (3) best yet, different people will draw entirely different conclusions from the project, and (4) in any event, most people will fail to understand the truth that the science has revealed. That would be called *miscommunication,* and if you wish to be sure that you know how to communicate, you must also know how to miscommunicate and understand the potential for misunderstanding.

> **If you wish to be sure that you know how to communicate, you must also know how to miscommunicate.**

A Brief History

In the beginning, there was the spoken word. Presumably, communication was first conducted through grunts and other noises, then later, through symbolic sounds, sounds that stood for concepts and objects. Not all of this, of course, was science communication—much of it was gossip, threats, warnings, emotional utterances, and the like. However, those early human noises devoted to information gathering and the quest for new ideas were certainly the first efforts at science communication. In those prehistoric times, there must have been a great deal of misunderstanding, of miscommunication.

The evolution of transmitting science information, new discoveries, new thoughts about the world, and the nature of things can be looked at as a kind of refining process toward common understanding. Western science is a process of group think, a communal effort at discovering physical truth, and, clearly, that process is enhanced through clear communication. Therefore,

scientists developed a specialized language to express precision and reduce the chances for misunderstanding and miscommunication.

There must have been all sorts of barriers to communication in the beginning: language difficulties (amplified enormously with the multitude of spoken dialects around the world) and time and space difficulties (messengers and minstrels had to carry information from place to place and formal meetings had to be scheduled months and years in advance to allow for travel time). For formal disciplines such as science, protocols had yet to be developed to specify the ground rules for transparency, experimental design, replicability, and the other requisites of scientific process.

Then came the written word, far more permanent than the spoken word and susceptible to scientific dispute resolution—papers could be drafted and circulated, albeit inefficiently, through crude and uncertain delivery systems. Then came the journals—the earliest journal in English was published by The Royal Society of London in the mid 17th century, a good 250 years after Gutenberg's famous improvement of mechanical publishing.[1] Newspapers and a formalized journalistic structure helped to disseminate scientific discoveries and theories and popularize them.

Subsequent 19th-century revolutions in transportation, communication, and electronics technology have expanded science and other forms of communication exponentially. However, the explosion of technological innovation in the 20th (and, so far, the 21st) century has dwarfed all previous progress in communication. What this means is that communication potential for science is now an order of magnitude greater than ever before, but the potential for miscommunication is equally great.

Miscommunication: A Definition

Merriam-Webster's online dictionary defines *communication* as "a process by which information is exchanged between individuals through a common system of symbols, signs, or behavior."[2] It follows that *miscommunication* is "a process by which information is *not* exchanged . . ." or, better yet, "a process by which information is exchanged in a faulty, incomplete, or incorrect way, resulting in a failure to understand on the part of the communication recipient." *Miscommunication* can also mean "a process by which incorrect information is communicated, perhaps a series of faulty research conclusions or findings that rest on a faulty research design, data collection process, or other research failure." If the recipient of the information misunderstands the truths purportedly being communicated, then the communication must be faulted.

Guidelines for communicating science have focused not only on communication practices themselves but also on strategies to avoid public misunderstanding of the supposed truths being communicated. The question that needs to be asked is not so much about the actual act of communicating the science, but rather, do the public audiences appropriately understand the scientific truths being communicated?

A number of good guidelines exist for best practices in communicating—that is, how to not miscommunicate. *Improving Public Understanding—Guidelines for Communicating Emerging Science on Nutrition, Food Safety, and Health*[3] from the International Food Information Council Foundation, for one, sets down some basic rules for ensuring that research results are understood, suggesting that scientists do a good deal of explaining when communicating their science: laying out, for example, all details of the study including the purpose, hypothesis, type and number of subjects, research design, methods of data collection and analysis, and the primary findings but also suggesting a kind of self-analysis somewhere in the written report analyzing the propriety of the methods of inquiry employed as well as any shortcomings or limitations of the research, including methods of data collection. We would like to focus on a key point in the guidelines not generally highlighted when science communication is discussed: *how consistent the study's findings are with the original purpose of the data collection.*

At a government-sponsored conference for science communicators several years ago, participants concluded that the simple skills of the past are no longer sufficient to communicate with contemporary audiences: "Today's science and technology communicators need a much broader array of skills. They need to understand both the technologies and the aesthetics of multimedia, interactivity, and the Web."[4] In this article, we would like to focus on 2 key points raised at the conference—points not normally highlighted in communication guidelines.

It is vital to tailor communications to specific audience and remember the needs of the audience, not the needs of the researchers.

- There is no such thing as a "general audience" for science and technology communication; rather, there are many people with many different uses for science and technology information and many different levels of understanding. Communication programs should be designed to address and serve the needs of each group; there is no "one-size-fits-all" message or method of communication.
- Science and technology communication programs should be directed to addressing an audience's needs and interests, not by the research enterprise's ideas about what the public "should know."

A picture of how to best miscommunicate science is emerging: even if scientific protocol is followed, the study design is strong, the data collection is sound and sufficient, analysis is transparent, and so forth, it is still possible to transmit the findings in such a way that the public will fail to understand the truth.

Formula for Misunderstanding

- Operate from a preconceived idea of conclusions you want out of the research—forget about having a specific purpose for the formal data collection; you can see what pops up later in support of your preconception.
- Do not worry about targeting any specific audience for the research findings—the most famous scientific projects are the ones that seem earth shattering and universally applicable.
- Proceed with projects that have your desires and needs in mind (future research funding, book and television appearance potential, etc) rather than any public need—let congress take care of public needs.
- In running the final analyses of your data, disregard any and all discrepancies that militate against your preconceived conclusions and cover yourself by including language disclaiming inaccuracies or apparent public policy implications of your work so that your work will appear above board.

You get the idea—this is just a short list of how miscommunication can erode good work or make less honest work seem credible.

It is possible to do unassailable research yet communicate it so inadequately that the public misses all the important points.

In fact, there is an inextricable association between how science is conducted and how it is communicated; is it possible to execute absolutely shoddy research yet communicate it perfectly so as to improve public understanding of the underlying truth? We think not. However, it is possible to do unassailable research yet communicate it so inadequately that the public misses all the important points. Most of us know of cases when the scientific community, in its zeal for creating correct protocol, may have forgotten to allow for communication to the public. Consider the following: there are formulas for submitting research papers; there is peer review to provide scientific feedback and appropriate editorial control; there are rules to safeguard ownership of intellectual discovery and rules to protect publishing rights. Yet, there is nothing in the protocols to guarantee public understanding in terms of the way we live, of emerging science.

Too often, the communication of science amounts to a battleground of would-be public policy advocacy, instead of public understanding. This, too, amounts to miscommunication, and what are the forces that promote miscommunication?

- sheer numbers
- sheer speed of transmission
- sheer velocity of calculation
- sheer greed (or, to put it less crudely, heightened competition for ownership)

Let us break these categories down.

Sheer numbers: sheer numbers of scientists competing for attention,[5] numbers of Web sites,[6] numbers of scientific journals,[7] number of scientific conferences[8]—the proliferation of all of these puts mounting pressure on good communication.

Sheer speed of transmission: sheer speed of transmission of scientific information, both at the university level and among professional scientists and science societies—what used to take weeks or months to get around is now transmitted electronically in minutes or seconds, offering markedly less time to catch errors or edit thoughtfully.

Sheer velocity of calculation: the speed at which scientists can run trials, calculate results, generate data, and reach mathematical conclusions—to offer just a crude example, early computers in 1942 were able to perform roughly 40 operations per second; the latest supercomputers work at a speed better than 6 trillion times faster.[9] This improvement in calculation speed came in just 65 years; before the invention of computers, human calculations were somewhat slower. The speed at which scientific conclusions can be reached adds to the pressure of communicating those results adequately.

Heightened opportunities for ownership: heightened opportunities and heightened demands for ownership of both information and the practical applications that derive from the information are enormous and increasing, placing ever greater challenges on the public communication of that science.

The Uncertain Road Ahead

Furthermore, in this Internet era, there is a widespread belief that information is or should be free and freely accessible; there is no hierarchy as to the accuracy of the thousands or millions of informational Web sites; news reports spread word of scientific discovery nearly instantaneously and often uncritically; communication often takes on the appearance of a battle for

Internet eyeballs, nothing more. In other words, if you wish to miscommunicate your scientific research, it is now easier than it has ever been before.

In addition, that is not all—not just the communication of science but also the science itself is surely affected by the new speed, the new facility of research, calculation, and data analysis, as well communications. It is not necessary to dream up hypotheses to test when computer programs can be written to order up analysis of already available data and generate likely associations from which hypotheses can be inferred. The whole scientific process can now be stood on its ear, so to speak, and modern-day researchers can work backward, from computer-generated analyses to the hypotheses that used to be necessary before designing a study and collecting data (in effect, putting the scientific cart before the horse).

We would argue that publicizing such work amounts to miscommunication of science—miscommunication by computer— because the public is misled into thinking that the conclusions are the result of the normal scientific process.

The preceding comments are intended not to judge or cast aspersion on the current state of science communications but rather to bring attention to an issue that is growing more troubling by the day. If public understanding of science and, more importantly, emerging nutrition and health science is the objective, then the scientific community may be at a crucial crossroad—there needs to be a clear understanding not only of the best ways to communicate science but also of the increasing complexity of science miscommunication.

References

1. Brief History of the Society. The Royal Society Web site, http://royalsociety.org/page.asp?id=2176. Accessed February 10, 2008.
2. Merriam Webster.com. Definition of *communication*. http://www.merriam-webster.com/dictionary/communication. Accessed February 10, 2008.
3. International Food Information Council (IFIC) Foundation. http://www.ific.org/publications/brochures/guidelinesbroch.cfm. Accessed February 10, 2008.
4. Communicating the future: best practices for communication of science and technology to the public [proceedings summary]; National Institute of Standards and Technology (NIST): Gaithersburg, MD; March 6–8, 2002. http://www.nist.gov/public_affairs/bestpractices/conf_summary.htm. Accessed February 12, 2008.
5. Science Departments [Google search] (each listed agency presumably employing multiple scientists). Retrieved 13,000,000 listings. http://www.google.com/search?hl=en&rls=RNWE%2CRNWE%3A2006-40%2CRNWE%3Aen&q=science+departments&btnG=Search. Accessed February 13, 2008.
6. Science Web sites [Google search]. Retrieved 45,300,000 listings. http://www.google.com/search?hl=en&rls=RNWE%2CRNWE%3A2006-40%2CRNWE%3Aen&q=science+web+sites&btnG=Search. Accessed February 13, 2008.
7. Scientific journals [Google search]. Retrieved 4,420,000 listings. http://www.google.com/search?hl=en&rls=RNWE%2CRNWE%3A2006-40%2CRNWE%3Aen&q=2008+scientific+journals&btnG=Search. Accessed February 13, 2008.

8. 2008 Scientific conferences [Google search]. Retrieved 56,600 listings. http://www.google.com/search?sourceid=navelient&ie=UTF-8&rls=RNWE,RNWE:2006-40,RNWE:en&q=2008+scientific+conferences. Accessed February 13, 2008.

9. Wikipedia. Definition of *supercomputer.* http://en.wikipedia.org/wiki/Supercomputer. Accessed February 13, 2008.

SYLVIA ROWE, MA, is an adjunct professor at Tufts Friedman School of Nutrition Science and Policy and at the University of Massachusetts Amherst. She is also the president of SR Strategy, a health, nutrition, food safety, and risk communications and issue management consultancy located at Washington, DC. Previously, Ms Rowe served as president and chief executive officer of the IFIC and IFIC Foundation, nonprofit organizations that communicate science-based information of food safety and nutrition issues to health professionals, journalists, government officials, educators, and consumers. NICK ALEXANDER, BA, is former senior media counselor for the International Food Information Council Foundation, Washington, DC. He holds a Bachelor of Arts degree from Harvard University. A former network correspondent with ABC News, Mr Alexander has been, for the past 7½ years, tracking and writing about science communications issues and the evolving challenge to public acceptance of credible science.

Shaping up the Dietary Supplement Industry

With public safety at stake, some organizations are developing initiatives to better protect consumers from false claims and potentially dangerous products.

SHARON PALMER, RD

The dietary supplement industry seems to be a magnet for controversy. It's not uncommon to find your e-mail inbox flooded with spam on supplements claiming to enlarge choice body parts or spy best-selling diet books peddling an array of dietary supplements aimed at weight loss, antiaging, and beauty. What's a soul to do but cave in and pop a few pills? And this is just what people are doing. The Office of Dietary Supplements reports that in 2004, consumers spent $20.3 billion on dietary supplements.

Daniel Fabricant, PhD, vice president of scientific affairs at the Natural Products Association, says in defense of dietary supplements, "A smart buyer doesn't confuse the e-mail spammers making egregious claims with the legitimate dietary supplement industry [any] more than they would confuse the spammers claiming to give away cars with the legitimate automotive industry."

Sure, smart consumers could simply install a better spam protector to fend off spurious supplement e-mails or ignore ads promoting dubious products, but there will be a certain number of people suckered into wasting their cash on products with little scientific evidence to support them. And of greater concern is the potential for people to be harmed due to fraudulent supplements. When it comes to life-threatening diseases such as cancer, even one consumer who falls prey to a supplement suggesting that it cures cancer in lieu of traditional treatments such as chemotherapy and radiation is too many.

In a study published in *Family Medicine* in 2002, researchers from the Scripps Center for Integrative Medicine in La Jolla, Calif., conducted Internet searches using the linked terms *herb* and *cancer,* resulting in matches for each of the six primary search engines of between 11,730 and 58,605. Further cross matching with the three master search engines revealed that prevention, treatment, and cure were discussed at rates of 92%, 89%, and 58%, respectively. Researchers concluded that although the Dietary Supplement Health and Education Act of 1994 (DSHEA) was enacted to decrease unlawful claims of disease prevention, treatment, and cure, such claims on commercial Internet sites are prevalent.[1]

"The Internet has had a mixed effect on the supplement industry. It has allowed a lot of bad and misleading products to be promoted very effectively through spam e-mails or professional-looking Web sites. People tend to believe what they see and are trying products that don't have much evidence behind them," says Tod Cooperman, MD, president of ConsumerLab.com, a Web site that provides independent testing and reviews of dietary supplements.

The Upside of the Supplement Biz

In the midst of today's concern over questionable dietary supplements comes a wave of health professionals speaking out on behalf of supplements, reminding us that not all are created equally. Complementary nutrition is growing, with a number of studies being funded and published that address efficacy of various herbs and supplements.

Take omega-3 fatty acid supplements. Research has supported the heart-healthy benefits of omega-3 fatty acids in supplemental form, suggesting that it may not be possible to get adequate amounts of the omega-3 fatty acids docosahexaenoic acid (DHA) and eicosapentaenoic acid (EPA) necessary to effect health change in those with coronary heart disease through diet alone. In addition, some supplement manufacturers remove heavy metals and other contaminants from fish oil, which increases purity, potency, and safety of the product compared with dietary sources of DHA and EPA.[2] Even heart health guru Dean Ornish, MD, recommends omega-3 fatty acid supplements in his Lifestyle Program.

And let's not forget that good, old-fashioned multivitamin and mineral preparations fall under the dietary supplement category.

What dietitian hasn't recommended a standard multivitamin and mineral supplement for a patient with less than desirable nutrient intake? "We don't have a problem with vitamins and minerals in general, but they are lumped in with the herbal and other questionable products used in the United States," says Ilene Ringel Heller, senior staff attorney at the Center for Science in the Public Interest (CSPI).

The National Center for Complementary and Alternative Medicine (NCCAM) is busy funding studies on a number of supplements such as echinacea and glucosamine/chondroitin. The NCCAM's position is that there is scientific evidence for the effectiveness of some complementary and alternative medicine treatments, but for most, there are key questions yet to be answered through well-designed scientific studies, such as whether they are safe and work for the diseases or conditions for which they are used.

Consumer Perceptions Surrounding Supplements

Consumer attitudes are all over the place when it comes to dietary supplements, but one thing is for sure: people are using them. Fabricant reports that more than 70% of American consumers use dietary supplements and that these consumers are typically well-educated, both in general and about the products they're buying.

Douglas S. Kalman, PhD candidate, MS, RD, FACN, director of nutrition and applied clinical research at Miami Research Associates and chair of the Nutrition in Complementary Care Dietetic Practice Group (NCC-DPG), says, "Customers believe in the industry. A recent study found that 34% of consumers looking to lose weight first turn to a dietary supplement as their adjunct in the battle against obesity."

But consumers are also confused. According to a recent national survey, American adults believe weight-loss supplements are safer and more effective than they really are. More than 60% of 1,444 telephone respondents in the survey, all of whom had made significant efforts to lose weight, said weight-loss supplements have been tested and proven safe and effective. More than one half stated that these supplements are approved by the FDA.[3]

"Things are really out of control," says Heller, who reports that some customers don't notice the FDA disclaimer required on dietary supplements (stating that the FDA has not reviewed the statements made) and interpret it as an FDA approval for the product. Other consumers band together in groups such as Save Our Supplements to rail against further regulation of the dietary supplement industry.

"Over the last five years, it seems that consumers have become more interested in information about dietary supplements as opposed to taking promotional material at face value. It seems that more people are realizing that this industry is not well-regulated by the government, although many still think supplements are as well-regulated as prescription medications and over-the-counter medicines," says Cooperman.

The Regulatory Backdrop for Dietary Supplements

So how did an environment evolve that allowed dubious supplements such as breast enhancers to flourish? Flash back to the enactment of DSHEA in 1994. Dietary supplements were defined as products intended to supplement the diet; containing one or more dietary ingredients (including vitamins, minerals, herbs or other botanicals, amino acids, and other substances) or their constituents; intended to be taken by mouth as a pill, capsule, tablet, or liquid; and labeled on the front panel as being a dietary supplement.[4]

Dietary supplements are regulated by the FDA but differently than other foods and drugs. A dietary supplement cannot claim on its label that it will diagnose, cure, mitigate, treat, or prevent a disease. The label of a dietary supplement may contain one of three types of claims: a health claim, nutrient content claim, or structure/function claim. Health claims describe a relationship between a food, food component, or dietary supplement ingredient and reducing risk of a disease or health-related condition. Nutrient content claims talk about the relative amount of a nutrient or dietary substance in a product. And structure/function claims are statements about how a product may affect the organs or systems of the body without mentioning a specific disease. The latter claims do not require FDA approval, but the manufacturer must provide the FDA with the text of the claim within 30 days of putting the product on the market. Product labels containing such claims must also include a disclaimer that reads, "This statement has not been evaluated by the FDA. This product is not intended to diagnose, treat, cure, or prevent any disease." The label of a dietary supplement product is required to be truthful and not misleading. If the label does not meet this requirement, the FDA may remove the product from the marketplace or take other action.[4]

Supplement ingredients sold in the United States before October 15, 1994, are not required to be reviewed by the FDA for their safety before they are marketed because they are presumed to be safe based on their history of use. For a new dietary ingredient (not sold as a dietary supplement before 1994), the manufacturer must notify the FDA of its intent to market a dietary supplement containing the new dietary ingredient and provide reasonable evidence for safe human use of the product.[4]

Dietary supplement makers do not have to provide the FDA with evidence that dietary supplements are effective or safe. Once a dietary supplement is marketed, the FDA has to prove that the product is not safe to restrict its use or remove it from the market. The quality control of dietary supplements depends on the manufacturer, supplier, and production process.[4]

A Whole Batch of Problems

"There are lots of problems with dietary supplements. There are no regulations that dictate appropriate serving recommendations. There is no organized collection of adverse events so that safety problems can be spotted early," says Cooperman. "The area that we focus most on is product quality. We are seeing one fourth of the products that we select for testing to have a quality problem. We find products with none or little of their claimed ingredients, products contaminated with lead or pesticides, [and] tablets that won't break apart to release their ingredients. Many products don't even specify a dose that is known to work." Cooperman gives an example of zinc lozenges for colds. Three fourths of the products that ConsumerLab.com tested did not have or suggest the amount of zinc that has been shown to be effective.

So what happens to all the products that don't contain what they are supposed to contain? Cooperman reports, "It is very rare that a manufacturer recalls a supplement, even after a report comes out on a product. The retailer is not required to recall the supplement. Only when people are really being hurt does [the] FDA take serious action against a manufacturer."

Heller agrees: "[The] FDA does not have recall authority over supplements. If there are fly-by-night supplements being made, they are not going to get off the market or off of shelves." Heller also believes the structure/function claims allowed on dietary supplements are close to disease claims and that many dietary ingredients in supplements on the market are grandfathered in, so there's a presumption of safety rather than the actual determination of safety.

Protecting Consumers

A movement is growing aimed at better protecting consumers. One leader of the pack is Sen Richard J. Durbin (D-Ill.), who introduced legislation to require dietary supplement manufacturers to ensure their products are safe before they are sold.

"Sen Durbin has orchestrated the adverse effects reporting legislature," says Heller, who reports that this legislature would obligate dietary supplement manufacturers to report adverse effects. "This goes back to the ephedra case in which there were about 16,000 adverse effects, but the manufacturers had no obligation to turn them over to [the] FDA. One percent of all adverse events are reported to [the] FDA under the current voluntary system," adds Heller. Dietary supplements containing ephedra have been banned in the United States since April 2004.

Edward Blonz, PhD, FACN, FNAASO, a newspaper nutrition columnist and author, has also taken up the cause. Blonz reports, "I now have three cases with the Federal Trade Commission [FTC], and I work for a group of 11 DAs [district attorneys] in California. All these efforts involve issues of questionable advertising claims being made for dietary supplements." Blonz also teaches a class at the University of California, Berkeley titled "Dietary Supplements: What Every Health Professional Needs to Know" and is seeking funding for a stand-alone non-profit organization that will aim to analyze dietary supplement advertising claims to provide information about products and their associated claims to consumers.

CSPI has worked extensively on making dietary supplements safe and honestly labeled. Quackwatch, Inc. is a non-profit corporation whose purpose is to combat health-related frauds, myths, fads, fallacies, and misconduct that often involve dietary supplements. Founded by Stephen Barrett, MD, in 1996, Quackwatch, Inc. works to investigate questionable claims,

advise quackery victims, report illegal marketing, and attack misleading advertising on the Internet. ConsumerLab.com includes review articles on various supplements to help educate consumers and healthcare professionals. Many NCC-DPG members work on forwarding progress in manufacturing practices, clinical research, and open communication with the FTC, the FDA, and other agencies. Numerous credible Web sites offer scientific information on herbs and supplements.

Tired of suffering a tarnished reputation at the hands of shady supplement makers, those in the dietary supplement industry are also banding together to clean up the industry. "The supplement industry has had bad press in recent years. Some of the industry supports adverse event reporting as a way of repairing that image," says Heller. The Natural Products Association, along with several other dietary supplement organizations and consumer groups, is supporting legislation in both the House and Senate that would require the reporting of serious adverse experiences for dietary supplements and over-the-counter drugs. (The Senate recently passed this legislation.) Kalman, who performs clinical trials for the food and supplement industry, also finds more and more companies working on independent research for supplements.

The American Herbal Products Association, the Consumer Healthcare Products Association, the Council for Responsible Nutrition, and the Natural Products Association recently announced a voluntary industrywide protocol, Standardized Information of Dietary Ingredients, to facilitate the exchange of information between ingredient suppliers and finished product manufacturers to help identify and qualify supplement ingredients from trustworthy sources.

Good Manufacturing Practices

One action eagerly awaited is Good Manufacturing Practices (GMP) for supplements. The FDA is authorized to create GMP regulations describing conditions under which dietary supplements must be prepared, packed, and stored. The FDA published a proposed rule in March 2003, but until this proposed rule is finalized, dietary supplements must comply with food GMPs that are primarily concerned with safety and sanitation rather than quality.

"It's been 12 years since they have been promised, and there are still no established GMPs for supplements. There is a lot of talk about them coming out this year, but they say that every year. If GMPs are approved, manufacturers will be required to make the products the same way from lot to lot. This would be a step in the right direction," says Cooperman. "To be even more meaningful, GMPs would include standards around what is supposed to be in the product. For example, what levels of specific plant chemicals should be in a product claiming to be gingko, garlic, or ginseng."

Fabricant reports that rather than waiting for the federal GMPs to be issued, his association developed its own GMP certification program in 1999. The Natural Products Association has certified nearly 60 companies and provided education for representatives from more than 350 dietary supplement companies. Their standard is used by other organizations as the basis of their dietary supplement GMP program. "GMPs mean understanding, analyzing, controlling, and documenting the manufacturing process. It is a third party audit system," says Fabricant.

Dietary Supplement Certification

Voluntary certification can offer supplement consumers some quality assurance. ConsumerLab.com, which offers a voluntary certification program, is finding more and more manufacturers interested in certification. They allow manufacturers and distributors to use specific "CL Seals" to identify products that have met ConsumerLab.com standards based on its product reviews.

NSF International, a public health and safety company, also developed an independent product evaluation program to address dietary supplements. Their voluntary testing and certification program verifies the identity and quantity of dietary ingredients listed on the product label; ensures the product does not contain undeclared ingredients or unacceptable levels of contaminants; and demonstrates conformance to currently recommended industry GMPs for dietary supplements.

Enforcement Action

"There is a little bit of action, a joint program between [the] FTC and FDA, to go after products on the Web," says Heller. "[The] FDA is increasing enforcement on dietary supplements, but it's not at the level it should be."

The FTC and FDA work together against fighting dietary supplement fraud. The FDA has primary responsibility for claims on product labeling and the FTC has primary authority over advertising claims. The FDA can identify fraudulent products through market surveys, inspections, Internet searches, adverse event reports, consumer complaints, informants, and referrals from other government agencies. The highest priority for the FDA are products that pose direct health hazards to consumers. When a problem arises with a supplement, the FDA can act by working with the product's marketer to correct the problem voluntarily. If that doesn't work, the FDA may bring a lawsuit to seize the product and enjoin the firm marketing it. The FDA can also seek criminal penalties against parties breaking the law.

Although it may seem like a drop in the bucket, many examples do exist in which the FDA and FTC went after supplement makers that broke the law. Recently, it made news when the FDA and FTC sent warning letters to dozens of U.S.- and foreign-owned Web sites selling or advertising dietary supplements that claimed to cure, treat, or prevent diabetes. These were discovered through an Internet sweep for fraudulent sites and products.

Finding a Safe Place for Complementary Nutrition

While fraudulent dietary supplements may sully the industry's reputation, it's important for dietitians to be objective and equip themselves with knowledge to better guide their patients. After all, many of your patients are probably taking supplements, whether or not they tell you. Numerous reputable sources of information on dietary supplements are available to guide your patients to making safe choices.

"Our goal is to educate dietitians about complementary nutrition. Some of our members have written articles in *USA Today*. There is good, solid information out there," says Kalman. "Unfortunately, a lot of dietitians' quest for information is limited to what they are exposed to. They are unaware of academic, NIH [National Institutes of Health]-approved nutrition education on complementary nutrition."

In today's world of healthcare, there is room for both traditional and alternative therapies. For cancer patients visiting the Duke Center for Integrative Medicine in North Carolina, the health team may recommend specific vitamins, Chinese herbs, and acupuncture in addition to chemotherapy. The healthcare team takes into consideration the whole person, including support systems, spiritual practices, and stress reduction in an effort to help patients better tolerate chemotherapy.

Integrating complementary and alternative therapies seems to be the wave of the future. Perhaps dietitians can help their patients wade through the sea of supplements to find the true treasures.

References

1. Bonakdar RA. Herbal cancer cures on the Web: Noncompliance with The Dietary Supplement Health and Education Act. *Fam Med.* 2002;34(7):522–527.
2. Kris-Etherton PM, Harris WS, Appel W, et al. AHA Scientific Statement: Fish Consumption, Fish Oil, Omega-3 Fatty Acids, and Cardiovascular Disease. *Circulation.* 2002;106:2747.
3. Americans Fall Prey to Weight-Loss Supplement 'Hype.' *HealthDay.* October 27, 2006. Available at: http://www.nlm.nih.gov/medlineplus/news/fullstory_40638.html
4. Dietary Supplement Health and Education Act of 1994. FDA, Center for Food Safety and Applied Nutrition, December 1, 1995. Available at: http://www.fda.gov/opacom/laws/dshea.html#sec3

SHARON PALMER, RD, is a contributing editor at *Today's Dietitian* and a freelance food and nutrition writer in southern California.

Why People Use Vitamin and Mineral Supplements

Motivations for dietary supplement use and current trends in the market for vitamin and mineral supplements are described.

ELIZABETH SLOAN, PhD

Although levels of vitamin and mineral supplement use are similar to what they were 6 years ago in similar surveys, use of condition specific supplements more than doubled between 1999 and 2005, up to 49% in 2005.[1] The increasing use of condition-specific supplements reflects 2 trends. First, consumers are switching from single-nutrient supplements to treat and prevent health issues to combination and condition-specific formulas. They see this as a way of taking an easier and less costly route toward one-stop shopping for health. Second, Americans are more confident of their ability to take care of their own health and are looking to dietary supplements as a way to manage and treat specific health issues.

Over the past 5 years, prevention of specific health issues and medical conditions has become the number one reason why 57% of consumers took a vitamin-mineral supplement for the first time: 37% did so for enhancing performance or energy, and 35% did so for treatment.[1] Only 16% of Americans were satisfied with their energy level.[1]

Condition-specific supplements for a specific disease or condition are increasingly popular.

Improving physical performance is particularly important as a motivator for initiating vitamin and mineral supplement use among young people. In fact, the number one reason that the 43 million Generation Y adults—aged 18 to 29 years—go on a vitamin-mineral regimen or make a dietary change is to enhance performance; weight control is the second reason.[2] With the 29 million younger Generation Y members aged 12 to 18 years, who are still heavily influenced by their older siblings' behaviors, this motivational factor will become even more prevalent.

Belief in vitamin-mineral supplements as an effective means of treating and preventing health problems and conditions has shown steady growth over the past 3 years. Almost three-quarters (74%) of consumers believe that vitamins and minerals are effective in the prevention of certain health conditions, up 6% from 2003 to 2005. Some 69% of consumers use them for the treatment of specific health conditions.[1]

Concerns about vitamin-mineral supplements are growing. About 2 (43%) of 5 users are concerned about interactions with their prescription medications. One (21%) in 5 users is dissatisfied with the quantity of pills taken, up by 4% in the past 2 years. About 1 (18%) in 5 has difficulty swallowing pills, up by 11%.[1]

In total, vitamins represented a $7.1-billion market in 2005, or 34% of the $20.9 billion US supplement market.[3] Multivitamins accounted for 58% of sales in 2005, increasing in share as sales of single vitamins—especially vitamins E and C—have dropped since 2000. For example, vitamin E sales fell from $860 million in 1999 to $440 million in 2005. Multivitamin sales have continued to grow, albeit at fairly modest annual rates of 3% to 6% from 1999 to 2004.

Lastly, consumers still take vitamin-mineral supplements because they believe that their diets lack vitamins and minerals. Just over half (56%) name nutrients that they believe are missing from their diet: a vitamin (52%), a mineral (about one third), antioxidants, fiber, and calcium (Table 1).[4] Calcium and Vitamin C are the most frequently taken vitamin supplements (Figure 1). Phytochemicals are increasingly being mentioned as nutritional substances missing from the diet.

Condition-Specific Supplements

Of the 44% who used a condition-specific supplement in 2005, joint pain was the most frequently mentioned condition (24%), followed by heart health, osteoporosis, and arthritis—all at 18%.[1] Use of vitamins and mineral supplements for osteoporosis and memory concentration is also on the rise.

Table 1 Nutrients That Consumers (56%) Believe Are Missing from Their Diet

	2005
Vitamins	52%
Minerals (Net)	34%
Antioxidants (Net)	28%
Dietary Fiber	26%
Calcium	22%
Carotenoids	20%
B-vitamins	18%
Vitamin C	17%
Iron	17%
Fish oil/omega-3	12%
Potassium	12%
Vitamin E	11%
B-complex	10%
Vitamin D	8%
Folic Acid	8%
Zinc	7%
Beta Carotene	7%
Vitamin A	6%
Niacin	4%
Magnesium	4%
Vitamin K	4%
Lutein	3%
Lycopene	3%
Polyphenol	2%
Flavonoids	1%

Reprinted with permission from Multi-sponsor Surveys, Inc.[4]

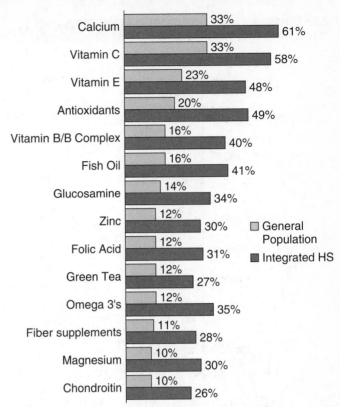

Figure 1 Type of supplements used in addition to multi-vitamin for general population versus heavy users (Integrated H.S.).[1]

Condition-specific supplements are the fastest growing sector of the supplement business. In 2005, 44% of all US supplements sold emphasized a specific health condition.[5] The 14 conditions listed in Table 3 account for 84% of condition-specific supplement sales. Sports/Energy/Weight loss and general health supplements, which rank 1 and 2, respectively, account for almost half of sales. Sales growth of gut health, heart, and anticancer supplements were significantly higher than the condition-specific category overall.

Looking Ahead

With the 22 million members of Generation X group being a 30% smaller group than the 76 million Baby Boomers now aged 42 to 60 years and the 72 million Generation Y members, it is the latter groups who will be the audiences for supplement marketers to target—and they will draw further attention to condition-specific supplements. Those who are not currently using a supplement say they are most likely to do so to prevent/treat arthritis (Table 2).

By 2010, 98 million Americans will be 50 years and older.[6] The age bracket that has traditionally had the highest supplement

Table 2 Percentage of General Population Indicating That They Are Likely to Use Supplements in Both Preventing and Treating the Following Conditions

	Prevent	Treat
Arthritis/joint disease	68%	69%
Osteoporosis	65%	64%
Frequent cold and flu	63%	62%
Lack of energy	58%	56%
Menopausal issues	56%	58%
Memory/concentration problems	56%	56%
High blood pressure	48%	52%
Acid reflux/heartburn	47%	50%
Heart disease	48%	50%
Vision problems	46%	47%
High cholesterol	43%	49%
Intestinal irregularity	40%	43%
Obesity/overweight	35%	39%
Diabetes	34%	41%
Blood sugar imbalance	31%	37%

Reprinted with permission from Molyneaux, Copyright 2006, Natural Marketing Institute.

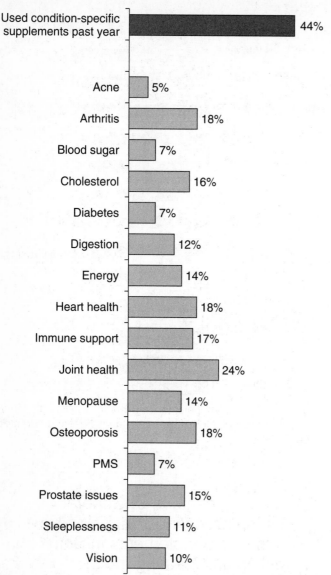

Figure 2 Conditions targeted by those taking condition-specific supplements (2005).

use, (those 50–64) is now being entered by the Boomers. With many Boomers experiencing age-associated conditions for the first time, they are likely to opt for supplements directed at conditions, including arthritis, cholesterol, wrinkles, eye health, acid reflux, and hypertension, whose incidence jumps dramatically among this age group (Table 4). They also will remain strong supporters of supplements directed toward enhancing energy, lessening stress, and controlling weight.[7]

One of the most high-potential new marketing practices is to cross-promote supplements and foods with sales of prescription medications for specific conditions. Information Resources, Inc, observed that 56% of consumers who fill a prescription at a supermarket, drug store, or mass merchandiser pharmacy also purchase related connector products while in the store.[8] For example, 1- and 2-letter vitamins, multivitamins, and minerals are among the items most frequently purchased with a heart-related prescription in a drugstore or grocery store.[7] Information Resources, Inc, estimates that cross-marketing heart-healthy

Table 3 US Sales of Condition-Specific Supplements: 2003–2005

	2003 Sales	2004 Sales	2005 Sales	2005 Growth	% of Total in 2005
Sports/Energy/ Weight Loss	5,760	5,664	5,683	0.3%	27%
General health	4,340	4,453	4,580	2.8%	22%
Joint health	1,097	1,105	1,138	3.0%	5%
Cold/Flu- Immune	957	996	1,028	3.2%	5%
Anticancer	858	926	1,006	8.6%	5%
Heart health	884	957	1,002	4.7%	5%
Bone health	1,022	980	972	−0.8%	5%
Gastrointestinal health	536	591	633	7.0%	3%
Diabetes	466	501	519	3.7%	2%
Menopause	297	289	273	−5.4%	1%
Brain mental	210	228	239	4.7%	1%
Mood	196	196	200	1.6%	1%
Sexual health	186	200	186	−6.9%	1%
Insomnia	105	112	117	3.8%	1%
Top conditions	16,915	17,199	17,575	2.2%	84%
Others	2,887	3,125	3,268	4.5%	16%
Total supplements	19,803	20,324	20,842	2.5%	100%

Reprinted with permission from the *Nutrition Business Journal*.[3] Copyright 2007, Penton Media, Inc.

Table 4 Health Conditions Reported by Consumers, by Age

Personally Affected by	All Shoppers	18–29 Years	30–39 Years	40–49 Years	50–64 Years	65+ Years
Tiredness/ lack of energy	45%	64%	53%	49%	39%	30%
Stress	42%	60%	52%	50%	37%	19%
Overweight for myself	36%	35%	41%	35%	41%	29%
Arthritis	31%	10%	15%	24%	39%	54%
High cholesterol	25%	7%	13%	18%	33%	42%
Wrinkles/ other signs of aging	25%	9%	20%	26%	30%	30%
Eye health	24%	23%	17%	21%	25%	31%
Acid reflux disease	24%	24%	18%	21%	28%	25%
Hypertension/ high blood pressure	23%	6%	10%	14%	30%	44%
Depression	22%	31%	23%	24%	22%	12%

Reprinted with permission from HealthFocus International.[7]

Table 5 Sales Projections for Prescription Centric Marketing by Category and Top Connector Products in Drug and Food Stores

US Ailments	Projected Prescription Scripts (in millions)	Frequency	Projected Dollars, Frontend Spending, Total US ($ billions)
Allergies/Asthma/Bronchitis	93	3.1	$44
Anxiety and Depression	61	3.6	$26
Arthritis	24	2.9	$14
Birth Control/Contraceptives	22	3.1	$13
Cholesterol (High)	39	3.1	$21
Diabetes	39	4.7	$14
Headaches and Migraine	16	3.1	$ 9
Heart Health	39	4.4	$15
Heartburn/Gastrointestinal/Reflux	36	2.9	$21
High Blood Pressure/Hypertension	98	4.4	$35
Infection (ear and UR)	39	1.5	$37
Menopause and Osteoporosis	30	3.3	$16
Pain Management, Muscular/Joint	71	2.8	$40
Skin conditions	23	2	$19
Total Heart	176	5.4	$71

Heart Condition "Connectors" in Food Stores		Heart Condition "Connectors" in Drugstores	
Nonprescription Products Purchased by "Heart Health" Consumers	**Index of Purchase**	**Nonprescription Products Purchased by** "Heart Health" Consumers	**Index of Purchase**
Mineral supplements	186	Low calorie soft drinks	205
Internal analgesic tablets	142	1- and 2-Letter vitamins	200
1- and 2-Letter vitamins	137	Internal analgesic tablets	192
Margarine/Spreads/Butter blends	118	Multivitamins	178
Antacid tablets	116	Mineral supplements	177
Low-calorie soft drinks	113	Antacid tablets	175
Skim/low fat milk	103	Skim/low fat milk	166

Reprinted with permission from Information Resources, Inc. (8).

products with prescriptions is a virtually untapped sales opportunity for supermarkets ($71 billion), with gastrointestinal reflux ($21 billion), menopause ($16 billion), diabetes ($14 billion), and arthritis ($14 billion) products (Table 5).

Vitamin and mineral supplement users will continue to keep pace with the incidence of chronic degenerative disease. Osteoporosis, heart disease, and cancer top the list of the fastest growing conditions afflicting women.[9] In men, from 2003 to 2013, heart disease is projected to increase by 24%; cancer, by 21%; prostate cancer, by 20%; and diabetes, by 20%.[9]

Generation Y, the children of the Baby Boomers, will be moving into the age range where they will be heavy users of sports nutrition products and supplements because of their keen interest in performance and weight control, sending sales of sports and weight loss supplements soaring. In 7 to 10 years, a critical mass of Generation Y reaches childbearing age, which, coupled with the growth of large family households among Hispanics, is expected to result in a baby boom that will dwarf the Baby Boomers and drive explosive sales of prenatal and infant supplements skyrocketing.

In the next few years, we will also see more lifestyle issues driving use, with increased vitamin-mineral supplementation. A Yankelovich study[10] found that 85% of Americans did not feel healthy at least 1 day during the past 30 days; 60% were kept from normal activity. Low energy affected 58%; colds, 49%; back-neck pain, 32%; depression, anxiety, or sadness, 28%; joint pain, 27%; and arthritis, 18%.

The proprietary TrendSense model of Sloan Trends, Inc, which has been used since 1993 to help predict the timing of nutrition trends and their potential magnitude and to differentiate fads from trends, indicates that bioavailability reached mass market status (commercialization) in 2003-2004. Bioavailability is going to be a strong factor in the supplement marketplace in future years.[11] As consumers embrace the concept of bioavailability, they will stimulate the production of supplements with greater absorbability. Based on similar TrendSense modeling, vitamin C, antioxidants, iron, phosphorus, vitamin D, omega-3, docosahexaenoic acid, and magnesium have strong potential as up-and-coming supplements.[11]

ACNielsen[12] projects that products that carry an antioxidant claim will enjoy double-digit growth in 2006 and be second only to the glycemic index among the next big blockbuster trends. Sales of antioxidants increased by 19% in 2006. From 2004 to 2005, ACNielsen's leading-edge Health Activist group spent more on antioxidants than any other health-related category. More important, 52% of their hard-to-attract Health Neglectors, whose support is also essential for a blockbuster trend, used more antioxidant foods than the year before.

As risk factors in children begin to rise, more than likely, many mothers will turn to supplements to help get their children back on the health track, opening yet another new set of issues in the years ahead. One in 8 children has more than 1 risk factor for heart disease, and 10% of teens have high cholesterol levels.[13] The incidence of high blood pressure has tripled in children during the past decade, and the American Academy of Pediatrics has urged physicians to begin monitoring blood pressure at age 3 years.[14] One million teens are afflicted with metabolic syndrome—multiple risk factors for health disease and type 2 diabetes—and 1 in 3 children born in 2000 is expected to become diabetic.[15] With 7 of 10 teenage boys and 9 of 10 girls not getting enough calcium and the American Academy of Pediatrics recommending that physicians monitor calcium nutriture at age 3 years, calcium is likely to be an even stronger nutritional issue in the future than it is today.[16]

Conclusion

Prevention of undesirable medical conditions and health issues is the top reason Americans opt to take a vitamin-mineral supplement, followed in rank order by a sense of feeling better and having more energy and treatment of a health issue or condition. To reach these goals, consumers are switching from single-nutrient supplements to combination and condition-specific formulae. Condition-specific supplements are the fastest growing segment of the US supplement business. Of the 44% who used a condition-specific supplement in 2005, joint pain was the most frequently targeted condition, followed by heart health, osteoporosis, and arthritis. Over the past 4 years, use of supplements for menopause enjoyed the largest growth in the likelihood of supplement use for prevention and treatment, followed by arthritis, osteoporosis, and enhancement of memory and concentration. Arthritis, osteoporosis, frequent cold or flu, lack of energy, and menopausal issues are the conditions most likely to be targeted for condition-specific supplements in the future. In the years to come, older Baby Boomers aged 50 to 64 years and Generation Y members aged 18 to 29 years will be prime targets because of demographics. Older Boomers are likely to opt for supplements specific to arthritis, cholesterol, wrinkles, eye health, acid reflux, and hypertension—conditions all increasing markedly after age 50 years. Generation Y members will drive a dramatic increase in the sports nutrition-performance

segment. Bioavailability; cross-marketing of supplements with prescription medications in grocery, drug, and mass merchandiser stores; lifestyle issues, including energy, stress, and depression-anxiety; and interest in specific nutrients, including antioxidants, vitamin D, omega-3, docosahexaenoic acid, iron, phosphorus, potassium, and magnesium, will boost vitamin and mineral sales.

References

1. Molyneaux M. *The 2005 Health & Wellness Trends Database*™. Harleysville, Pa: The Natural Marketing Institute; 2005.
2. Multi-Sponsor Surveys. *Gallup Study of Teen Eating Behaviors 2004*. Princeton, NJ: Multi-Sponsor Surveys, Inc.
3. Anonymous. Segment profile: vitamins & minerals. *Nutr Bus J.* 2006;XI(2):1, 3–11.
4. Multi-Sponsor Surveys. *Gallup Multi-sponsor Study of Nutrient Knowledge and Consumption 2005*. Princeton, NJ: Multi-Sponsor Surveys, Inc.
5. Anonymous. Condition-specific supplements. *Nutr Bus J.* 2006;XI(1):1, 3–13.
6. US Census Bureau. Data from U.S. Census Bureau. Economic and Statistics Administration. Washington, DC: US Department of Commerce. Available at: http://www.census.gov.
7. HealthFocus, International. *HealthFocus 2005 Trends Report*. St Petersburg, Fla: HealthFocus International.
8. Information Resources, Inc. *RI, Rx-Shopping Centric Retailing. Times & Trends*. Chicago IL: Information Resources Inc; November 2004.
9. Multi-Sponsor Surveys. *Gallup Focus Report 2004*. Princeton, NJ: Multi-Sponsor Surveys.
10. Yankelovich. *Preventative Healthcare and Wellness in America*. Chapel Hill, NC: Yankelovich; 2006.
11. Sloan Trends, Inc. *TrendSense Trend Report*. Escondido, Calif: Sloan Trends, Inc; 2006.
12. ACNielsen. ACNielsen unveils predictions for 2006 [press release]. January 30, 2006. Available at: http://us.acnielsen.com/news/20060130.shtml. Accessed March 6, 2006.
13. American Heart Association. *Heart Diseases and Stoke Statistics—2006 Update*. Dallas, Tex: American Heart Association; 2006.
14. American Academy of Pediatrics. Blood pressure screening should start by age 3, according to new guidelines [press release]. August 2, 2004. Available at: http://www.aap.org/advocacy/releases/augbloodpressure.htm. Accessed March 6, 2006.
15. Centers for Disease Control and Prevention. *Epidemiology of Type 1 and Type 2 Diabetes Mellitus Among North American Children and Adolescents. Diabetes Projects*. Atlanta, Ga: Centers for Disease Control and Prevention; 2006.
16. AAP. AAP updates guidelines for stronger bones [press release]. February 6, 2006. Available at: http://www.aap.org/pressroom/aappr-feb06mailing.htm. Accessed March 6, 2006.

ELIZABETH SLOAN, PhD, is President, Sloan Trends, INC., a food/nutrition trends consultancy and contributing editor, *Food Technology* magazine and *Functional Foods & Nutraceuticals*.

"Fountain of Youth" Fact and Fantasy

What you really need to know about antioxidants and your health.

Are antioxidants the new "fountain of youth"? Media reports and nutritional products promote the idea that these vitamins and nutrients can reduce or even reverse the damage caused to the body by "free radicals," combating chronic disease and the ravages of aging. In a new book, *Understanding the Antioxidant Controversy: Scrutinizing the Fountain of Youth* (Praeger, $49.95), Tufts scientist Paul E. Milbury, PhD, and co-author Alice C. Richer, RD, explore what science really does—and doesn't—know about the benefits of antioxidants. Milbury is a scientist at Tufts' Jean Mayer USDA Human Nutrition Research Center on Aging and an assistant professor at the Friedman School. Richer is a Registered/Licensed Dietitian in private practice at Spaulding Rehabilitation Hospital outpatient centers and a medical writer.

In this excerpt from their book, Milbury and Richer look at the bottom line on antioxidants and what the latest research findings mean to you and your health.

Research studies to date in vitro and in animals show consistent evidence supporting antioxidant health benefits, yet human trials have been disappointing. There is also recent evidence that suggests, under certain circumstances, supplementation may actually do more harm than good. Individual antioxidants in the form of dietary supplements are more potent and bioavailable than they are in foods, and they do not exhibit the **synergistic effects** with other compounds found within natural food sources. Therefore, supplements most likely do not possess all the physiologically active components needed to be truly effective in preventing disease incidence and progression. In addition, individual genetics and/or physical status may have as significant an effect on health as antioxidant nutrients do.

We saw in the early years of America that poor diets caused many nutrition-related, life-threatening and debilitating diseases. Food fortification programs, such as vitamin D and iodine, proved to be beneficial and improved public health by eradicating or preventing most associated illnesses. Today nutrition deficiencies are rare in America. Poor diet is usually the result of individual choice, lack of knowledge, extreme poverty, or illness. The average American has the opportunity to obtain his or her **daily nutrient needs from diet alone.** Nevertheless, many Americans do not achieve optimal levels of vitamin C and E and perhaps the flavonoids (see box, next page).

Possible decreased nutrient value of crops and an aging population that is living longer, has more disposable income, believes supplements to be safe and effective, and is willing to self-medicate in an effort to feel better and decrease health care costs has driven the popularity

and increased use of antioxidant supplement sales. Almost daily media reports extolling the virtues of antioxidants for increased longevity and improved health have steadily increased this trend in use of **antioxidant dietary supplements** and functional foods/nutraceuticals.

Deflating the Hype

Years of self-promoting lobbying efforts by the dietary supplement industry urged Congress to preserve consumer freedom of choice and Congress, believing that all supplements were safe, allowed passage of the **Dietary Supplement Health and Education Act** (DSHEA) in 1994. DSHEA effectively deregulated supplements and weakened the FDA's ability to safeguard the public by allowing harm to occur before action can be taken to protect the public. As to the safety of these products "caveat emptor" is the rule of the day—the exact opposite of what the consumers assume is the case. Surveys of older Americans find that approximately 75% want the government to review and approve supplements for safety and verify all marketing claims *before* they are sold in the market. In many ways we have returned to pre-1906 legislation days when unproven and harmful patent medicines and cures were rampant.

Consumers are beginning to realize that many claims made about supplements and functional foods are marketing "hype" designed to increase product sales and manufacturer bottom lines, not necessarily to improve the health and safety of the consumer. Judy Foreman, a writer for the *Boston Globe,* sums up this growing disenchantment with supplements in her May 14, 2007, "Health Sense" column. She writes her "love affair with vitamins and supplements is over: with a few exceptions . . . I'm tossing them out." She further explains that reports about vitamins and minerals influenced her to take specific supplements, mostly antioxidants. But as scientific studies began to accumulate disputing previous claims of improved health or showed they could be dangerous, she stopped taking most of them. She does admit that multivitamins will remain a part of her daily regime for now because she fails to eat enough fruits and vegetables. But even this has her concerned after reading the recent ConsumerLab .com analysis that revealed many multivitamins are either contaminated with lead, do not dissolve properly, or do not contain the ingredients or amounts listed on the label. She notes one benefit of not taking these supplements is "the handful of twenties I'm not spending on supplements!"

As food manufacturers enhance foods to enter the **functional foods/nutraceuticals** market, concerns about **"hypersupplementation"** will rise. The majority of supplement users are better educated, have higher incomes, are older, and take an active and preventive approach toward their health. However, antioxidant vitamin and mineral intakes from the available American diet provide sufficient, and at times more than, Dietary Reference Intakes (DRI) levels of these essential micronutrients. In addition, dietary supplements and functional foods/nutraceuticals support the concept that food is medicine and may sway individuals from eating a balanced diet from natural food sources, believing that they can acquire the same or superior benefits from supplementation at a lower overall cost. Instead of improving eating patterns to include more fruits, vegetables and whole grains, people tend to eat the same foods they have always eaten (often processed and high in sugars and fats) with the "insurance" of a supplement to "fix" all that is wrong with their diet. Aging Americans, who also tend to have an increased use of pharmaceutical medications, have a tendency to incorporate supplements and functional foods/nutraceuticals into what may already be a nutritionally adequate diet. Nutrient and drug interactions, toxicities, and overdoses may contribute to a potential public safety disaster.

Antioxidant Guidelines

The antioxidant nutrients—**vitamins C and E, carotenoids, selenium** and **polyphenols**—do appear to have a positive correlation in chronic disease reduction and better overall health. But lifestyle factors (exercise, tobacco and alcohol use, and diet choices key among them) and genetic factors also factor heavily into disease incidence. Scientific evidence is insufficient to prove that antioxidant nutrients are the exclusive reason for benefits observed from high phytochemical intake of fruits and vegetables. Antioxidants also do not appear to be a quick fix in prevention or treatment of chronic health problems that may have taken decades to develop, despite the hopes of so many Americans.

Finding Flavonoids

Most people are familiar with the antioxidant vitamins and minerals—vitamin C, E, the carotenoids like beta-carotene, selenium—and have some idea how to obtain them from food. If not, you can always check Nutrition Facts labels. But what about the antioxidants collectively known as flavonoids, which have been associated with a wide variety of possible health benefits?

Flavonoids are a subclass of plant polyphenols that represent over 6,000 compounds identified to date. Flavonoids are compounds that plants have conserved and diversified over a billion years of evolution. These polyphenolic compounds fulfill many different functions for plants, including protecting the plant from predators and environmental stresses. Plants also use flavonoids as both deterrents and attractants for insects and fruit-eating animals. During pollination, plants attract insects and birds to their flowers by using the anthocyanin flavonoids. When seeds need protection, bitter-tasting flavonoids in seed husks deter fruit-eating animals and insects. When seeds are ready for dispersal, plants add sugar to mask the bitter flavonoids and again add anthocyanins to signal birds and animals that the fruits are ripe.

But it is not just fruits that contain flavonoids. Flavonoids are ubiquitous, although in differing forms and concentrations, throughout all plant parts. So it is not unexpected that catechins, well-known flavonoids, are found in both the tender leaves of the tea plant, the fruits of the apple tree and the root bulbs of the onion.

Despite the ubiquitous presence of flavonoids in our plant-based foods, the determination of flavonoid intakes has only recently been undertaken. The task of analyzing the great variety of flavonoids present in foods is challenging, and existing food databases are incomplete.

But you can start finding foods rich in flavonoids with this quick guide to common dietary sources:

Anthocyanidins—Berries (red, blue, purple), cherries, grapes (red, purple), plums, red wine, rhubarb

Flavanols—Apples, berries, chocolate, grapes (green, red), red wine, teas (green, white, black, oolong)

Flavanones—Citrus fruits and juice (orange, grapefruit, lemon)

Flavonols—Apples, berries, broccoli, kale, scallions, teas, yellow onions

Flavones—Celery, hot peppers, parsley, thyme

Isoflavones—Legumes, soy foods, soybeans

Catechin, Epicatechin—Apples and cider, apricots, beans, blackberries, cherries, grapes, peaches, red wine, teas (black, green)

Hydroxybenzoic acids—Black currants, blackberries, raspberries, strawberries

Proanthocyanidins—Apples, apricots, avocados, bananas, beans (red kidney, pinto, black), beer, berries, cherries, chocolate, cinnamon, curry, grapes (green, grape seed), Indian squash, juices (cranberry, apple, grape), kiwis, mangos, nectarines, nuts, peaches, pears, plums, red wine

The leading causes of death in the United States—coronary heart disease, cancer, stroke, and diabetes—have been associated with poor diet choices. Many positive health outcomes have been associated with increasing dietary intake of fruits, vegetables, legumes and whole grains—all high in naturally occurring antioxidant nutrients. Combining different fruits and vegetables has also been discovered to have an even greater disease-fighting potential (for example, mixing tomatoes with broccoli instead of consuming separately has been shown to provide a much more potent combination in prostate cancer reduction).

In 1991, the National Cancer Institute and the Produce for Better Health Foundation partnered to create the **5 A Day For Better Health Program.** The 5 A Day Program focuses on increasing public awareness about eating a diet high in fruits and vegetables for better health and reduction of stroke, high blood pressure, diabetes and cancer risks. Despite this national marketing effort, fruit and vegetable consumption appears to have remained below recommended levels. The **Healthy People 2010** objectives for our nation recommended increasing fruit and vegetable consumption of at least two daily servings of fruit to 75% of the population, and at least three daily servings of vegetables to 50% of the population. But "The State of Aging and Health in America 2007 Report," which is submitted by the CDC, stated that approximately 29.8% of all Americans are currently meeting these goals. However, a *Journal of the American Dietetic Association* study, using data from the NHANES 1999–2000 and 1994–1996 CSFII, reported 40% of Americans ate the recommended amount of at least five servings of fruits and vegetables daily between 1999 and 2000. Despite these discrepancies in study results, which highlight just how difficult it is to really accurately assess food and nutrient intakes, the bottom line still reveals that Americans continue to eat below optimal levels of fruits and vegetables (although consumption was estimated to have increased by 3% between 1990 and 2000). Cultural food preferences, environmental barriers, cost, convenience, advertising and lack of education are just some of the barriers affecting fruit and vegetable consumption in the United States.

The clearest answer about what to do when advising others about antioxidants appears to be what mothers and home-economic teachers have recommended for years: eat a healthy and well-balanced diet with an emphasis on intake of fruits, vegetables, legumes and whole grains. Obviously, exercise and lifestyle habits (avoiding tobacco, alcohol and drug abuse) and genetic legacy factor into our prospective overall health. But controlling what we eat and making healthy, nutrient-dense food choices (not gulping down a dietary supplement pill in place of them) appear to be the best choice when trying to prevent or delay chronic illnesses and improve quality of life as we age.

It should be kept in mind, however, that there is a function and role for dietary supplements. Specific at-risk populations—such as those who live in poverty, the elderly who have changing gastric secretions that may affect how much of a nutrient is absorbed, those consuming below 1,600 calories per day, and those who suffer from diseases that affect nutrient absorption—benefit from supervised dietary supplementation. Supplements are a relatively inexpensive form of nutrients that can be administered, if taken consistently, in a more precise and reliable dose than through fruits and vegetables. As such, they may be beneficial for certain life stage groups, such as during pregnancy and the elderly years when appetite and nutrient intake or absorption are diminished.

Two Smart Eating Plans

Based on the growing body of evidence that using foods to meet nutrient needs is safer and more beneficial to our health, the Department of Health and Human Services (HHS) and the USDA published dietary guidelines that promote health and reduce risk for chronic disease. These guidelines, reviewed every five years, take into account current research and the state of health in America, seeking to provide an overall pattern of eating that will improve health and that the general public can easily follow. The **Dietary Guidelines for Americans 2005** promotes the need for all healthy Americans to choose meals and snacks high in variety and that are nutrient-dense but low in excess calories, saturated and trans fat, added sugars, and alcohol.

At-risk populations have specific nutrition risks. People over age 50 are often low in vitamin B12, pregnant women are often low in iron, women of childbearing age need to fortify their daily diet with folic acid (from functional foods or supplements) to prevent birth defects, and older adults or people who are dark-skinned (or get very little exposure to sunlight) are often deficient in vitamin D.

HHS and USDA recommend two food guides for better health: the **USDA Food Guide** and the **DASH Eating Plan.** These guides allow individuals to meet their daily DRIs without the need of additional supplementation. But if a person's diet is not varied, doesn't include enough fruits, vegetables and whole grains, or is below 1,600 calories, then functional foods or multivitamins may be of benefit.

In general, it appears that most American adults consume less than recommended amounts of calcium, potassium, fiber, magnesium and vitamins A (carotenoids), C and E, even though the Institute of Medicine draws different conclusions. Children and adolescents consume less than recommended amounts of calcium, potassium, fiber, magnesium and vitamin E. At-risk populations tend to consume less of vitamin B12, iron, folic acid and vitamins E and D. Americans generally consume too many calories and too much saturated fat, cholesterol, added sugars and salt.

The first key point the USDA Food Guide and the DASH Eating Plans stress is the inclusion of more dark green and orange vegetables, fruits, legumes, whole grains and low-fat milk and milk products and less refined grains, total fats, added sugars and calories in the daily diet. The second point they stress is picking foods that are nutrient-dense. Nutrient-dense foods provide substantial amounts of vitamins and minerals in few calories. For example, fruits and vegetables are nutrient-dense foods because they contain antioxidants (vitamins, minerals and phytochemicals) and fiber at low calorie levels. In comparison, processed foods often high in sugar, fat and salt—such as cookies and potato chips—are poor nutrient-dense food choices because they contain very little (and sometimes no) nutrient values at a high calorie level.

In addition to the HHS and USDA dietary guidelines, the CDC partners with other government agencies and not-for-profit and industry groups to increase public awareness about the benefits of fruits and vegetables and increasing their consumption through the **National Fruit & Vegetable Program** (formerly the 5 A Day For Better Health Program). They support the HHS and USDA dietary guidelines and provide a Web site <www.fruitsandveggiesmorematters.org> that helps people learn about the benefits of eating these natural antioxidants and also gives tips, ideas and recipes to assist people to increase them in their diet.

Individuals may also want to incorporate more organic produce into their diets as well. Although organic produce is more expensive, one study indicates their value may be worth the extra expense. Studies are still ongoing to determine whether there is a significant difference between organic and conventional produce. Nevertheless, organic products are becoming more popular and available. As demand continues to increase, more suppliers will enter the market and prices should come down.

What about Supplements and Nutraceuticals?

In general, all vitamin and mineral needs should be consumed via natural food sources. But because most Americans do not eat the recommended amounts of fruits and vegetables, eat on the run (therefore eating at fast food restaurants or not balancing meals), and/or follow weight-reducing diets, taking a multivitamin/multimineral is an appropriate choice to compensate for possible nutrient deficits in the diet. To date the evidence neither supports nor opposes taking a daily multivitamin as "insurance." Even if a healthy diet is eaten, which follows all recommendations, taking an additional multivitamin/multimineral supplement as an inexpensive "insurance" is unlikely to exceed the ULs for nutrients. Natural or synthetic brands make no difference in absorption of most nutrients and it is best to purchase the least-expensive brand that is free of fillers and other additives (such as sugar, yeast or artificial colorings) that conform to **US Pharmacopeia** (USP) guidelines. Multivitamin/multimineral supplements should be taken within 30 minutes before or after meals.

Concerns about quality of multivitamins on the market surfaced when a recent **ConsumerLab.com** analysis found some products were contaminated with lead, did not have the correct amounts of listed nutrients, and/or did not dissolve properly. (Both ConsumerLab.com and the USP are independent agencies that test health products and pharmaceuticals, including supplements.) This study supports the concept that ingesting daily nutrients from foods is the best option. However, adding functional foods/nutraceuticals and multivitamins/multiminerals to adequate diets may become problematic and may lead to hypersupplementation. With a nutraceutical that provides 100% of most daily nutrients—such as Kellogg's SmartStart Antioxidant Cereal—including this cereal every day along with a balanced and adequate diet plus a multivitamin/multimineral can quite possibly lead to taking in excess recommended nutrient intakes.

When considering functional foods/nutraceuticals, the following questions should be asked before consuming them:

- **Should I be eating this?** Don't add this food just for its medicinal value.
- **How meaningful is the claim?** When a product claims that it affects the body, that is, "supports the immune system" or "enhances mood," what scientific evidence backs up the claim? Beware ORAC (oxygen radical absorbance capacity) claims. Marketers often suggest a high ORAC value "proves" superior antioxidant value. The ORAC assay, however, is only one of many assays that measure the capability of a product or food to "quench radicals" and are useful in the lab setting and in vitro only. All these assays, including the ORAC, are limited and none truly measure "radical quenching" of all radicals. They do not predict health effects of antioxidants in humans. Marketing claims about product antioxidant capacity are often overstated, unscientific and written out of context.
- **Do I need this(these) nutrient(s)?** Healthy people who eat well-balanced diets do not need to add these products to their diet. If an individual is in an at-risk category or has diseases that may affect nutrient absorption, then their diet must be carefully evaluated before adding them into a daily diet.
- **Am I overdosing?** Be sure to know what the maximum amount of any nutrient is safe to take and the sources of the nutrient to avoid toxicities.

(Healthletter *editor's note: Consult with your physician before beginning any supplement regimen.*)

There is some evidence that free radicals can cause oxidative damage to cells. Antioxidants appear to reduce this damage and are worth incorporating into our daily diets, although supporting evidence has been conflicting. But the source of antioxidants should come from a balanced diet that includes a variety of fruits, vegetables, legumes and whole grains.

Much more research needs to be done and the media and the average American need to take a wait-and-see approach, rather than jump on the latest fad, which could endanger their health. The media should also give more publicity to the government programs that have been already been put into place to help Americans improve their health. Lastly, health-care professionals need to be better informed about current self-care trends that Americans are embracing and actively query their patients about what they are doing, educating them on the benefits and dangers.

Hippocrates seems to have summed it up best: "Let food be thy medicine, thy medicine shall be thy food."

To Learn More

US Pharmacopeia, www.usp.org.
Consumer Lab, www.consumerlab.com.
HHS & USDA Dietary Guidelines, www.health.gov/dietaryguidelines.
Fruit & Veggies Matter, www.fruitsandveggiesmorematters.org.
DASH eating plan, www.nhlbi.nih.gov/health/public/heart/hbp/dash.

Brain Food

Linda Milo Ohr

Cognitive health is a growing concern for consumers of all ages. Parents are continually learning about the importance of omega-3 fatty acids for their babies, toddlers, and adolescents. Teenagers and adults need to stay mentally sharp and focused for school and work. And baby boomers and seniors face conditions such as Alzheimer's and cognitive decline as they age.

This increased interest in brain health is evident in the growing number of brain-related products and brain-healthy ingredients that are available in the market. For example, *Minute Maid® Enhanced Pomegranate Blueberry Juice Blend* from Coca-Cola Co., Atlanta, Ga. (www.thecoca-colacompany.com, www.minutemaid.com), contains omega-3/DHA—50 mg/8 oz. It also contains choline and vitamin B-12, which "play a role in brain and nervous system signaling"; vitamin E to "help shield the omega-3s in the brain from free radicals"; and vitamin C, which is "highly concentrated in brain nerve endings."

In addition to these ingredients, other brain boosters include fruits, botanicals, walnuts, and more. Here is information on some of these "foods for thought."

Omega-3 Fatty Acids

A proven ingredient for brain health for all ages, omega-3 fatty acids such as docosahexaenoic acid (DHA), arachidonic acid, and eicosapentaenoic acid aid in development as well as benefit certain mental conditions. Most recently, Ryan and Nelson (2008) indicated that higher DHA levels are associated with improved listening comprehension and vocabulary skills in preschool children. They gave 400 mg/day of DHA (n = 85) or matching placebo (n = 90) to 4-year-old children for 4 mo. A preplanned regression analysis yielded a statistically significant positive association between a higher DHA level in the blood and higher scores on the Peabody Picture Vocabulary Test, a cognitive test designed to measure listening comprehension and vocabulary skills.

Omega-3 fatty acids have also been linked to improving various clinical and behavioral conditions involving mental function, including depression, bipolar disorder, schizophrenia, aggression, attention deficit hyperactivity disorder, Alzheimer's, and Parkinson's disease. Ma et al. (2007) showed that DHA decreased an important risk factor for late-onset Alzheimer's disease. Using a mouse model, a diabetic rat model, and

cultured human cells, the study found that DHA increased the production of LR11, a protein vital to clearing the brain of the enzymes that make amyloid beta plaques often associated with Alzheimer's disease.

Currently, a National Institutes of Health-funded study is studying the effects of DHA in slowing the progression of Alzheimer's disease. Patients with mild-to-moderate Alzheimer's disease will be treated for 18 mo, taking either 2 g/day of DHA or a placebo. The results are anticipated by December 2009. The DHA is produced by Martek Biosciences Corp., Columbia, Mo. (phone 410-740-0081, www.martek.com).

Blueberries

High in antioxidants, blueberries are gaining recognition as brain-healthy foods. U.S. Dept. of Agriculture Agricultural Research Service scientists studied the effect of a blueberry extract on mice that carried a genetic mutation for promoting increased amounts of amyloid beta plaque in the brain (Bliss, 2007). They found increased activity of a family of enzymes, called kinases, in the brains of amyloid-plaqued mice that were fed blueberry extract. Two of the kinases found are important in mediating cognitive function.

Other research has shown that Alaskan wild-bog blueberries contain compounds that can reduce inflammation in the central nervous system that is associated with the progression of neurodegeneration (Society for Neuroscience, 2007). Another study at the Center for Aging and Brain Repair at the University of South Florida College of Medicine, Tampa, Fla., showed that supplementing the diet of old rats with blueberries for 8 weeks resulted in maintenance and rejuvenation of brain circuitry.

Grapes

Wang et al. (2008) found that grape-seed-derived polyphenolics, *MegaNatural®-AZ* from Polyphenolics, Madera, Calif. (phone 559-661-5556, www.polyphenolics.com), significantly reduced Alzheimer's disease-type cognitive deterioration. They gave mice with Alzheimer's disease either water containing grape seed extract or plain water for 5 mo and found that the mice treated with grape seed extract had significantly reduced Alzheimer's disease-type cognitive deterioration compared to the mice in the control group. This was due to the prevention of amyloid beta plaque forming in the brain.

Another study suggested that Concord grape juice in the diet may provide benefits for older adults with early memory decline (Welch, 2008). Subjects drank a total of 15–21 oz of either Concord grape juice or a placebo for 12 weeks. Those who drank the grape juice showed significant improvement in list learning, and trends suggested improved short-term retention and spatial memory.

Walnuts

Walnuts, already associated with a reduced risk of coronary heart disease, contain alpha-linolenic acid, an essential omega-3 fatty acid, and other polyphenols. Researchers at the USDA Human Nutrition Research Center at Tufts University, Boston, Mass., showed that diets containing 2%, 6%, or 9% walnuts were found to reverse several parameters of brain aging, as well as age-related motor and cognitive deficits in old mice (Society for Neuroscience, 2007).

Walnuts, already associated with a reduced risk of coronary heart disease, contain alpha-linolenic acid, an essential omega-3 fatty acid, and other polyphenols.

Researchers from Baldwin-Wallace College, Berea, Ohio, showed that walnut extracts may play a role in developing novel treatments for Alzheimer's disease. The enzyme acetylcholinesterase has been shown to induce amyloid beta plaque formation. Using chemical techniques in the absence of living cells, the researchers showed that walnut extract and two of its major components, gallic and ellagic acids, not only inhibit the site of acetylcholinesterase associated with amyloid beta protein aggregation, but also inhibit the site of acetylcholinesterase responsible for the breakdown of acetylcholine.

Botanicals and Botanical Blends

Ginseng is one of the most widely used medicinal herbs in the world. According to the National Center for Complementary and Alternative Medicine, Bethesda, Md. (www.nccam.nih .gov), traditional and modern uses of ginseng include increasing a sense of well-being and stamina, as well as improving both mental and physical performance.

In February 2008, Naturex, South Hackensack, N.J. (phone 201-440-5000, www.naturex.com), announced that it would be participating in "New Technologies for Ginseng Agriculture and Product Development," a program oriented to validating

several health claims on North American ginseng. Research will focus on various medical and health areas, including metabolic syndrome, stress, physical endurance, cardiovascular diseases, immuno-modulation, reproductive health, and neuroprotective and psychiatric disorders.

A novel dietary supplement, *Think Gum*™, from Think Gum LLC, Los Angeles, Calif. (www.thinkgum.com), includes a blend of botanicals touted to enhance mental performance. The chewing gum contains peppermint, rosemary, ginkgo biloba, vinpocetine from periwinkle plants, and the Indian herb bacopa. The company's Web site cites studies backing each herb's mental benefit, like improving mental clarity and protecting brain cells.

A wild green-oat extract, *Neuravena*®, from Frutarom USA Inc., North Bergen, N.J. (phone 201-861-9500, www.frutarom .com), has been shown to enhance stress-coping abilities as well as learning performance. The extract's phytonutrients are thought to affect the activity of cerebral enzymes closely related to mental health and cognitive function.

Phospholipids

Phospholipids are building blocks in the brain and are often linked to improving memory and mental health. Phosphatidylcholine is a major source of choline, which is used to produce the neurotransmitter acetylcholine, a chemical messenger molecule that seems to be involved in neuron networks.

A Food and Drug Administration-approved qualified health claim for dietary supplements states that soy-derived phosphatidylserine (PS), another phospholipid, may reduce the risk of cognitive dysfunction in the elderly. Earlier this year, a commercial form of PS, *Sharp-PS*™, from Enzymotec, Israel (phone +972-4-654-5112, www.enzymotec.com), received "No Questions" from FDA for its GRAS notification. The company also offers *Sharp-PS*™ *Silver*, a blend of PS and DHA for improving mental and cognitive ability, and *Sharp-PS*™ *Gold*, a PS and DHA conjugate for better memory and mental performance.

L-Carnitine

L-carnitine is essential for transporting long-chain fatty acids across the mitochondrial membrane for subsequent fat breakdown and energy production. Known to benefit exercise and weight management, L-carnitine has also been shown to aid in mental function in the elderly.

Malaguarnera et al. (2007) reported that L-carnitine lessened fatigue and boosted mental function. They gave 66 males and females age 100 years and older either 2 g of L-carnitine or a placebo once daily. After 6 mo, researchers concluded that oral administration of L-carnitine facilitated an increased capacity for physical and cognitive activity by reducing fatigue and improving cognitive functions.

The acetyl derivative of L-carnitine, acetyl L-carnitine (ALC), is found throughout the central nervous system. According to information from Lonza Inc., Allendale, N.J. (phone 201-316-9200, www.lonza.com, www.carnipure.com), ALC plays a broad role in central nervous system metabolism as a source of acetyl groups both for the synthesis of acetylcholine and for energy-producing reactions.

Citicoline

Citicoline is a naturally occurring, water-soluble molecule that is used by the brain to make phospholipids. Information from Kyowa Hakko, New York (phone 212-319-5353, www.kyowa-usa.com), explains that one way citicoline supports brain health is by increasing the activity of the mitochondria in neurons to produce energy, particularly high-energy ATP. Silveri et al. (2007) recently confirmed the ability of *Cognizin*® citicoline to improve brain energy by increasing levels of specific markers for ATP and increasing activity in the frontal-lobe region of the brain. The frontal lobe directs complex thought, decision-making, and attention. Age-related declines in cognitive abilities are also related to deteriorating frontal-lobe function.

Phytosterols

Mother Nature's Cholesterol Fighters

Foods fortified with phytosterols, naturally occurring compounds found in plant cells, are a relatively new weapon in the struggle to lower high low-density lipoprotein cholesterol levels.

JILL WEISENBERGER, MS, RD, CDE

Orange juice, granola bars, oatmeal, cheese, and chocolates. With the flurry of new phytosterol-containing products on the market, we have one more tool to help our patients reach the strict low-density lipoprotein (LDL) cholesterol goals recommended in the 2004 update to the National Cholesterol Education Program (NCEP).

Nicole Brown, a Virginia-based RD, often recommends phytosterol-fortified foods to her patients. They frequently eat cheeses, orange juice, and granola bars anyway, she says. Switching brands is "a simple way to attack the LDL levels."

As their name suggests, plant sterols are cousins of cholesterol. Cholesterol helps form the structure of mammalian cell membranes, whereas plant sterols are important to the structure of the plant's cell membranes. Various plants synthesize more than 40 sterols, with the most common being sitosterol, campesterol, and stigmasterol.

Compared with taking medication, the overall cost and safety of phytosterol-containing foods is favorable.

The typical diet varies from approximately 167 to 437 milligrams per day of naturally occurring plant sterols. One tablespoon of corn oil contains 132 milligrams and 1 ounce of almonds provides 34 milligrams of plant sterols. Saturated plant sterols, or phytostanols, are naturally present in the diet in even smaller amounts. At these levels, they have no effect on serum cholesterol. However, in quantities of 800 milligrams to 2 grams per day, plant sterols and stanols interfere with the absorption of both exogenous and endogenous cholesterol, thus shunting cholesterol into the stool and effectively lowering serum levels. Typically, LDL cholesterol levels drop 10% to 14%. Plant sterols and stanols are themselves absorbed in only minute amounts. They are collectively called *phytosterols*. The cholesterol-lowering effects of phytosterols are additive to drug and other dietary treatments.

Pumped-Up Margarine-Like Spreads

Fifty-five years ago, researchers showed that beta-sitosterol decreased serum cholesterol in chickens during a cholesterol load. That finding started a series of studies in both animals and humans. Initial attention was focused on beta-sitosterol in doses of 10 to 15 grams per day, resulting in as much as a 20% reduction in total serum cholesterol. Study participants tolerated the various doses well; however, there was no additional cholesterol-lowering benefit above 3 grams daily. Further studies demonstrated the efficacy of stanols. Today, both stanols and sterols are added to foods in both their esterified and unesterified forms.

Perhaps the most commonly recognized phytosterol-enriched foods are the Benecol spreads (McNeil Nutritionals) and Take Control spreads (Unilever Bestfoods). Benecol spreads contain plant stanol esters made from the oils of pine trees and soy and Take Control products contain plant sterol esters from soybeans. Both have been shown to reduce total and LDL cholesterol when eaten in the recommended quantities. A study sponsored by Unilever and published in the *European Journal of Clinical Nutrition* in 1998 found that plasma total and LDL cholesterol concentrations were reduced by 8% to 13% for margarines enriched in soybean oil sterol-esters or sitostanol-ester compared with a control margarine. There was no effect on high-density lipoprotein (HDL) cholesterol levels. The authors concluded that the margarine products were equally effective.

One of Many Tools

Phytosterols have an additive or synergistic effect when combined with other positive dietary changes, says David Jenkins, MD, PhD, DSc, research chair in nutrition and metabolism at the

University of Toronto. Dietary restriction of cholesterol, saturated fats, and trans fats likely provides a 10% decrease in LDL cholesterol. Add phytosterols to the mix for an additional drop of 10%. Study volunteers consuming an NCEP Step II diet with a reduced-fat stanol ester-containing margarine lowered their total and LDL cholesterol as much as 18.3% and 23.6%, respectively. Control subjects following the Step II diet with no added phytosterols saw only a 7.7% reduction in their total cholesterol and a 9.9% drop in LDL cholesterol. Again, there were no significant changes in HDL cholesterol levels from baseline in any of the study groups.

For Some, an Easy Fix

For Kathe Jefferson, one of Brown's clients, adding phytosterols gave her LDL cholesterol the push she had been trying to get with other dietary strategies. Prior to adding the phytosterols to her diet, Jefferson had worked with Brown to improve her food choices. She kept a food record, followed an exchange-based meal plan, exercised daily, and began trying new foods. All combined, these efforts rewarded her with an 85-pound weight loss. With great disappointment, however, she saw that her LDL cholesterol barely moved. It fell from 143 milligrams per deciliter in December 2004 to 140 milligrams per deciliter in April 2005.

It wasn't until Jefferson added plant sterols to her diet that she saw a dramatic reduction in her LDL cholesterol. She's had a glass of phytosterol-containing orange juice daily since November 2005 and watched her LDL cholesterol fall from 140 to 127 milligrams per deciliter in only a few weeks after beginning the orange juice regimen.

Strategy to Reduce Low-Density Lipoprotein (LDL) Cholesterol	Approximate LDL Lowering
Moderate weight loss	5%
Dietary addition of viscous fibers, almonds, and soy	5% to 6%
1 to 2 grams phytosterols daily	10%
Dietary restriction of cholesterol, saturated fat, and trans fat	10%
Statin drugs	20% to 50%

Source: David Jenkins, MD, PhD, DSc, University of Toronto.

In some patients, drug therapy may be avoided or continued at a lower dose. Thus far, Jefferson has avoided cholesterol-lowering medications, which is an important goal for her. "Why risk damaging my liver if I could do it [lower cholesterol] on my own?" she says. The fortified foods are readily accessible, they taste good, and it's easy to do, she adds.

Since statin drugs and phytosterols lower cholesterol levels with different mechanisms, they can be used together. A phytosterol-containing spread reduced LDL cholesterol by 10% to 15% in both hypercholesterolemic patients taking a statin drug and those not taking cholesterol-lowering medication, according to a 2001 study published in *Atherosclerosis*.

Is There a Downside?

"Plant sterols are nonabsorbable, so there are minimal side effects," says Robert Nicolosi, PhD, CSN, professor and director of the Center for Health and Disease Research at the University of Massachusetts, Lowell. Compare that with statin drugs, the most widely prescribed cholesterol-lowering medications, which may cause muscle aching and intestinal discomfort. Occasionally, statins cause muscle cells to break down or liver enzymes to increase. The downside to phytosterols, says Nicolosi, is that "because they prevent the absorption of cholesterol, they can have an effect on the fat-soluble vitamins." Researchers have observed decreased plasma levels of alpha-carotene, beta-carotene, alpha-tocopherol, and lycopene.

As dietetic professionals, we need to assess our clients' intakes of fat-soluble vitamins and phytonutrients when making recommendations about phytosterols. Increasing the usual intake of fruits and vegetables may be enough to offset the negative effects of the phytosterols. Consider a 2002 study published in the *American Journal of Clinical Nutrition*. Investigators measured the plasma beta-carotene concentrations of volunteers eating a spread either with or without added phytosterols. The subjects in each group were advised to eat at least five servings of fruits and vegetables daily, of which one or more was to be broccoli, carrots, spinach, tomatoes, sweet potatoes, pumpkins, or apricots. The researchers concluded that an average of one extra daily serving of carotenoid-rich fruits and vegetables maintains plasma carotenoid concentrations.

Health Claim

The FDA permits a health claim for phytosterols and coronary heart disease. The regulations require that the health claim specify that the daily intake of phytosterols should be consumed in two servings at different times of the day and with other foods. The total daily dose must be at least 800 milligrams free sterols or stanols. There is no restriction in the types of foods that may contain the phytosterols and bear the health claim. However, there are qualifying criteria. A serving must do the following:

- contain at least 0.4 grams plant sterols or stanols;
- meet the criteria for a low-saturated fat and low-cholesterol food;
- not provide more than 13 grams of total fat and 480 milligrams of sodium per serving or per 50 grams (Exceptions for the fat restriction are made for margarine-type spreads, salad dressings, and vegetable oils.); and
- contain at least 10% of the Daily Value for one or more of the following nutrients: calcium, iron, protein, dietary fiber, vitamin A, and vitamin C. (Salad dressings are exempt from this requirement.)

Stock Your Pantry

Below is a list of phytosterol-containing foods. The FDA recently granted approval for the addition of plant sterols to a variety of other foods, including coffee, baked goods, cereals, vegetarian meat analogues, pasta, salty snacks, and soups. So watch your grocer's shelves.

Food with at Least One Half the Daily Dose	Serving Size	Comments
Smart Balance Omega Plus Buttery Spread	1 T	Contains marine-based fish oils; 80 calories, 9 grams fat, 2.5 grams saturated fat, 0 grams trans fat, 3.5 grams monounsaturated fat, 0 milligrams cholesterol, 10% Daily Value (DV) for vitamin A, 10% DV for vitamin E
Benecol Regular Spread	1 T	Can be used in cooking and baking. 70 calories, 8 grams fat, 1 gram saturated fat, 0 grams trans fat, 4.5 grams monounsaturated fat, 0 milligrams cholesterol, 10% DV for vitamin A, 20% DV for vitamin E
Benecol Light Spread	1 T	Not recommended for cooking and baking. 50 calories, 5 grams fat, 0.5 grams saturated fat, 0 grams trans fat, 2.5 grams monounsaturated fat, 0 milligrams cholesterol, 10% DV for vitamin A, 20% DV for vitamin E
Take Control Regular Spread	1 T	Can be used in cooking and baking and can be frozen. 80 calories, 8 grams fat, 1 gram saturated fat, 4.5 grams monounsaturated fat, <5 milligrams cholesterol, 10% DV for vitamin A, 20% DV for vitamin E
Take Control Light Spread	1 T	Not strongly recommended for cooking. 45 calories, 5 grams fat, 0.5 grams saturated fat, 2 grams monounsaturated fat, <5 milligrams cholesterol, 10% DV for vitamin A, 15% DV for vitamin E
Minute Maid Premium Heart Wise Orange Juice	8 fluid ounces	Added vitamins E, B_6, B_{12}, and beta-carotene
Rice Dream Heartwise Rice Drink	No information available	No information available
Nature Valley Healthy Heart Chewy Granola Bar	1 bar	Available in two flavors: oatmeal raisin and honey nut. 150 to 160 calories, 2 to 4 grams fat, 0.5 grams saturated fat, 0 grams trans fat, 28 to 30 grams carbohydrate, 3 grams fiber
CocaVia Chocolate Bar	1 bar (20 to 22 grams)	Provides a higher-than-usual amount of plant sterols: 1.1 grams plant sterols, 90 to 100 calories, 5 to 6 grams fat, 3 to 3.5 grams saturated fat, 0 grams trans fat, 11 to 12 grams carbohydrate, 2 grams fiber, 20% to 25% DV for calcium, >10% DV for vitamins E, B_6, B_{12}, C, and folate
CocaVia Snack Bar	1 bar (22 to 23 grams)	Provides a higher-than-usual amount of plant sterols: 1.5 grams plant sterols, 70 to 80 calories, 2 grams fat, 1 gram saturated fat, 0 grams trans fat, 13 grams carbohydrate, 1 gram fiber, 20% to 25% DV for calcium, >10% DV for vitamins E, B_6, B_{12}, C, and folate
CocaVia Chocolate Covered Almonds	1 pack (28 grams)	Provides a higher-than-usual amount of plant sterols: 1.1 grams plant sterols, 140 calories, 11 grams fat, 3.5 grams saturated fat, 0 grams trans fat, 12 grams carbohydrate, 3 grams fiber, 20% DV for calcium, 10% DV for vitamins E, B_6, B_{12}, C, and folate
Sturns Instant Oatmeal	1 packet	Also contains flaxmeal
Lifetime Low-Fat Cheese Slices	1 slice (19 grams)	If not available locally, order at www.lifetimecheese.com. Available in cheddar flavor only. 30 calories, 1 gram fat, 0.5 grams saturated fat, 0 grams trans fat, 5 milligrams cholesterol, 180 milligrams sodium
Lifetime Low-Fat Cheese Blocks	1 ounce	Also available at the company's Web site. Four flavors: Cheddar, sharp cheddar, jalapeno jack, and mozzarella. 55 calories, 2.5 grams fat, 1 gram saturated fat, 0 grams trans fat, 10 milligrams cholesterol, 200 milligrams sodium

Sources: Food company Web sites, representatives, and package labels.

Putting It into Practice

Dietetic professionals have many practical considerations when advising clients on the use of these functional foods. Some products are costlier than their unfortified counterparts. However, compared with taking medication, the overall cost and safety of phytosterol-containing foods is favorable, says Kathryn Kolasa, PhD, RD, LDN, of the Brody School of Medicine at East Carolina University.

Adding calories and fat to the diet can also present problems. Substituting a fortified food for a nonfortified food avoids extra calories and may increase compliance. One CocoaVia chocolate bar (22 grams) provides 100 calories and 3.5 grams of saturated fat. Added to the diet, it would eventually cause weight gain and possibly affect blood lipids. But to replace a larger, more calorie- and fat-laden dessert with one CocoaVia bar may have the desired effects.

Ease of use and availability are other considerations. Kathy Dwyer, also one of Brown's clients, watched her LDL cholesterol plummet from 178 to 140 milligrams per deciliter in approximately four months by following a reduced-calorie Therapeutic Lifestyles Changes diet incorporating phytosterol-containing orange juice and yogurt and walking for exercise. She found it easy to incorporate the new products into her diet, though some clients may wish for a wider selection of foods.

After several months of enjoying the yogurt daily, Dwyer could no longer find it in any grocery store. Changing the diet once is hard enough, but after successfully following a new, healthier plan, it can be frustrating to some clients to have to change again. Weeks passed before Dwyer found the time and made an effort to include another serving of phytosterol-fortified product. She settled on Nature Valley Healthy Heart granola bars.

Although still under debate, current recommendations suggest that the total daily dose be divided into two smaller doses. For many, this will mean having to find more than just one or two products they like. It's a good idea to consume the phytosterols in two doses, says Jenkins. "Most things do better when spread out over the day." He also says that phytosterols are more effective when consumed with fat because of increased bile excretion into the small intestine.

Some of your clients may ask whether it is safe and advisable for family members to use these products, too. Studies have been conducted in normocholesterolemic adults and hypercholesterolemic children. Phytosterol-containing foods appear to be safe in both populations. However, the decreased absorption of fat-soluble vitamins and phytochemicals may be of greater importance in children and others with increased nutrient needs.

Although the vast majority of the population absorbs only tiny amounts of phytosterols, a small number of people are homozygous for hyperphytosterolemia. In these individuals, large amounts of circulating phytosterols may contribute to premature atherosclerosis. Thus, they should avoid products with added phytosterols. Because they tend to develop multiple xanthomas, their condition is recognized early in life, so this should not be a concern to our typical clients or the public at large. These functional foods are very important, says Jenkins. We wouldn't take bread off the grocery shelves because some people have celiac disease or remove peanut butter because many children have allergies, he adds. However, some researchers prefer the use of plant stanol esters over plant sterol esters because the latter may increase serum plant sterol levels and possibly the risk of coronary heart disease.

The increasing variety of phytosterol-containing foods provides our clients a fairly inexpensive adjunct to other lifestyle and pharmaceutical therapies. To assist them in using this tool, we can offer taste testings, a list of products and their availabilities, an interpretation of their laboratory results, and our continued support.

JILL WEISENBERGER, MS, RD, CDE, is a research dietitian and certified diabetes educator for Hampton Roads Center for Clinical Research in Norfolk, Va., and a freelance writer.

For references, view article on our archive at www.TodaysDietitian.com.

The Benefits of Flax

Flax products have been popping up all over grocery-store shelves lately, with claims such as "special protection for women's health" and "fights the blues." Here's our take on the seed's potential benefits, as well as some advice on how to incorporate it into your diet.

As Good as Fish Oil?

Flax products come in three forms: supplements, oil, and the seed itself. All of those, like fish oil, contain omega-3 fatty acids. In fish oil, those substances protect the heart in several ways, notably thinning the blood and lowering levels of LDL (bad) cholesterol and triglycerides. Moreover, those fatty acids might offer other health benefits, including protection against mild depression, Alzheimer's disease, and macular degeneration.

But it's unclear if the fatty acids in flax, which come in the form of alphalinolenic acid (ALA), provide the same benefits. That's because the body has to convert ALA into the two fatty acids, eicosapentaenoic acid (EPA) and docosahexaenoic acid (DHA), found in fish oil. And to get meaningful amounts of those compounds you may have to consume lots of flax, according to a September 2008 study in the American Journal of Clinical Nutrition. It found that even large doses of flax oil—four to six 600-milligram capsules—boosted blood levels of EPA by only about 35 percent and had no effect on DHA.

Benefits Beyond the Heart

Still, flax oil might provide at least some coronary protection. And flaxseeds, especially crushed or ground, may offer certain benefits that fish oil does not. For example, they are rich sources of lignans, compounds that alter the way the body handles estrogen. That may explain why preliminary research hints

---

How to Get more into Your Diet

- Add a tablespoon of crushed or ground flaxseed to your hot or cold breakfast cereal or yogurt.
- Add a teaspoon of crushed or ground flaxseed to mayonnaise or mustard when making a sandwich.
- Use crushed or ground flaxseed in place of eggs in baking. Mix 1 tablespoon with 3 tablespoons of water as a substitute for 1 large egg, and let it sit for a few minutes. Note that this will change the texture of the food.
- Look for products that contain flax, including cereals, granola bars, and breads.

---

that flaxseed can lower the risk of breast cancer. And one small study of women with mild menopausal symptoms found that about 3 tablespoons of flaxseed a day eased their hot flashes and night sweats as effectively as supplemental estrogen. Finally, the seeds contain lots of fiber, protein, magnesium, and thiamin.

Recommendation

Flax-oil supplements might be worth a try for people who want some of the benefits of fish oil but don't like the taste of fish or fish-oil pills, or avoid fish because they're vegetarians. But the supplements aren't good for people who can't take fish oil for safety reasons, because they may interact with the same blood-thinning drugs. And women with a history of breast, ovarian, or uterine cancers, as well as endometriosis or fibroids, should talk with their doctor before consuming flaxseeds because of their possible effect on estrogen. But most other people can safely add flaxseed to their diet.

UNIT 6

Food Safety/Technology

Unit Selections

38. **Is Your Food Contaminated?,** Mark Fischetti
39. **Dirty Birds: Even 'Premium' Chickens Harbor Dangerous Bacteria,** *Consumer Reports*
40. **Fear of Fresh: How to Avoid Food-Borne Illness from Fresh Fruits & Vegetables,** Bonnie Liebman and Robert Tauxe
41. **Irradiation of Fresh Fruits and Vegetables,** Xuetong Fan et al.
42. **The *E. Coli* Outbreak: Lettuce Learn a Lesson,** Sharon Palmer
43. **Produce Safety: Back to Basics for Producers and Consumers,** *Food Insight*

Key Points to Consider

• What action should you take to minimize your risk from exposure to environmental contaminants in the food chain?

• Describe the new technologies developed to protect our food supply from intentional contamination.

• How does antibiotic resistance develop in humans?

• What steps are you going to take to prevent food-borne illness while processing meat and produce at home?

• Discuss the pros and cons of fresh fruit and vegetable contamination.

Student Website
www.mhhe.com/cls

Internet References

American Council on Science and Health (ACSH)
www.acsh.org
Centers for Disease Control and Prevention (CDC)
www.cdc.gov
FDA Center for Food Safety and Applied Nutrition
http://vm.cfsan.fda.gov
Food Safety Project (FSP)
www.extension.iastate.edu/foodsafety
USDA Food Safety and Inspection Service (FSIS)
www.fsis.usda.gov

Food-borne disease constitutes an important public health problem in the United States. The U.S. Centers for Disease Control has reported 76 million cases of food-borne illness each year, out of which 5,000 end in death. The annual cost of losses in productivity ranges from 20 to 40 billion dollars. Food-borne disease results primarily from microbial contamination, and also from naturally occurring toxicants, environmental contaminants, pesticide residues, and food additives.

The first Food and Drug Act was passed in 1906 and was followed by tighter control on the use of additives that might be carcinogenic. In 1958, the Delaney Clause was passed and a list of additives that were considered as safe for human consumption (GRAS list) was developed. The Food and Drug Administration (FDA) controls and regulates procedures dealing with food safety, including food service and production. The FDA has established rules (Hazard Analysis and Critical Control Points) to improve safety control and to monitor the production of seafood, meat, and poultry.

Agricultural trade between nations has led to a truly globalized food supply. This globalization meets the demand of wealthy nations for year round access to foods grown in tropical environments and strengthens the economies of poorer, underdeveloped countries. One detriment of the global food supply is the translocation of biological contaminants via food. Less than 1 percent of foods imported into the United States are inspected each year. Although U.S. demand for variety of foods has driven the worldwide food trade, our nation has not established an effective method to regulate the safety of foods shipped in from other countries. The current regulatory agency for U.S. food, the Food and Drug Administration, is faced with many challenges of trying to regulate the U.S. food and pharmaceutical industries, much less the newly introduced challenges of the safety of food imports.

Imported foods are not the only concern for biological contaminants. Changes in food production and farming in the United States has led to an increase in the spread of bacterial contamination of our foods. Many conventional poultry and livestock farms raise their animals in crowded, unsanitary conditions. The crowded conditions make the spread of bacteria very likely; therefore, conventional farmers must inoculate their animals with antibiotics to prevent bacteria from spreading throughout the entire stock. An example of the poor regulation of foods grown in the United States is the dramatic increase in *Salmonella* and *Campylobacter* bacteria in chickens over the few last years as reported by *Consumer Reports*. The U.S. Department of Agriculture has no standards for *Campylobacter* and only tests for *Salmonella* in a small sample of animals.

Surveys show that over 95 percent of the time people do not follow proper sanitation methods when working with food. Thus our best defense is to have safe food-handling practices at home. The U.S. government, therefore, launched the Food Safety Initiative program to minimize food-borne disease and to educate the public about safe-handling practices.

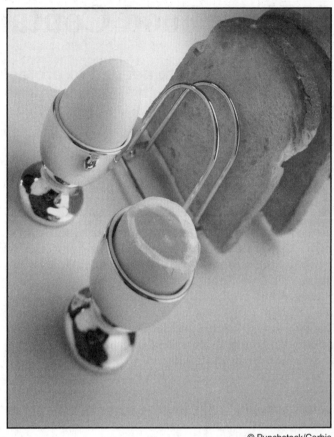

© Punchstock/Corbis

Even though animal foods are more likely to be contaminated, there has been an increase of food-borne illness from fruit and vegetable consumption. Articles in this unit present and discuss why food-borne illnesses are on the rise, major outbreaks, and farming practices such as irrigation, animal husbandry, and feeding that may directly affect contamination. Food processors and growers are taking steps to eliminate new outbreaks. Meat products go through thermal treatment to kill bacteria and pathogens before consumption, but fresh fruits and vegetables are not treated and are often consumed raw. Irradiation could offer a solution to this problem, inactivating the pathogens on fresh produce. Different types of radiation and its positive and negative effects on different characteristics of produce are discussed.

New technologies are being developed in order to protect our food supply from bacterial or even intentional contamination. Radio-frequency identification tags is one of the newest technologies described in this article. However, widespread adoption of this new equipment will not happen until government regulations are enacted. The last article in this unit informs the readers of the ways to protect themselves against food-borne illness and the steps they can take to reduce their chances of disease. It also summarizes what food producers and regulators are doing to protect their customers from harm.

Is Your Food Contaminated?

New approaches are needed to protect the food supply.

MARK FISCHETTI

Given the billions of food items that are packaged, purchased and consumed every day in the U.S., let alone the world, it is remarkable how few of them are contaminated. Yet since the terrorist attacks of September 11, 2001, "food defense" experts have grown increasingly worried that extremists might try to poison the food supply, either to kill people or to cripple the economy by undermining public confidence. At the same time, production of edible products is becoming ever more centralized, speeding the spread of natural contaminants, or those introduced purposely, from farms or processing plants to dinner tables everywhere. Mounting imports pose yet another rising risk, as recent restrictions on Chinese seafood containing drugs and pesticides attest.

Can the tainting of what we eat be prevented? And if toxins or pathogens do slip into the supply chain, can they be quickly detected to limit their harm to consumers? Tighter production procedures can go a long way toward protecting the public, and if they fail, smarter monitoring technologies can at least limit injury.

Tighten Security

Preventing a terrorist or a disgruntled employee from contaminating milk, juice, produce, meat or any type of comestible is a daunting problem. The food supply chain comprises a maze of steps, and virtually every one of them presents an opportunity for tampering. Blanket solutions are unlikely because "the chain differs from commodity to commodity," says David Hennessy, an economics professor at Iowa State University's Center for Agricultural and Rural Development. "Protecting dairy products is different from protecting apple juice, which is different from protecting beef."

Even within a given supply chain there are few technology-based quick fixes. Preventing contamination largely comes down to tightening physical plant security and processing procedures at every turn. Each farmer, rancher, processor, packager, shipper, wholesaler and retailer "has to identify every possible vulnerability in the facility and in their procedures and close up every hole," says Frank Busta, director of the National Center for Food Protection and Defense at the University of Minnesota. The effort begins with standard facility access controls, which Busta often refers to as "gates, guns and guards," but extends to thoroughly screening employees and carefully sampling products at all junctures across the facility at all times.

That advice seems sound, of course, but the challenge for operators is how best to button down procedures. Several systems for safeguarding food production have been rolled out in recent years. Though these are not required by any regulatory agency, Busta strongly recommends that producers implement them. In the U.S., that impetus has been made stronger by legislation such as the 2002 Bioterrorism Act and a 2004 presidential directive, both of which require closer scrutiny of ingredient suppliers and tighter control of manufacturing procedures.

The primary safeguard systems Busta recommends borrow from military practices. The newest tool, which the FDA and the U.S. Department of Agriculture are now promoting, carries the awkward name of CARVER + Shock. It is being adapted from Defense Department procedures for identifying a military service's greatest vulnerabilities. "CARVER + Shock is essentially a complete security audit," says Keith Schneider, associate professor at the University of Florida's department of food science and human nutrition. The approach analyzes every node in the system for factors that range from the likely success of different kinds of attacks to the magnitude of public health, economic and psychological effects (together, the "shock" value) that a given type of infiltration could cause.

Track Contaminants

No matter how tightly procedures are controlled, determined perpetrators could still find ways to introduce pathogens or poisons. And natural pathogens such as salmonella are always a

Detect, Track and Trace

If a natural pathogen, or a perpetrator, contaminates food, lives will be saved if the tainted product can be quickly detected, then traced back to its point of origin so the rest of the batch can be tracked down or recalled. The following technologies, in development, could help:

- **Microfluidic Detectors**—Botulinum bacteria produce the most poisonous toxin known. They and similar agents, such as tetanus, could be detected during food processing by microfluidic chips—self-contained diagnostic labs the size of a finger. The University of Wisconsin–Madison is crafting such a chip, lined with antibodies held in place by magnetic beads, that could detect botulism during milk production. The chip could sample milk before or after it was piped into tanker trucks that leave the dairy and before or after it was pasteurized at a production plant. Other chips could detect other toxins at various fluid-processing plants, such as those that produce apple juice, soup or baby formula.
- **Active Packaging**—*E. coli,* salmonella and other pathogens could be detected by small windows in packaging, such as the cellophane around meat or the plastic jar around peanut butter. The "intelligent" window would contain antibodies that bind to enzymes or metabolites produced by the microorganism, and if that occurred the patch would turn color. The challenge is to craft the windows from materials and reactants that can safely contact food. Similar biosensors could react if the contents reached a certain pH level or were exposed to high temperature, indicating spoilage. And they could sense if packaging was

tampered with, for example, by reacting to the pressure imposed by a syringe or to oxygen seeping in through a puncture hole.
- **RFID Tags**—Pallets or cases of a few select foods now sport radio-frequency identification (RFID) tags that, when read by a scanner, indicate which farm or processing plant the batch came from. Future tokens that are smaller, smarter and cheaper could adorn individual packages and log every facility they had passed through and when. The University of Florida is devising tags that could be read through fluid (traditional designs cannot) and thus could be embedded inside the wall of sour cream or yogurt containers. The university is also developing active tags that could record the temperatures a package had been exposed to.
- **Edible Tags**—Manufacturers often combine crops from many growers, such as spinach leaves, into a retail package, so tags affixed to bags might not help investigators track contamination back to a specific source. ARmark Authentication Technologies can print microscopic markers that indicate site of origin directly onto a spinach leaf, apple or pellet of dog food using a spray made from edible materials such as cellulose, vegetable oil or proteins. Also, the tiny size would be hard for terrorists to fake, making it harder for them to sneak toxin-laced counterfeit foods past inspectors and into the supply. As an alternative, DataLase can spray citrus fruits or meats with an edible film in a half-inch-diameter patch that is then exposed to a laser beam that writes identification codes within the film.

concern. Detecting these agents, tracing them back to the spot of introduction, and tracking which grocery stores and restaurants ended up with tainted products are therefore paramount. Putting such systems in place "is just as important as prevention," Schneider says.

Here new technology does play a major role, with various sensors applied at different points along the chain. "You can't expect one technology to counter all the possible taintings for a given food," notes Ken Lee, chairman of Ohio State University's department of food science and technology.

A variety of hardware is being developed [see box on top of this page], although little has been deployed commercially thus far. Radio-frequency identification (RFID) tags are furthest along, in part because the Defense Department and Wal-Mart have required their main suppliers to attach the tokens to pallets or cases of foodstuffs. The Metro AG supermarket chain in Germany has done the same. The ultimate intent is for automated readers to scan the tags at each step along the supply chain—from farm, orchard, ranch or processor, through

packaging, shipping and wholesale—and to report each item's location to a central registry. That way if a problem surfaces, investigators can quickly determine where the batch originated and which stores or facilities might have received goods from that batch and when. Retailers can also read the tags on their items to see if they have received a product later identified as suspicious.

As RFID tags get smaller and cheaper, they will be placed directly on individual items—on every bag of spinach, jar of peanut butter, container of shrimp and sack of dog food. "That way if a recall is issued, the items can be found as they run past a scanner at the checkout counter," says Jean-Pierre Émond, professor of agricultural and biological engineering at the University of Florida.

Universities and companies are developing all kinds of other tags, some that are very inexpensive and others that cost more but supply extensive information. Some tokens, for example, can sense if food has been exposed to warm temperatures and thus might be more likely to harbor *Escherichia coli* or

Intentional Poisonings

U.S., 1984,
salmonella in salad bars, by Rajneeshees cult,
751 sickened

China, 2002,
rat poison in breakfast foods, by competitor to the vendor,
400 sickened, over 40 killed

U.S., 2002,
nicotine sulfate in ground beef, by disgruntled worker,
111 sickened

salmonella. Other tags could track how long items spent in transit from node to node in the supply chain, which could indicate unusually long delays that might raise suspicion about tampering. So-called active packaging could detect contamination directly and warn consumers not to eat the product they are holding.

The big impediment for any marker, of course, is the price. "Right now it costs 25 cents to put an RFID tag on a case of lettuce," Émond notes. "But for some growers, that equals the profit they're going to make on that case."

To be embraced widely, therefore, he says tags will have to provide additional value to suppliers or buyers. His university has been conducting an ongoing project with Publix Super Markets and produce suppliers in Florida and California to assess the possibilities. In initial trials, tags tracked crates and pallets that were shipped from the growers to several of Publix's distribution centers. Information gleaned from scanning tags at various points was available to all the companies via a secure Internet site hosted by VeriSign, the data security firm. The compilation allowed the participants to more quickly resolve order discrepancies, to log how long food sat idle, and to reveal ways to raise shipping efficiency. The group plans to extend the test to retail stores.

The U.S. imports 50 percent more food than it did just five years ago.

Control Suppliers

Costs will not drop until new technologies are widely deployed, but food defense analysts say adoption is unlikely to occur until clear, streamlined regulations are enacted. That prospect, in turn, will remain remote until the highest levels of government are reformed. "There are more than a dozen different federal agencies that oversee some aspect of food safety," Lee points out, noting that simple coordination among

Making Imports Safer

Alarming warnings about Chinese products in recent months have shown how dangerous imported edibles can be. In March some 100 brands of pet food were recalled after they were found to contain melamine, a toxic chemical used as a cheap replacement for wheat gluten. Then in June the U.S. Food and Drug Administration issued alerts about five types of seafood that contained antibiotic residues, pesticides and salmonella.

After the seafood scare, Senator Charles Schumer of New York declared that the federal government should establish an import czar. He blamed poor control of imports on a lack of inspection and poor regulation, telling the *Washington Post* that "neither the Chinese or American government is doing their job."

Regardless of how safe domestic production is, "imports are our Achilles' heel," says Ken Lee, chairman of Ohio State University's department of food science and technology. "There is no global food regulator. If the Chinese want to put an adulterant into food, they can do it until they get caught. I'll wager it will happen again, because it's driven by the profit motive."

Realistically, no technology can ensure that imports are safe. The food in every shipping container entering a U.S. port or border crossing could be pulled and irradiated, and some comestibles such as spices are already processed this way. But industry says the step would add significant cost for producers and shipping delays for middlemen. And the public continues to be wary of the technology. Furthermore, although irradiation would kill pathogens, it would have no effect on poisons or adulterants.

Inspecting all incoming food would also require vast increases in FDA and U.S. Department of Agriculture budgets; the agencies currently inspect a meager 1 percent of imports. As a partial alternative, in June the FDA said it intended to conduct more inspections of products from countries it deems to have poorer food-safety controls, such as China, offset by fewer inspections of products from countries with stronger standards, such as Britain and Canada. The agency also said it might require importers and U.S. manufacturers that use imported ingredients to provide more detailed information about production processes at foreign suppliers.

The best recourse, Lee says, is for companies to insist that suppliers impose strict standards and that the companies send inspectors overseas to verify compliance. Other experts agree, adding that government edicts are not as effective. "Too often import requirements are used as trade barriers, and they just escalate," says David Hennessy, an economics professor at Iowa State University. "The food companies themselves have a lot to lose, however. When they source a product in a country, they ought to impose tough procedures there."

—M.F.

The Vigilant Kitchen

If contaminated food does make it into your grocery bag, smart appliances could still prevent it from reaching your mouth. Innovations that could reach commercial introduction are described here by Ken Lee of Ohio State University. "None of this technology would be visually obtrusive," he says, "and all of it would be easy to clean."

Pulsed Light

When homeowners are asleep, fixtures underneath cabinets emit pulses of ultraviolet light that kill germs on counter-tops and other surfaces.

Microwave

An infrared sensor gauges internal food temperature and compares it with safety guidelines, indicating when the proper value has been reached. Instead of entering a cooking time, a user enters the food type or target temperature.

Refrigerator

A built-in reader scans RFID tags on food and checks for recalls over a wireless Internet connection. (A homeowner could hold nonrefrigerator items under it, too.) The reader also notes expiration dates written into the tags and tracks when containers such as milk cartons are removed and put back, to see if they have been out for too long and therefore might be spoiled. A red light warns of trouble.

them is difficult enough, and efficient approval of sensible requirements is even harder to come by. The FDA regulates pizza with cheese on it, but the USDA regulates pizza if it has meat on it, quips Jacqueline Fletcher, professor of entomology and plant pathology at Oklahoma State University. "The requirements for organic farmers are different from those for nonorganic farmers."

Spurred by recent recalls, members of Congress have called for streamlining the regulation system. Illinois Senator Richard Durbin and Connecticut Representative Rosa DeLauro are advocating a single food-safety agency, but turf wars have hampered any progress toward that goal.

Concerned that more effective government is a long shot, experts say the responsibility for improved vigilance falls largely on food suppliers. "The strongest tool for stopping intentional contamination is supply-chain verification," says Shaun Kennedy, deputy director of the National Center for Food Protection and Defense. That means a brand-name provider such as Dole or a grocery store conglomerate such as Safeway must insist that every company involved in its supply chain implement the latest security procedures and detection, track and trace technologies or be dropped if it does not. The brand company should also validate compliance through inspections and other measures. The impetus falls on the brand-name provider because it has the most to lose. If a natural or man-made toxin is found in, say, a bag of Dole spinach or a container of Safeway milk, consumers will shun that particular label. "If a brand-name company wants to protect its products," Kennedy says, "it should validate every participant in the chain, all the way back to the farm."

Dirty Birds

Even 'Premium' Chickens Harbor Dangerous Bacteria

If you eat undercooked or mishandled chicken, our new tests indicate, you have a good chance of feeling miserable. CR's analysis of fresh, whole broilers bought nationwide revealed that 83 percent harbored campylobacter or salmonella, the leading bacterial causes of foodborne disease.

That's a stunning increase from 2003, when we reported finding that 49 percent tested positive for one or both pathogens. Leading chicken producers have stabilized the incidence of salmonella, but spiral-shaped campylobacter has wriggled onto more chickens than ever. And although the U.S. Department of Agriculture tests chickens for salmonella against a federal standard, it has not set a standard for campylobacter.

Our results show there should be. More than ever, it's up to consumers to make sure they protect themselves by cooking chicken to at least 165° F and guarding against cross-contamination.

Think premium brands are safer? Overall, chickens labeled as organic or raised without antibiotics and costing $3 to $5 per pound were more likely to harbor salmonella than were conventionally produced broilers that cost more like $1 per pound.

Moreover, most of the bacteria we tested from all types of contaminated chicken showed resistance to one or more antibiotics, including some fed to chickens to speed their growth and those prescribed to humans to treat infections. The findings suggest that some people who are sickened by chicken might need to try several antibiotics before finding one that works.

In the largest national analysis of contamination and antibiotic resistance in store-bought chicken ever published, we tested 525 fresh, whole broilers bought at supermarkets, mass merchandisers, gourmet shops, and natural-food stores in 23 states last spring. Represented in our tests were four leading brands (Foster Farms, Perdue, Pilgrim's Pride, and Tyson) and 10 organic and 12 nonorganic no-antibiotics brands, including three that are "air chilled" in a newer slaughterhouse process designed to reduce contamination. Among our findings:

- Campylobacter was present in 81 percent of the chickens, salmonella in 15 percent; both bacteria in 13 percent. Only 17 percent had neither pathogen. That's the lowest percentage of clean birds in all four of our tests since 1998, and far less than the 51 percent of clean birds we found for our 2003 report.
- No major brand fared better than others overall. Foster Farms, Pilgrim's Pride, and Tyson chickens were lower

in salmonella incidence than Perdue, but they were higher in campylobacter.

- There was an exception to the poor showing of most premium chickens. As in our previous tests, Ranger—a no-antibiotics brand sold in the Northwest—was extremely clean. Of the 10 samples we analyzed, none had salmonella, and only two had campylobacter.
- Among all brands, 84 percent of the salmonella and 67 percent of the campylobacter organisms we analyzed showed resistance to one or more antibiotics.

How the Bugs Get to You

Chickens become contaminated in many ways, among them by pecking at insects that pick up bacteria from the environment, pecking at droppings that carry germs, or drinking contaminated water. Both salmonella and campylobacter colonize the birds' intestines (usually without harm), but birds typically harbor more campylobacter than salmonella, and it spreads through flocks faster.

Among the measures taken to limit bacteria in chicken houses: disinfecting coops that may hold as many as 30,000 birds, shielding against bacterial carriers such as insects and rodents, ensuring that feed is clean, and using powerful ventilation systems to keep the chickens' bedding drier and less inviting to germs. But when a chicken is slaughtered, bacteria in its digestive tract can wind up on its carcass, where some hide in feather follicles.

To keep contamination in check, processors follow procedures collectively known as HACCP (pronounced hass-ip). The initials stand for Hazard Analysis and Critical Control Point, the consumer's main protection against contaminated chicken. HACCP requires companies to spell out where contamination could be controlled during processing, then build in procedures—such as scalding carcasses—to prevent it.

But our tests show the current practices aren't enough. Bell & Evans, producer of broilers raised without antibiotics, spent $30 million to modernize its processing plant in 2005, including $9 million for a high-tech air-chill system designed in part to reduce cross-contamination. The system whisks carcasses on two miles of track through chambers in which they're misted and chilled with air, then submerged in an antimicrobial dip. Tom Stone, the company's marketing director, says the measures helped reduce the rate of salmonella to less than 3 percent in recent in-house tests of chickens done before packaging. But in our tests of 28 store-bought chickens, 5 of the Bell & Evans samples had salmonella and 19 had campylobacter.

When contaminated chickens arrive at supermarkets, problems can multiply. Just one slip-up in storage, handling, or cooking, and you're at risk. Both salmonella and campylobacter can cause intestinal distress, and campylobacter can also lead to meningitis, arthritis, and Guillain-Barré syndrome, a neurological disorder. Campylobacter and salmonella from all food sources sickened more than 3.4 million Americans and killed more than 700, according to the latest estimates from the federal Centers for Disease Control and Prevention, dating from 1999.

The CDC notes that the rate of laboratory-confirmed infections has decreased somewhat since 2001. However, the toll may be far higher than the numbers indicate because only a small percentage of foodborne illnesses are reported to public-health authorities. The CDC said that in 2004, poultry was involved in 24 percent of outbreaks in which a single product was identified, up from 20 percent in 1998. Also in 2004, the CDC noted, 53 percent of campylobacter samples and 18 percent of salmonella samples were resistant to at least one antibiotic.

What the Numbers Showed

Contamination. Among the major brands, campylobacter incidence ranged from 74 percent, in Perdue, to 89 percent, in Tyson. Samples from organic and no-antibiotics brands, as a group, averaged within that range.

Salmonella incidence in Foster Farms, Tyson, and Pilgrim's Pride was 3 percent, 5 percent, and 8 percent, respectively—notably lower than in the organic and no-antibiotics types, which had an overall incidence of roughly 25 percent.

None of Ranger's 10 samples harbored salmonella. We questioned Rick Koplowitz, chief executive officer of Draper Valley Farms, which raises Ranger chickens, but he revealed no unusual measures to prevent contamination.

Antibiotic resistance. When we took bacteria samples from contaminated broilers and tested for sensitivity to antibiotics, there was evidence of resistance not just to individual drugs but to multiple classes of drugs. That indicates there may be fewer to choose from, and infections may be more stubborn. We didn't have enough data to assess whether there were differences in resistance among brands.

It's not surprising that we found antibiotic-resistant bacteria even in chickens that were raised without antibiotics: Those germs are widespread and can persist in the environment.

Twenty percent of campylobacter samples were resistant to ciprofloxacin (Cipro), a drug similar to the one the U.S. Food and Drug Administration banned chicken producers from using as of September 2005 to protect its effectiveness in people.

Holes in the Safety Net

Inspectors for the USDA's Food Safety and Inspection Service (FSIS) check carcasses in each plant and reject those with visible fecal matter, defects, and signs of illness. They also collect one broiler on each of 51 consecutive days of chicken production and have it tested for salmonella. Asked if the agency has enough funds to inspect chickens adequately, FSIS spokesman Steven Cohen said it did.

Germ Count

Levels of Contamination

Below, the percentages of tested broilers that harbored campylobacter or salmonella. We analyzed 78 chickens for each major brand and a total of 86 chickens for USDA organic brands and 125 for no-antibiotics brands. Figures are averages for brands and types. Ranking is based on contamination with campylobacter, more prevalent than salmonella.

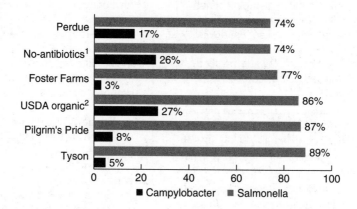

[1]Bell & Evans (air-chilled), Buddy's, Coleman, MBA Brand Smart Chicken (air-chilled), Murray's, North Country Farms, Ranger, Rocky, Rocky Jr., Springer Mountain Farms, Wegman's, and Whole Foods.

[2]Coastal Range, Coleman, D'Artagnan, Eberly's, Maverick Ranch, MBA Brand Smart Chicken (air-chilled), Organic Raised Right, Rosie, Whole Foods, and Wise.

Resistance to Antibiotics

We took a random selection of 162 bacteria samples from chicken that tested positive for campylobacter and 80 that tested positive for salmonella and determined how many samples resisted antibiotics that are usually effective against those pathogens. **Resistant** indicates the percentage of samples in which bacteria beat the antibiotic. You might end up taking a drug for longer or trying several before finding one that clears the infection. Differences among brands couldn't be evaluated because the sample size was small.

Salmonella	Resistant	Campylobacter	Resistant
Kanamycin	19%	Azithromycin	7%
Streptomycin	38	Erythromycin	7
Amoxicillin/ clavulanic acid	30	Telithromycin	4
		Clindamycin	3
Ampicillin	30	Ciprofloxacin	20
Cefoxitin	35	Nalidixic acid	19
Ceftlofur	31	Tetracycline	57
Ceftriaxone	0	One or more drugs	67
Nalidixic acid	3		
Sulfisoxazole	28		
Tetracycline	70		
One or more drugs	84		

[1]31 percent of samples were somewhat resistant: The antibiotic inhibited bacterial growth but did not stop it.

Among more-effective drugs on salmonella (0 or 1 percent bacteria samples were resistant): amikacin, gentamicin, chloramphenicol, ciprofloxacin, trimethoprim/sulfamethoxazole.

Among more-effective drugs on campylobacter: gentamicin, florfenicol.

Plants that produce more than 12 salmonella-positive samples during that time fail to meet the minimum federal standard. When a plant fails, the USDA can suspend chicken production, but it has no authority to levy fines and can't close plants by withdrawing inspectors solely because a plant doesn't meet the federal salmonella standard, a federal court ruled in 2001. To get processors to clean up their act, the USDA threatened in February 2006 to publicly disclose processors' salmonella test results.

A nonprofit group beat the agency to it. In July 2006, Food & Water Watch, an environmental health organization based in Washington, D.C., published the names of 106 chicken processing plants—including some operated by the four leading brands we tested—that failed federal salmonella standards in at least one test period between 1998 and 2005. When we contacted those four companies for comment, all said they've taken steps to reduce salmonella contamination.

In August 2006, the USDA reported that the rate of positive salmonella tests in broilers had jumped to 16.3 percent in 2005, up from 11.5 percent in 2002. Richard Lobb, a spokesman for the National Chicken Council, a trade group, said it's not clear why the rate went up in 2005, but he cited preliminary government data indicating that it has since declined. Cohen of the FSIS added that the agency has begun an initiative aimed at curbing salmonella by focusing on plants that failed the federal standard or had problems meeting it.

That leaves campylobacter. Now that a test method was recently validated, Cohen said, the USDA has announced it will begin collecting data on campylobacter in broilers in processing plants nationwide. It's too soon to say whether data collection will lead to a federal limit and routine testing, he added.

Based on our tests, that's what needs to happen. All indications are that it won't be easy to banish campylobacter, but the government can start by implementing a realistic standard, then start testing and monitoring in processing plants. Some of the chicken producers we asked said they already target campylobacter in HACCP plans. Others said they assume that what works against salmonella will also work against campylobacter. Clearly, it doesn't.

"The USDA has moved at glacial speeds on controlling campylobacter in the chicken industry," says Caroline Smith De Waal, director of food safety for the Center for Science in the Public Interest.

What You Can Do

Make chicken one of the last items you buy before heading to the checkout line. If you choose organic, no-antibiotics, or air-chilled chicken, do so for reasons other than avoiding bacteria.

- In the supermarket, choose well-wrapped chicken, and put it in a plastic bag to keep juices from leaking.
- Store chicken at 40°F or below. If you won't use it for a couple of days, freeze it.
- Thaw frozen chicken in a refrigerator (in its packaging and on a plate), or on a plate in a microwave oven. Cook chicken thawed in a microwave oven right away.
- Separate raw chicken from other foods. Immediately after preparing it, wash your hands with soap and water, and clean anything you or raw chicken touched.
- To kill harmful bacteria, cook chicken to at least 165°F.
- Don't return cooked meat to the plate that held it raw.
- Refrigerate or freeze leftovers within two hours of cooking.

Fear of Fresh

How to Avoid Food-Borne Illness from Fruits & Vegetables

BONNIE LIEBMAN AND ROBERT TAUXE

Q: Is it riskier to eat produce these days?

A: Yes. The outbreaks are bigger and more frequent than they were 20 or 30 or even 15 years ago. Even though we can identify and control outbreaks better than we used to, when contamination occurs with lettuce, spinach, cantaloupe, or tomatoes, we can have a big problem on our hands.

The headlines about *E. coli* O157:H7 in spinach tell the story. Since some produce is very conveniently packed in a bag and prewashed, there is nothing consumers can do to lower their risk. In many cases, you don't cook it. You don't blanch it. You don't do much except eat it. So it's critically important that it not be contaminated from the beginning.

Q: Why are outbreaks in produce on the rise in North America?

A: One reason is that people are eating more fresh fruits and vegetables than they did 30 years ago. That's a good thing. We want people to eat fresh produce. Before fresh spinach went off the market in the United States following the recent outbreak, something like a third of people we called had eaten fresh spinach in the previous week. That's great news.

Q: Are greens in bags causing more outbreaks?

A: Conceivably. Rather than just one head of lettuce or a bunch of spinach, there could be leaves from many different plants in one bag. Bacteria from one contaminated leaf in a bag, you can just imagine, would be over all the leaves in the bag by the end of the distribution chain.

It's a pooling issue, like ground beef. How many cows are in one patty of ground beef? How many cows contribute to one glass of milk? It means that procedures have to be in place to make sure that none of it is contaminated.

Q: Does the bacteria come from nearby animals?

A: Possibly. We know that feedlots have *E. coli* O157:H7. How wise is it to grow spinach or lettuce plants, which are very close to the ground, just downwind or downstream or down the hill from a feedlot or cow pasture? Doesn't sound like a good idea to me.

The produce industry has to figure out how to prevent contamination. Maybe we need a half-mile buffer between feedlots and produce farms.

Q: Does it help to wash produce?

A: We recommend washing produce in general, even if you plan to peel it. When you slice a melon, for example, the knife can transfer bacteria from the surface to the inside.

But it's tough to get bacteria off greens. Those germs are very sticky. This triple-washed stuff that comes out of the bag—if it's got contamination on it, there's no way to wash it off, even if you use bleach or detergent.

And you can't wash off germs if they're inside the melon, mango, or apple. For example, bacteria can creep in through the apple core. Germs can go in the hole at the very bottom of the apple where the flower was—it's called the calyx.

Q: Is organic produce less likely to have E. coli?

A: No. I don't see this as an organic versus conventional issue, just like it's not a domestic versus imported issue. There's room for improvement with both kinds of production and on both sides of the border.

Q: Which produce is most likely to have E. coli O157:H7?

A: The recurrent outbreaks have come from leafy greens— especially lettuce—sprouts, and unpasteurized juices and cider. It's not all fruits and vegetables. And apple cider might be a special case because it's sometimes made from apples that have fallen from the tree.

What those fruits and vegetables have in common is that they're grown fairly close to the ground, they're not cooked, and they're not acidic. In general, the bacteria that cause food-borne disease don't like acid. But North Americans have a phenomenal sweet tooth, and my understanding is that apples and tomatoes are getting sweeter and less tart and acidic.

Q: Is all food-borne disease rising?

A: No. Over the last ten years, we've witnessed important decreases, 29 to 32 percent, in infections that are related to meat and poultry—like *E. coli* O157:H7 linked to ground

Bugs Are Breaking out All Over

The Public Health Agency of Canada estimates that 11 million Canadians are sickened each year from food-borne bugs. The price tag: close to $600 million in hospitalization costs, medical expenses, and other "direct" costs, and some $100 million in premature deaths, lost productivity, and other "indirect" costs.

Here are some of the foods that are most likely to cause food-borne illness. The list is drawn from a database of some 5,000 outbreaks that sickened more than 150,000 people from 1990 through 2004. The database is maintained by the Centre for Science in the Public Interest (publisher of *Nutrition Action*). A few caveats from CSPI director of food safety Caroline Smith DeWaal:

- The database includes outbreaks that occurred entirely in the United States or in both Canada and the United States. It doesn't include outbreaks that were confined to Canada.
- Most food-borne illnesses are isolated cases, so outbreaks (two or more people sickened by the same food) are the exception.
- Many outbreaks and illnesses are never investigated or reported to authorities.
- Foods with multiple ingredients (like tacos, lasagna, cheeseburgers, chili, egg salad, stuffing, and some sandwiches) are in the database but most aren't listed here.

All Bugs (includes *E. coli* O15 :H)

Food	Outbreaks	Cases*
Greens-based salad	199	7,555
Turkey	109	5,832
Chicken	215	3,979
Ground beef	171	3,425
Shellfish	155	3,399
Berries	20	3,330
Tomatoes	19	2,852
Lettuce	56	2,380
Eggs	74	2,117
Ham	46	2,107
Sprouts	30	2,018
Ice cream	44	1,807
Cheese	50	1,791
Melon	29	1,683
Juice & cider	22	1,514
Unpasteurized milk	56	1,457
Scallions	9	1,221
Potatoes	40	1,099
Luncheon meat	50	1,014
Bread	32	980
Fresh tuna	193	824
Fruit salad	17	538
Mahi mahi	71	422
Fresh salmon	14	195

***E. coli* O157 :H7**

Food	Outbreaks	Cases*
Ground beef	107	2,028
Lettuce	12	336
Unpasteurized milk	4	222
Greens-based salad	9	216
Coleslaw	3	194
Apple cider/juice	6	142
Alfalfa sprouts	3	120
Potato salad	2	49
Melon	2	36

*Number of people sickened. (For the latest report from the CSPI outbreak database, see www.cspinet.org/foodsafety/outbreak_report.html.)
Source: *Outbreak Alert! 2005*, Centre for Science in the Public Interest.

beef; or *Listeria* infections, which are often linked to processed meats; or *Campylobacter,* which is linked to poultry.

We haven't eliminated them, but we're certainly headed in the right direction.

[There are no comparable statistics for Canada.]

Q: What about Salmonella?

A: It's down 9 percent. [Illnesses from *Salmonella* are also down in Canada.] *Salmonella* is complicated, because it can come from a number of foods and even non-food sources like pet turtles or lizards. And antibiotic-resistant *Salmonella*—much of it from ground beef—has become more of a problem over the last decade.

When to Call the Doctor

Q: Which symptoms should alert people to call the doctor?

A: The red flag is diarrheal illness that's not resolved in three days or that's accompanied by a fever over 38.6°C [101.5°F] or by blood in the stools.

If a very young child seems lethargic or doesn't seem to be making much urine or tears, that could be a sign of dehydration and is another reason to seek medical attention. Any young child with diarrhea should start drinking pediatric electrolyte solution—it's in all the drugstores—to prevent dehydration.

Q: How soon do the symptoms of E. coli O157:H7 show up?

A: They usually appear within 3 to 4 days, but it could be anywhere from 1 to 10 days. Most people have bloody diarrhea and severe abdominal cramps, but sometimes the infection causes non-bloody diarrhea or no symptoms at all. Usually the person gets little or no fever, and the illness resolves in 5 to 10 days.

Q: How many people end up with life-threatening complications?

A: About 3 to 8 percent get hemolytic uremic syndrome, or HUS. Some don't have complete kidney failure, but most do.

There are two parts to HUS. One is the kidney failure—that's uremia, the 'U.' The other is hemolysis, the 'H.' That's when red blood cells look like they've been through a blender.

The Dirty Dozen

Bug	Major Symptoms	Some Foods That Have Caused Outbreaks	How Soon It Typically Strikes	How Soon It Typically Ends
Campylobacter (bacteria)	diarrhea (can be bloody), cramps, fever, vomiting	undercooked poultry, unpasteurized (raw) milk, contaminated water	2 to 5 days	2 to 10 days
Ciguatera (toxin)	*within 2 to 6 hours:* abdominal pain, diarrhea, general pain and weakness, nausea, temperature reversal (hot things feel cold and cold things feel hot), tingling, vomiting *within 2 to 5 days:* slow heartbeat, low blood pressure	large reef fish like barracuda, grouper, red snapper, and amberjack	2 hours to 5 days	days to months
Clostridium botulinum (bacteria)	vomiting, diarrhea, blurred vision, double vision, difficulty swallowing, muscle weakness that spreads from the upper to the lower body	home-canned foods, improperly canned commercial foods, herb-infused oils, potatoes baked in aluminum foil, bottled garlic	12 to 72 hours	days to months (get treatment immediately)
Cyclospora (parasite)	diarrhea (usually watery), loss of appetite, substantial weight loss, stomach cramps, nausea, vomiting	imported berries, lettuce	1 to 14 days (usually at least 1 week)	weeks to months
E. coli O157:H7 (bacteria)	severe diarrhea that is often bloody, abdominal pain, vomiting (usually accompanied by little or no fever)	undercooked beef, unpasteurized (raw) milk or juice, raw produce, salami, contaminated water	1 to 8 days	5 to 10 days (get treatment immediately, especially for a child or elderly person)
Hepatitis A (virus)	diarrhea, dark urine, jaundice (yellow "whites" of the eyes), flu-like symptoms	shellfish, raw produce, foods that are not reheated after coming into contact with an infected food handler	15 to 50 days	2 weeks to 3 months
Listeria (bacteria)	fever, muscle aches, nausea, diarrhea (pregnant women may have mild flu-like symptoms; can lead to premature delivery or stillbirth)	fresh soft cheeses, unpasteurized (raw) or inadequately pasteurized milk, ready-to-eat deli meats and hot dogs	9 to 48 hours for gastrointestinal symptoms, 2 to 6 weeks for infections in the blood, brain, or uterus	days to months (get treatment immediately)
Noroviruses (virus)	nausea, vomiting (more common in children), abdominal cramping, diarrhea (more common in adults), fever	poorly cooked shellfish, ready-to-eat foods touched by infected food handlers, salads, sandwiches	12 to 48 hours	12 to 60 hours
Salmonella (bacteria)	diarrhea, fever, abdominal cramps, vomiting	eggs, poultry, unpasteurized (raw) milk or juice, cheese, raw produce	1 to 3 days	4 to 7 days
Scombrotoxin (toxin)	flushing; rash; burning sensation in skin, mouth, and throat; dizziness; hives; tingling	fresh tuna, bluefish, mackerel, marlin, mahi-mahi	1 minute to 3 hours	3 to 6 hours
Vibrio parahaemolyticus (bacteria)	watery diarrhea, abdominal cramps, nausea, vomiting	undercooked or raw seafood	2 to 48 hours	2 to 5 days
Vibrio vulnificus (bacteria)	vomiting, diarrhea, abdominal pain, bacteria in the blood, wounds that become infected	undercooked or raw shellfish (especially oysters), other contaminated seafood	1 to 7 days	2 to 8 days (get treatment immediately)

Source: Adapted from *Diagnosis and Management of Foodborne Illnesses: A Primer for Physicians and Other Health Care Professionals* (www.cdc.gov/mmwr/preview/mmwrhtml/rr5304a1.htm), by the American Medical Association, American Nurses Association, U.S. Centers for Disease Control and Prevention, U.S. Food and Drug Administration, and U.S. Department of Agriculture.

Safe at Home

How you handle food matters. With enough warmth, moisture, and nutrients, one bacterium that divides every half hour can produce 17 million progeny in 12 hours.

Putting food in the fridge or freezer stops most bacteria from growing. Exceptions: *Listeria* (typically found in soft cheese, lunch meats, and hot dogs) and *Yersinia enterocolitica* (typically found in undercooked pork and unpasteurized milk) grow at refrigerator temperatures.

Rules for Leftovers
2 Hours—2 Inches—4 Days

2 Hours from oven to refrigerator

Refrigerate or freeze leftovers within 2 hours of cooking. Otherwise throw them away.

2 Inches thick to cool it quick

Store food at a shallow depth—about 2 inches—to speed chilling.

4 Days in the refrigerator—otherwise freeze it

Use leftovers from the refrigerator within 4 days. Exception: use stuffing and gravy within 2 days. Reheat solid leftovers to 74°C (165°F) and liquid leftovers to a rolling boil. Toss what you don't finish.

- Buy **fresh-cut produce** like half a watermelon or bagged salad greens only if it's refrigerated or surrounded by ice.
- Store **perishable fresh fruits and vegetables** (like strawberries, lettuce, herbs, and mushrooms) or **precut or peeled produce** in a clean refrigerator at a temperature of 4°C (40°F) or below.
- Wash your hands for 20 seconds with warm water and soap before and after preparing **any food.**
- Wash **fruits and vegetables** under running water just before eating, cutting, or cooking, even if you plan to peel them. Don't use soap (it leaves a residue). Produce washes are okay. (Exception: triple-washed bagged lettuce or other produce needs no further washing.)
- Scrub **firm produce,** like melons and cucumbers, with a clean produce brush. Let them air dry before cutting.
- Remove the outer leaves of **heads of leafy vegetables** like cabbage and lettuce.
- Don't eat **raw sprouts** (alfalfa, bean, clover, or radish).
- Cooking a food at 71°C (160°F) will kill any *E. coli* O157:H7.
- Neither **processed spinach** (frozen or canned) nor **other fresh or processed leafy greens** (like lettuce or kale) were implicated in the recent *E. coli* outbreak.
- Drink only pasteurized **milk, juice, or cider.**
- For more information on handling produce safely: www.canfightbac.org, www.foodsafetynetwork.ca, food safety hotline (866-503-7638).
- For information on *E. coli* O157:H7: www.inspection.gc.ca/english/fssa /concen/cause/ecolie.shtml.

Sources: Canadian Food Inspection Agency, Canadian Partnership for Consumer Food Safety Education, U.S. Centers for Disease Control and Prevention, U.S. Department of Agriculture, U.S. Food and Drug Administration, Centre for Science in the Public Interest.

The *E. coli* toxin damages blood vessels by creating small strands across the insides, so when the red blood cells go through them, it's like they're going through a cheese cutter. It just slices up the red cells.

So people may need transfusions and dialysis before the blood vessels get better. They're destroying their own red blood cells. Even with intensive care, 3 to 5 percent of these patients die.

Q: Should doctors send a stool sample to the local health department?

A: That's absolutely vital to our tracing the outbreaks. But the doctor may wait to see if the diarrhea goes away in a few days. We recommend a stool specimen if it's a severe illness, bloody diarrhea, high fever, or if the illness is lasting.

A stool sample can also tell the doctor whether the infection will respond to an antibiotic and to which antibiotic. With so much resistant bacteria around, that could be especially important. But often the patient will get better with no antibiotics.

Q: Can antibiotics make E. coli O157:H7 infections worse?

A: There's a real paradox. The *E. coli* harms people by producing a toxin that destroys blood vessels in the gut, kidney, and brain. An antibiotic drug kills the *E. coli,* but it also can provoke them to make a lot more toxin. So it may make the patient worse. Antidiarrheal agents like Imodium should also be avoided.

What's Next?

Q: What new food-borne illnesses are emerging?

A: Some new and highly resistant strains of *Salmonella* have appeared in recent years. In Japan, they've seen cases of hepatitis E from pork sushi.

And in Finland, they're seeing outbreaks of *Yersinia pseudotuberculosis*. It's a second cousin to the bug that causes the plague. Finland recently realized that the outbreaks of what looks like appendicitis were due to this bug, which was traced to eating local lettuce.

Q: So people there may have unnecessary surgery for appendicitis?

A: Yes. Doctors perform surgery and find no problem with the appendix, but they see big swollen nodes all over the intestines. That's what the gastrointestinal tuberculosis looks like.

The working assumption is that *Yersinia* causes disease in deer and rabbits, which are getting into the lettuce and carrot fields and contaminating them. It's not a problem in this country, but there are other problems elsewhere in the world, and I expect that we'll be finding more of them in our food supply.

Q: What about in North America?

A: Some investigators have raised the possibility that the *E. coli* that causes urinary tract infections comes from the animals we eat, but the link is by no means proven.

Q: Have antibiotics made some Salmonella resistant?

A: Yes. Anytime an antibiotic is used in a hospital, in a child with an earache, or in animals on a farm, there are winners and losers in the local bacterial population. You hope that the losers are the bacteria that were making the patient, child, or animal sick. But if there's a bacterium there that's resistant, it's a winner.

The bacteria in food that make us ill—like *Salmonella* or *Campylobacter*—have their natural home in animals, not people. So antibiotic use in those animals can make those bacteria resistant.

Q: Are bacteria that live in people also becoming resistant?

A: Yes. The antibiotics we use in people cause resistance in the bacteria that cause pneumonia and tuberculosis. We have to try to reduce unnecessary antibiotic use for people who have colds. Antibiotics aren't going to make them better. Likewise, we have to promote prudent antibiotic use in animals.

Q: And the farm is where contamination starts?

A: Right. Most of the progress we've made with *E. coli, Listeria,* and *Campylobacter* has been at the slaughterhouse. The process is cleaner than it was before. But many of the animals coming in off ranches and farms are still contaminated.

And I'm concerned that back on the farm, bugs are transferring from animals to plants or cycling back and forth from animals to plants. You can't slaughter a spinach plant in a way that guarantees that it comes out clean. So the effort has to be focused on the farm, and that includes the animal farm.

Q: Should people stop eating leafy greens?

A: No. We want to encourage people to eat fresh fruits and vegetables. But obviously, the spinach problem—and previous problems with lettuce, tomatoes, and other fresh produce—show us that contamination is not under control.

ROBERT TAUXE is Acting Deputy Director of the Division of Foodborne, Bacterial and Mycotic Diseases at the U.S. Centers for Disease Control and Prevention. He spoke to *Nutrition Action*'s Bonnie Liebman by phone from his office in Atlanta, Georgia.

Irradiation of Fresh Fruits and Vegetables

Irradiation could provide a kill step to enhance safety of fresh and fresh-cut produce, but challenges remain for full commercial application.

Xuetong Fan, Brendan A. Niemira, and Anuradha Prakash

Consumption of fresh and fresh-cut fruits and vegetables in the United States has increased every year in the past decade, because of their convenience and nutritional benefits. Unfortunately, the increasing consumption of fresh produce has been accompanied with an increase in the number of outbreaks and recalls due to contamination with human pathogens.

Fresh fruits and vegetables carry the potential risk of contamination because they are generally grown in open fields with potential exposure to enteric pathogens from soil, irrigation water, manure, wildlife, or other sources. Unlike meat and meat products to which a kill step (thermal treatment) is applied before being consumed, fresh produce is often consumed without cooking or other treatments that could eliminate pathogens that may be present.

The recent *Escherichia coli* O157:H7 illness outbreaks and product recalls of spinach, lettuce, and other leafy greens, most notably in 2006 and 2007, have gained much media attention and raised public concerns over produce safety. The fresh produce industry is in need of a kill step to ensure the safety of produce. Ionizing radiation is known to effectively eliminate human pathogens such as *E. coli* O157:H7 on fresh produce.

This article reviews the latest knowledge about irradiation inactivation of human pathogens on and in fresh-cut produce and its impact on the quality of produce. It also highlights current developments in irradiation regulation and labeling, the challenge and opportunity for commercial application, and research needs.

Types of Ionizing Radiation

Radiation is in every part of our lives, and we encounter it every day in the natural environment. Common types of radiation include radio frequency, visible light, infrared light, microwave, and ultraviolet light. More energetic forms of radiation, such as gamma-ray, X-ray, and electron beams are called ionizing radiations because they are capable of producing ions, electronically charged atoms or molecules. All three types of ionizing radiation have the same mechanisms in terms of their effects on foods and microorganisms.

Water is the principal target of ionizing radiation. The radiolysis of water generates free radicals, and these radicals, in turn, attack other components such as DNA in microorganisms.

Water is the principal target of ionizing radiation. The radiolysis of water generates free radicals, and these radicals, in turn, attack other components such as DNA in microorganisms. Each type of ionizing radiation has its own advantages and disadvantages. For example, gamma rays and X-rays have higher penetration ability than electron beams. However, gamma rays are emitted by radioactive materials, such as cobalt-60 and cesium-137, while generation of X-rays is a relatively inefficient and energy-intensive process. Most energy (about 90%) is lost to heat during the conversion of electron beams into X-rays. Electron beams have a low penetration ability, even though the electron beam generators can be switched on and off and do not involve radioactive materials.

Effectiveness in Inactivating Pathogens

Historically, the high radiation doses used in attempts to produce a sterile or shelf-stable fruit or vegetable commodity have resulted in unpalatable products. Of specific interest within the context of modern produce processing is the potential for incorporating lower irradiation doses, lower than 3 kGy, as one of several "hurdles" in an otherwise conventional produce processing system. Recent research has consistently shown that irradiation effectively kills bacterial pathogens on fresh and fresh-cut produce (Smith and Pillai, 2004; Niemira and Fan, 2005). This efficacy holds for human bacterial pathogens such as *E. coli* O157:H7, *Salmonella,* and *Listeria monocytogenes,* as well as for bacterial phytopathogens and spoilage organisms.

Irradiation doses that will result in a 1-log reduction in bacterial pathogens are typically in the range of 0.2–0.8 kGy. In contrast, pathogenic viruses and fungi are generally more resistant to irradiation, often requiring 1–3 kGy to achieve 1-log reduction (Niemira and Fan, 2005). To achieve meaningful reductions of viruses and fungi, the doses required are typically above what most produce will tolerate.

In terms of food safety, it should be noted that on an annual basis, the majority of minor foodborne illnesses are caused by viruses (67%), while the majority of serious foodborne illnesses resulting in hospitalizations and deaths (60% and 72%, respectively) stem from bacterial pathogens (Mead et al., 1999). As an intervention, irradiation is thus most suited for elimination of the most serious safety threats for consumers of fruits and vegetables.

The antimicrobial efficacy of irradiation is influenced by a number of factors, including the pathogen being targeted as the primary safety concern, the type of produce being treated, the condition of the fruit or vegetable (whole vs cored, peeled, cut, chopped, etc.), the atmosphere in which it is packaged, and other commodity-specific factors (Niemira and Fan, 2005). Like any other industrial food processing technology, the methodological details of time, temperature, handling, and irradiation protocols must undergo process validation for the product being treated. For example, irradiation protocols developed for elimination of *E. coli* O157:H7 from leafy greens may not achieve the required food safety and quality benchmarks if applied for the elimination of *Salmonella* from tomatoes.

One area of recent research focuses on determining the ability of irradiation to kill internalized, biofilm-associated, or otherwise protected pathogens. These protective environments dramatically reduce the efficacy of chemicals and other conventional treatment options, often by orders of magnitude (Niemira and Fan, 2005). Initial data in this emerging field of research suggest that *Salmonella* and *E. coli* O157:H7 in biofilms are effectively eliminated by irradiation, although the specific response depends on the pathogen type and maturity (Niemira, 2007).

Cells of *E. coli* O157:H7 that are internalized appear to be more resistant to irradiation than surface-associated cells (Table 1). At 1 kGy, pathogens such as *E. coli* O157:H7 on the surface of fresh-cut produce can be reduced by 3–8 logs, while internalized pathogens are only reduced by 2–3 logs. Additional research is needed to more fully understand the influence of internalization on pathogens, and on the efficacy of irradiation and other treatments.

Table 1 Dose Required to Achieve a 1 Log Reduction for *E. coli* O157:H7 Inoculated on or in Fresh-Cut Produce, Then Irradiated with Gamma Rays

Product	D_{10} Value (kGy)	
	On Surface	Inside
Iceberg lettuce	0.14	0.30
Boston lettuce	0.14	0.45
Red leaf lettuce	0.12	0.35
Green leaf lettuce	0.12	0.37
Romaine lettuce	0.21	0.39
Baby spinach	0.24	0.45
Green onion, long cut	0.26	0.42
Green onion, short cut	0.28	0.42

From Niemira and Fan (2007).

Quality of Irradiated Fresh Produce

At low dose levels (1 kGy or less), most fresh-cut vegetables show little change in appearance, flavor, color, and texture, although some products can lose firmness. As an example, the appearance of irradiated spinach was similar to that of the non-irradiated samples after 14 days storage at 4°C. Some vegetables such as fresh-cut cilantro can tolerate 3.85 kGy of radiation (Foley et al., 2004). In fact, the destruction of spoilage organisms increases the shelf life of most fresh and fresh-cut vegetables (Prakash and Foley, 2004; Niemira and Fan, 2005). The response to irradiation is specific to product, and even similar varieties, as shown in studies on various lettuce types (Niemira et al., 2002), exhibit differences in texture and respiration rates.

Irradiation's effect on permeability and functionality of cell membranes can result in electrolyte leakage and loss of tissue integrity.

Appearance and leakage. Irradiation's effect on permeability and functionality of cell membranes can result in electrolyte leakage and loss of tissue integrity. These effects are limited at dose levels below 1 kGy, but at higher dose levels, electrolyte leakage may cause a soggy and wilted appearance. The increase in electrolyte leakage varies among vegetables (Table 2). In a study of 13 vegetables, Fan and Sokorai (2005) observed that red cabbage, broccoli, and endive had the lowest increases in electrolyte leakage, while celery, carrot, and green onion had the most increases in leakage.

Texture. Irradiation may induce the loss of firmness (softening) in some fruits (Gunes et al., 2000; Palekar et al., 2004).

Table 2 Electrolyte Leakage of Fresh-Cut Vegetables as a Function of Radiation Dose[a]

Vegetable	Leakage (%)							
	0 kGy	0.5	1	1.5	2.0	2.5	3.0	LSD$_{0.05}$[b]
Broccoli	0.6	0.7	0.7	0.8	0.7	1.2	1.1	0.4
Endive	1.5	1.7	1.8	2.3	2.2	3.2	3.1	0.6
Red cabbage	1.3	1.4	1.4	1.9	1.8	2.0	2.5	0.5
Green leaf lettuce	2.5	3.1	3.9	3.4	3.2	4.4	4.8	0.8
Parsley	2.1	2.1	2.6	3.0	3.7	3.7	4.7	1.1
Romaine lettuce	1.4	2.8	3.3	4.1	3.8	5.7	5.1	1.5
Iceberg lettuce	1.4	1.9	2.4	2.6	3.2	3.8	4.3	1.1
Spinach	2.8	3.4	3.3	3.8	4.1	5.4	6.2	1.2
Red leaf lettuce	3.5	3.7	4.6	5.0	5.0	6.8	8.5	1.3
Celery	2.1	3.4	3.3	4.9	6.9	8.4	9.8	1.3
Cilantro	1.4	1.8	2.1	2.4	3.1	4.3	4.1	0.9
Green onion	3.8	5.2	7.1	7.0	9.5	12.5	12.4	1.6
Carrots	2.8	3.1	3.8	4.4	5.7	6.1	8.6	1.0

[a]Vegetables were irradiated with 0, 0.5, 1.0, 1.5, 2.0, 2.5, and 3.0 kGy of gamma radiation at 5°C in air, then electrolyte leakage was measured.
[b]Least significant difference at $P<0.05$.
Modified from Fan and Sokorai (2005).

Irradiation-induced loss of firmness is related to partial depolymerization of cell-wall polysaccharides, cellulose, and pectin and to changes in activity of the cell-wall enzymes pectinmethylesterase and polygalacturonase that act on pectic substrates. However, the loss of firmness can be mitigated by dipping diced tomatoes and fresh-cut apples in a calcium solution prior to irradiation (Gunes et al., 2000; Prakash et al., 2007) and by storing the products in modified-atmosphere packaging (Boynton et al., 2006).

Irradiated (1 kGy) cilantro (Fan et al., 2003a) and lettuce (Fan et al., 2003b) showed some softening, but after a few days of storage, there was no significant difference between irradiated and non-irradiated samples. Other products, such as celery (Prakash et al., 2000), mushroom slices (Koorapati et al., 2004), and shredded carrots (Hagenmaier and Baker, 1998), also showed no change in firmness.

Flavor and aroma. At low dose levels (≤1 kGy), few if any effects on flavor and aroma are observed in fresh and fresh-cut vegetables. A decrease in characteristic aroma of cilantro (Fan et al., 2003a) and off-flavor of Bell peppers (Masson, 2002) has been observed at doses of ≥3 kGy. Changes in flavor and aroma of fresh vegetables are highly correlated with microbial spoilage. Thus, irradiation generally inhibits or delays development of off-flavors related to growth of spoilage organisms.

At low dose levels (≤1 kGy), few if any effects on flavor and aroma are observed in fresh and fresh-cut vegetables.

Nutritional quality. At low dose levels (≤1 kGy), the effects on nutritional quality are minimal. Irradiation can reduce ascorbic acid (vitamin C) in some vegetables, but the decrease is generally insignificant, given the natural variation observed in fresh produce, and does not exceed the decrease seen during storage (Fan and Sokorai, 2002). Irradiation converts ascorbic acid to dehydroascorbic acid, both of which exhibit biological activity and are readily interconvertible. Irradiation can also increase phenolic content of certain vegetables, thus increasing their antioxidant capacity (Fan, 2005). However, since phenolic compounds are also responsible for the browning reactions in vegetables, their increase is not a desired outcome.

In general, the effect of irradiation on quality of fresh and fresh-cut vegetables is minimal. In those cases where significant changes are seen at effective dose levels, effects on texture, color, or browning can be minimized by combining irradiation with other technologies such as calcium dips, modified-atmosphere packaging, or antibrowning agents.

Regulatory Approval, Labeling, and Safety

Currently in the U.S., irradiation of whole fruits and vegetables is approved only for insect control and shelf-life extension, with a maximum allowable dose of 1 kGy (Table 3). The use of irradiation for the purpose of enhancing microbial food safety has not been approved by the Food and Drug Administration. However, FDA is evaluating a petition, filed by the Food Irradiation Coalition, asking for the use of irradiation to enhance safety of fresh-cut produce at doses up to 4.5 kGy.

Table 3 Foods Permitted to Be Irradiated

Type of Food	Purpose	Maximum Dose (kGy)
Fresh, non-heated processed pork	Control of *Trichinella spiralis*	1
Fresh produce	Growth and maturation inhibition	1
Fresh produce	Arthropod disinfection	1
Dry or dehydrated enzyme preparations	Microbial disinfection	10
Dry or dehydrated spices/seasonings	Microbial disinfection	30
Fresh or frozen, uncooked poultry products	Pathogen control	3
Frozen packaged meats (solely NASA)	Sterilization	44
Refrigerated, uncooked meat products	Pathogen control	4.5
Frozen uncooked meat products	Pathogen control	7
Fresh shell eggs	Control of *Salmonella*	3.0
Seeds for sprouting	Control of microbial pathogens	8.0
Fresh or frozen molluscan shellfish	Control of *Vibrio* species and other foodborne pathogens	5.5

From FDA (2007c).

Under current FDA rules, foods that have been irradiated must bear both a "Radura" logo and a statement that the food has been "treated with radiation" or "treated by irradiation." Earlier last year, FDA proposed a change in the labeling of irradiated foods (FDA, 2007b). Under the proposed rule, only irradiated foods in which irradiation causes a material change in the food would need to be labeled with the Radura logo and either of those statements. The term "material change" refers to a change in the organoleptic, nutritional, or functional properties of a food. In addition, FDA would allow petitions for the use of alternative labeling, such as "pasteurized" or "pasteurization," for a food that has been treated by irradiation, where the irradiation results in the same level of pathogen reduction as thermal pasteurization. These changes are still under consideration by FDA, and a final ruling has not yet been made.

In multi-generational studies, animals fed irradiation-sterilized foods throughout their life were healthy and nutritionally satisfied, with no evidence of any negative nutritional or developmental effects. More recently, FDA has investigated the possibility that furan, a possible carcinogen present in canned meats, soups, and many other conventional thermally processed foods, might also be produced during irradiation. Studies demonstrated that irradiation at 5 kGy did not induce detectable levels of furan in most fresh-cut fruits and vegetables. In those few fruits where furan was detectable after irradiation, the levels were much lower than those in many thermally processed foods (Fan and Sokorai, 2007).

Consumer Acceptance

Adoption of irradiation for food applications has been a slow process. The limited number of foods approved by regulatory agencies, cost, consumer reluctance to accept irradiated foods, and the public's uncertainty of this technology may contribute to its minimal commercialization.

Studies on marketing of irradiated foods have demonstrated that consumers are more willing to buy irradiated foods after they are provided information about the process (Bhumiratana et al., 2007). Typically, fewer than half will buy the irradiated food if given a choice between an irradiated product and the non-irradiated product. If consumers are first educated about food irradiation and food safety, most of them will buy the product in these marketing tests.

In a survey conducted by *The Packer* (Anonymous, 2007), 63% of growers/shippers believe that the produce industry should push for irradiation or similar treatments if produce is not damaged in the process; 40% of packers think the industry should push for irradiation or similar treatments, with the same percentage undecided; more than 30% of growers/shippers think consumers are ready to buy irradiated produce, particularly leafy greens; but only 25% of retailers think consumers are ready to buy irradiated produce, leafy greens in particular—about 7% of retailers stock irradiated produce.

It seems that enthusiasm about the commercial application of irradiation on fresh produce decreases from growers/shippers, to packers, to retailers, and to consumers. Therefore, educating retailers and consumers about irradiation processing may be needed to advance the commercial applications of this technology.

Packaging

Packaging is another important aspect of food irradiation. FDA has approved about 10 polymeric packaging materials for use during irradiation of prepackaged foods. Package materials currently used by the produce industry are diversified. Most polymeric packaging materials that are used by the produce industry have been approved by FDA. The agency allows industry to submit requests for exemption from regulation if the use of the substance in the food-contact article results in a dietary concentration at or below 0.5 ppb. As a result, Proveit, on behalf of Sadex Inc., has successfully petitioned FDA to expand the packaging materials for irradiated foods (FDA, 2007a).

Specifically, FDA allows the use of all approved packaging materials to package food being irradiated, provided that the packaged food is already permitted by FDA, the packaging materials are subjected to radiation doses not exceeding 3 kGy, and the packaged food is irradiated in an oxygen-free environment or while the food is frozen and contained under vacuum.

Unfortunately, the exemptions cannot be applied for fresh-cut produce because fresh-cut produce cannot be frozen or processed in an oxygen-free environment (even though nitrogen is used for flushing some packages of leafy vegetables). Fresh-cut produce is usually packaged with oxygen levels of 1–20% and therefore does not qualify under the exemption.

The majority of fresh-cut produce is packaged in polyolefin film bags, which themselves are mostly approved under 21 CFR 179.45 without any limitation on oxygen environment. However, these polyolefins may contain additives that have not been approved for use during irradiation. Therefore, packaging materials intended for irradiation of prepackaged fresh-cut produce in the presence of oxygen may still need premarket approval.

In addition, packaging materials are very complex, and emerging new packaging materials present a challenge to FDA. For example, polyethylene terephthalate (PET) films are approved by FDA under 21 CFR 179.45, but rigid and semi-rigid PET polymers are not (Komolprasert, 2007). New materials such as degradable and antimicrobial packages, adjuvants (antioxidants, stabilizers, etc.), plasticizers, colorants, and adsorbent pads may need more research before being evaluated and approved by FDA (Komolprasert, 2007).

Additional Research Needed

More studies on sensory analysis of irradiated fresh produce are needed. In addition, similar to studies on consumer acceptance of ground beef and chicken, consumer acceptance of irradiated produce needs to be evaluated, especially within the context of recent outbreaks related to produce.

Fresh produce is unique because fresh-cut fruits and vegetables are promoted as fresh and nutritious. However, it is unknown whether the word "irradiation" will affect the consumer perception of "freshness" of irradiated produce. In its recent proposal of labeling changes, FDA (2007b) expressed interest in receiving information on whether the control of foodborne pathogens changes the characteristics of food in a way outside of normal variation, which would therefore require additional labeling to inform the consumer of such changes. Thus, studies are needed to determine irradiation conditions that would minimize changes in organoleptic, nutritional, or functional properties, if any, that would constitute a material change to the consumer.

Because the response of each type (cultivar, species, whole vs fresh-cut, etc.) of fruits and vegetables to irradiation varies, process validation is required for each. While much work has been done already, it is important to prioritize future studies and products that need to be evaluated by their implication in outbreaks and/or volume of consumption.

As mentioned above, radiation resistance of pathogens is influenced by their environment. More research is needed to determine radiation resistance of internalized and biofilm-associated pathogens. In addition, radiation resistance of pathogens is mostly determined by artificially inoculating fresh-cut produce to high populations before irradiation. Ideally, radiation resistance of pathogens should be determined using naturally contaminated produce and levels of pathogens similar to those found in naturally contaminated produce.

Furthermore, the effect of modified-atmosphere packaging on radiation resistance of pathogens requires more investigation. In most studies on determining radiation resistance of pathogens, the inoculated samples were irradiated in air, whereas many fresh-cut produce are packaged in modified atmosphere. The modified atmosphere (low O_2 and high CO_2 levels) may alter the radiation resistance of pathogens. Other areas, such as packaging materials, may need approval and research before irradiation is fully applied by the produce industry.

Thus, low-dose irradiation is a reliable technology capable of killing human pathogens such as *E. coli* O157:H7 and *Salmonella* by 2–8 logs without causing significant deterioration in product quality. There are many challenges ahead for commercial application of irradiation for fresh and fresh-cut produce, including regulatory approval, packaging materials, consumer acceptance, and lack of premarket studies.

References

Anonymous. 2007. Produce pulse. *The Packer* 114(6): A1, A4.

Bhumiratana, N., Belden, L.K., and Bruhn, C.M. 2007. Effect of an educational program on attitudes of California consumers toward food irradiation. *Food Protection Trends* 27: 744–748.

Boynton, B.B., Welt, B.A., Sims, C.A., Balaban, M.O., Brecht, J.K., and Marshall, M.R. 2006. Effects of low-dose electron beam irradiation on respiration, microbiology, texture, color, and sensory characteristics of fresh-cut cantaloupe stored in modified-atmosphere packages. *J. Food Sci.* 71: S149–S155.

Fan, X. 2005. Antioxidant capacity of fresh-cut vegetables exposed to ionizing radiation. *J. Sci. Food Agric.* 85: 995–1000.

Fan, X. and Sokorai, K.J.B. 2002. Sensorial and chemical quality of gamma irradiated fresh-cut iceberg lettuce in modified atmosphere packages. *J. Food Protect.* 65: 1760–1765.

Fan, X. and Sokorai, K.J.B. 2005. Assessment of radiation sensitivity of fresh-cut vegetables using electrolyte leakage measurement. *Postharvest Biol. Technol.* 36: 191–197.

Fan, X. and Sokorai, K.J.B. 2007. Formation of furan from fresh fruits and vegetables due to ionizing radiation. *J. Food Sci.* (in press).

Fan, X., Niemira, B.A., and Sokorai, K.J.B. 2003a. Sensorial, nutritional and microbiological quality of fresh cilantro leaves as influenced by ionizing irradiation and storage. *Food Res. Intl.* 36: 713–719.

Fan, X., Toivonen, P.M.A., Rajkowski, K.T., and Sokorai, K.J.B. 2003b. Warm water treatment in combination with modified atmosphere packaging reduced undesirable effects or irradiation on the quality of fresh-cut iceberg lettuce. *J. Agric. Food Chem.* 50: 1231–1236.

FDA. 2007a. Threshold of regulation exemptions. Food and Drug Admin. www.cfsan.fda. gov/~dms/opa-torx.html, accessed Oct. 25.

FDA. 2007b. Irradiation in the production, processing and handling of food. Proposed rules. Fed. Reg. 72: 16291–16306. www.cfsan .fda.gov/~lrd/ fr070404.html, accessed Oct. 25.

FDA. 2007c. Foods permitted to be irradiated under FDA's regulations (21 CFR 179.26). http://www.cfsan.fda.gov/~dms/ irrafood.html, accessed Oct. 25.

FDA. 2007d. Packaging materials listed in 21 CFR 179.45 for use during irradiation of prepackaged foods. http://www.cfsan.fda .gov/~dms/irrapack.html, accessed Oct. 25.

Foley, D., Euper, M., Caporaso, F., and Prakash, A. 2004. Irradiation and chlorination effectively reduces *Escherichia coli* O157:H7 inoculated on cilantro (*Coriandrum sativum*) without negatively affecting quality. *J. Food Protect.* 67: 2092–2098.

Gunes, G., Watkins, C.B., and Hotchkiss, J.H. 2000. Effects of irradiation on respiration and ethylene production of apple slices. *J. Sci. Food Agric.* 80: 1169–1175.

Hagenmaier, R.D., and Baker, R.A. 1998. Microbial population of shredded carrot in modified atmosphere packaging as related to irradiation treatment. *J. Food Sci.* 63: 162–164.

Komolprasert, V. 2007. Packaging for foods treated with ionizing radiation. In "Packaging for Non-Thermal Processing of Food," ed. J.H. Han, pp. 87–116. Blackwell Publishing, Ames, Iowa.

Koorapati, A., Foley, D., Pilling, R., and Prakash, A. 2004. Electron-beam irradiation preserves the quality of white button mushroom (*Agaricus bisporus*) slices. *J. Food Sci.* 69: S25–S29.

Masson, S. 2002. Effects of gamma irradiation on the shelf-life and quality characteristics of diced bell peppers. M.S. thesis. Chapman Univ., Orange, Calif.

Mead, P.S., Slutsker, L., Dietz, V., McCaig, L.F., Bresee, J.S., Shapiro, C., Griffin, P.M., and Tauxe, R.V. 1999. Food-related illness and death in the United States. *Emerg. Infect. Dis.* 5: 607–625.

Niemira, B.A. 2007. Irradiation sensitivity of planktonic and biofilm-associated *Escherichia coli* O157:H7 isolates is influenced by culture conditions. *Appl. Environ. Microbiol.* 73: 3239–3244.

Niemira, B.A., and Fan, X. 2005. Low-dose irradiation of fresh and fresh-cut produce: Safety, sensory and shelf life. In "Food Irradiation Research and Technology," ed. C. Sommers and X. Fan, pp. 169–181. Blackwell Publishing and the Institute of Food Technologists, Ames, Iowa.

Niemira, B.A., and Fan, X. 2007. Ionizing radiation enhances microbial safety of fresh and fresh-cut fruits and vegetables while maintaining product quality. Abstract# 042-03 Institute of Food Technologists Ann. Mtg., Chicago, IL.

Niemira, B.A., Sommers, C.H., and Fan, X. 2002. Suspending lettuce type influences recoverability and radiation sensitivity of *Escherichia coli* O157:H7. *J. Food Protect.* 65: 1388–1393.

Palekar, M.P., Cabrera-Diaz, E., KalbasiAshtari, A., Maxim, J.E., Miller, R.K., Cisneros-Zevallos, L., and Castillo, A. 2004. Effect of electron beam irradiation on the bacterial load and sensorial quality of sliced cantaloupe. *J. Food Sci.* 69: M267–M273.

Prakash, A., and Foley, D. 2004. Improving safety and extending shelf-life of fresh-cut fruits and vegetables using irradiation. In "Irradiation of Food and Packaging: Recent Developments," ed. V. Komolprasert and K.M. Morehouse, pp. 90–106. American Chemical Soc., Washington, D.C.

Prakash, A., Chen, P.C., Pilling, R., Johnson, N., and Foley, D. 2007. 1% Calcium chloride treatment in combination with gamma irradiation improves microbial and physicochemical properties of diced tomatoes. *Foodborne Pathogens Dis.* 4(1): 89–97.

Smith, J.S., and Pillai, S. 2004. Irradiation and food safety. An IFT Scientific Status Summary. *Food Technol.* 58(11): 48–55.

XUETONG FAN (xuetong.fan@ars.usda.gov) and **BRENDAN A. NIEMIRA** (brendan.niemira@ars.usda.gov) are, respectively, Research Food Technologist and Microbiologist, U.S. Dept. of Agriculture, Agricultural Research Service, Eastern Regional Research Center, 600 E. Mermaid Ln., Wyndmoor, PA 19038. **ANURADHA PRAKASH** (prakash@chapman.edu) is Professor, Chapman University, One University Dr., Orange, CA 92866. The authors are Professional Members of IFT. Send reprint requests to Xuetong Fan.

The *E. Coli* Outbreak

Lettuce Learn a Lesson

There are initiatives in place to guard against it—yet contaminated produce led to cases of illness and death. Are food safety regulations too soft or is it a matter of noncompliance?

SHARON PALMER, RD

When the *E. coli O157:H7* breakout related to fresh spinach hit the news last fall, it hit big. If people were looking for an excuse not to eat their dark, leafy greens, now they had one. Although people have grown accustomed to being buffeted by food poisoning reports on the evening news, this particular outbreak really hit home.

The sheer scope of the spinach outbreak was undeniable. An estimated 51 cases of illnesses per outbreak are linked with produce.[1] This outbreak was roughly four times that size. People wondered for weeks how something as supposedly healthy as fresh spinach could cause illness and death. In a survey by NBC11—which serves San Jose, San Francisco, and Oakland, Calif.—21% of voters to date have indicated that they will never eat spinach again unless it is locally grown.[2]

The FDA traced the spinach outbreak that sickened 204 people and killed three to four fields on four ranches located in Monterey and San Benito counties in California where the spinach was grown by third-party growers. The FDA reported on September 29, 2006, that all spinach implicated in the outbreak was traced back to the company Natural Selection Foods of San Juan Bautista, Calif.

Not Just a Meat Problem

While our food safety focus has often centered on the processing and handling of raw meat and poultry, this outbreak opened our eyes to a new era of food-borne illness dawning on produce farms. The fact that some consumers open bags of prewashed and prechopped fresh greens and dump them onto their dinner plates without cooking or washing them further increases the gravity of the situation.

For many, the *E. coli* outbreak in spinach came as no surprise. Since 1998, the FDA has warned fruit and vegetable producers about the potential of *E. coli O157:H7* contamination. A previous outbreak in October 2003 involving fresh spinach and *E. coli O157:H7* contamination in California resulted in 16 cases of illness and two deaths.

"Fresh produce was not a big source of food-borne illness. It was typically associated with meat items, but now the discussion is on fresh fruits and vegetables. It sounds an alarm for everyone in food safety practices," says John Krakowski, MA, RD, CDN, a food safety coach in Flanders, N.Y. An approximate 29% reduction in the number of *E. coli O157:H7* cases has occurred since 1996 to 1998, thanks to measures targeting ground beef safety and Hazard Analysis and Critical Control Point (HACCP).[3]

"The general impression among experts in the field is that the number and seriousness of outbreaks is greatest in produce, sprouts, and juices," says Charles Benbrook, chief scientist at The Organic Center in Enterprise, Ore. The Organic Center recently published a Critical Issue Report on *E. coli O157:H7* that discusses its relationship to agriculture.

Under the Microscope

There are more than 225 unique strains of *E. coli* and the majority of them are not dangerous. *E. coli* bacteria are essential to the healthy functioning of human and animal digestive systems, but some types have picked up extra genetic material that can turn harmless bacterium into a threat. *E. coli O157* is among the most dangerous strains when people are exposed to it. *E. coli O157:H7* doesn't harm cattle because it does not bind to the walls of their gastrointestinal tract. In humans, the bacterium causes diarrhea that is often bloody and can be accompanied by abdominal cramps or fever. Symptoms usually occur within two to three days following exposure. Healthy adults can typically shake *E. coli O157:H7*, but people at high risk, such as young children and older adults, can develop hemolytic uremic syndrome, which can lead to serious kidney damage and death.

> "The general impression among experts in the field is that the number and seriousness of outbreaks is greatest in produce, sprouts, and juices," says Charles Benbrook, chief scientist at The Organic Center in Enterprise, Ore.

E. coli O157:H7 is particularly pesky because it survives heat, drying, and acidic conditions and causes infections at very low doses. It has also been known to survive in soil for up to six months. The first case of *E. coli O157:H7* was reported in 1975 and the first outbreak followed in 1982. The 8,598 cases associated with 350 outbreaks of *E. coli O157:H7* reported to the Centers for Disease Control and Prevention from 1982 to 2002 accounted for less than one tenth of 1% of the total number of cases during those years.[4]

E. Coli's Link to the Land

As investigators tracked down the source of *E. coli O157:H7* contamination in fresh spinach, they discovered that all tests performed on Natural Selection Foods processing facilities by independent scientists and government investigators came up clean, indicating that the *E. coli* contamination occurred in the fields. The plant's triple washing procedure didn't appear to successfully remove the *E. coli O157:H7* from the spinach, prompting food safety experts to realize that produce needs to be clean at the time it enters processing.

Specific samples of cattle feces on one of the implicated ranches tested positive based on the genetic fingerprints for the same strain of *E. coli O157:H7* responsible for the outbreak. These results brought the whole connection of agriculture and food safety from the shadows. Since *E. coli* can survive in soil, water in troughs, and raw cattle manure for months, consider the myriad ways it could find itself onto a wrinkly leaf of spinach. The outbreak highlights how farming systems, cattle and dairy cow manure, animal husbandry and feeding practices, irrigation water quality, sanitation in field workers, fertilizers, and agricultural regulations play into food safety.

Perhaps it was a red flag when cases of *E. coli O157:H7* illness were reported due to children being infected at county fair petting zoos. Approximately 11% of the cattle fecal samples tested for *E. coli O157:H7* at Minnesota county fairs in 2000 and 2001 tested positive.[5]

The Farm, an Open Environment

Farms are all about wide open spaces—you can't seal them off into sterile biospheres. Issues of previous land use, adjacent land use practices, and water safety all come into play. And then there's that nagging problem of animal waste from nearby livestock or even wildlife.

Krakowski points out, "Fruits and vegetables are grown in nature's restroom." Agricultural experts believe that even wildlife and birds may play a role in spreading *E. coli*. Indeed, investigators found a positive match for *E. coli O157:H7* in the guts of a feral pig killed on the property of one of the identified ranches where the strain was found. There were signs that pigs had broken through a fence to eat the spinach. Although officials have not pinpointed feral pigs as the bacteria's carrier, this discovery has caused concerns about access of wildlife to crops.

Enough Bugs to Go Around

Just ponder the many ways *E. coli* could rear its ugly head on a farm and plenty of ideas pop into your head. "My first thought when I heard about the spinach outbreak was: Did a farmer change his [child's] diaper . . . before heading to the fields without first washing his hands?" says Amy Barr, MS, EdM, RD, cofounder of Marr Barr Communications, a strategic marketing and communications agency specializing in food, nutrition, health, lifestyle, and sustainability. Officials reported that the contamination route for the spinach outbreak may have been via wandering livestock, substandard worker hygiene, irrigation practices, or even wild boar.

One farming issue experts worry about is manure practices. Benbrook reports that there are clearly problems that arise as a result of manure lagoons and manure overflowing. Dairy farms using concrete alleys and flushing systems were eight times more likely to test positive for *E. coli O157:H7* than other manure removal systems. Benbrook suggests improvements can come from developing vegetative buffer strips along creeks and irrigation canals and having healthy, biologically active, organic soil with many different microbes that decrease pathogens due to competition.

A study looking at *E. coli O157:H7* cases in Canada found that the application to cropland of raw manure by a manure spreader or as liquid slurry was the second most significant variable explaining the geographic distribution of *E. coli* illnesses. (The strongest association was for the ratio of cattle to humans.)[6]

"We always need to control any run-off problems. Run-off can cause huge cross-contamination issues around both big and small farms," says Barr, who grew up on a small farm in the Midwest and recently observed a farmer in New England using a front-end loader to dump manure from a barn onto his land with a stream running through it.

The manure problem flows right into another big area of concern: water. The potential for irrigation ditches and canals to be contaminated is a serious risk. We know contaminated drinking water and water in lakes and pools have triggered cases of illness linked to *E. coli O157:H7* in the past.

"A big eye opener is water and how we use water and take care of water. When we pollute water in one part of the food system, it comes back to bite us in another part—it is all connected," says Alison H. Harmon, PhD, RD, LN, assistant professor of food and nutrition and director of the dietetics program at Montana State University and Sustainable Agriculture and Food Systems cochair of the Hunger and Environmental Nutrition Dietetic Practice Group.

The Great Cattle Debate

When samples of cattle fecal matter from one implicated ranch from the spinach outbreak tested positive for the same strain of *E. coli* bacteria that sickened people, the link between cattle and crops became significant. The fecal matter specimens were found one half mile to one mile from the produce field, which abutted the livestock pastures.

Most of *E. coli O157:H7* comes from the digestive systems of beef and dairy cattle. Less than 1% to more than 10% of cattle tested are found to shed *E. coli O157:H7*, which enters the environment when it is shed in the manure of infected cattle. Once unleashed in the environment, other animals can harbor it without apparently suffering from it.

"It is widely accepted that the antibiotics used in livestock accelerate the rate of genetic adaptation in bacteria. The evidence is overwhelming that antibiotics in pork and poultry lead to the emergence of new antibiotic-resistant strains of bacteria," says Benbrook.

"It is clear that cattle on forage diets are much less likely to shed *E. coli O157:H7* in manure than grain-fed cattle," says Benbrook. When cows are fed high-energy, grain-based diets, the pH in their digestive systems changes to favor *E. coli O157:H7*.

But Barr notes that while there's a lot to be said for avoiding feeding excessive amounts of grains to ruminants, after frost and before spring greening ranchers in most areas of the country can't rely on pasture. "Snow happens. Plus, most 'pasture-based' farmers, especially dairy farmers, also supplement their livestock's diets with grain," says Barr. "It's not black and white. If you feed cattle less grain, you're not going to eliminate *E. coli.*"

Some also argue that antibiotic use on livestock fosters genetic mutations capable of turning generic *E. coli* into a dangerous variant such as *E. coli O157:H7*. "It is widely accepted that the antibiotics used in livestock accelerate the rate of genetic adaptation in bacteria. The evidence is overwhelming

that antibiotics in pork and poultry lead to the emergence of new antibiotic-resistant strains of bacteria," says Benbrook. "If there's one antibiotic-resistant gene somewhere in the environment, there are numerous ways to get it into cattle. Agriculture has done far more than its fair share to create antibiotic-resistant bacteria and further spread it."

Research has found varying levels of antibiotic resistance in *E. coli O157:H7* serotypes. A study on isolates from cattle, humans, swine, and farms collected from 1985 to 2000 found that 39% of the *E. coli* isolates were resistant to one or more antimicrobials.[7]

One Big Salad Bowl

Here's a good question: Do people even think about where the leafy greens came from before they rip into a pretty, cellophane bag of precut salad purchased at their local supermarket? It was a shock when the spinach outbreak highlighted the fact that the spinach involved in making people sick in 26 different states and Canada all came from Natural Selection Foods in the Salinas Valley. To make matters worse, five other companies issued voluntary recalls since their products may have contained spinach from Natural Selection Foods. On top of that, Natural Selection Foods has 20 other brands—from Earthbound Farm and Dole Food Company, Inc. to Trader Joe's and Sysco—that were also recalled. Salinas Valley isn't called the "nation's salad bowl" for nothing—75% of the country's fresh spinach comes from this region.

Jennifer Wilkins, PhD, RD, senior extension associate at the division of nutritional sciences at Cornell University, pointed out in her "Food Citizen" column in the *Albany Times Union* on October 1, 2006, that the outbreak was amplified because the contaminated spinach from one or a few farms was mixed with spinach from numerous other farms, then bagged by a few processors, marketed under several brands, and distributed nationally and internationally.[8] This sort of centralized food system has more opportunities for contamination that can reach many people, while a smaller, local food system is easier to trace and does not offer such widespread consequences.

"One big problem is the traceability of foods. When people buy their food in a grocery store, they don't know how it got there. We do not know the history of the food and we have lost our connection to the land," says Harmon. "I see this as an encouragement to localize."

Regulations Down on the Farm

Experts feared the big one was coming. There had been 19 outbreaks of food-borne illness caused by *E. coli O157:H7* in lettuce or leafy greens. The FDA had written a letter to the lettuce industry in November 2005 warning about the ongoing risk for product contamination. The FDA developed the Lettuce Safety Initiative in response to recurring outbreaks of *E. coli O157:H7* in lettuce with the goal of reducing public health risk by focusing on the product, agents, and areas of greatest concern. In August 2006, the California Department of Health Services, the USDA, and the FDA met with industry and academia to further clarify the goals and plan the Lettuce Safety Initiative. Then all hell broke loose.

What sort of regulations are in place for produce growers? Farmers need to comply with FDA, Environmental Protection Agency, USDA, Occupational Safety & Health Administration, U.S. Department of Labor, and state and local regulations. The FDA also developed the voluntary Guide to Minimize Microbial Food Safety Hazards for Fresh Fruits and Vegetables in 1998, which offers the industry guidance on Good Agricultural Practices (GAPs). The guide covers agricultural water, wild and domestic animals, worker health and hygiene, the production environment, postharvest water quality, and sanitation of faculties and equipment.

"The current food safety program components or tools such as GAP, HACCP, and GMPs [Good Manufacturing Practices] are sound and effective at reducing risk of food-borne illness. But clearly everyone in the industry must know about these tools and understand how to use them effectively," says David Gombas, PhD, vice president of scientific and technical affairs at United Fresh Produce Association.

In reaction to the spinach outbreak, the FDA and the State of California now expect the industry to develop a plan that will minimize the risk of another outbreak, but the implementation of the plan will be voluntary. One big problem some complain about is the word *voluntary,* which shows up in guidelines to the industry.

Marion Nestle, PhD, MPH, reported in an editorial posted on October 23, 2006, in *The Mercury News* that the food safety system needs an overhaul, noting that Congress has not given the FDA the authority or resources to enforce safety procedures on farms.[9]

Building Farm Firewalls for Food Safety

Some produce growers and processors are taking charge of food safety. "The industry is evaluating and enhancing best practices, evaluating and recommending means of compliance, and, together with the government, academia, and industry experts, developing a long-term research agenda. We now must focus on ensuring industrywide compliance of current and future best practices," says Gombas.

Natural Selection Foods and Earthbound Farm set in place an unprecedented food safety program on September 28, 2006, that includes rigorous testing and analysis of field operations from the seed to harvest. They report that the seed, irrigation water, soil, soil amendments, plant tissues, and wildlife will be tested, monitored, and certified. The sanitation protocols for farm equipment, packaging supplies, and transportation vehicles will be enhanced and monitored. And they have installed a "firewall," which means that every lot of freshly harvested greens brought to their facility will be

---

Safe Produce Resource Guide

Centers for Disease Control and Prevention, http://www.cdc.gov

FDA, Center for Food Safety and Applied Nutrition, http://www.cfsan.fda.gov

Gateway to Government Food Safety Information, http://www.foodsafety.gov

International Food Information Council, http://www.ific.org

National Restaurant Association Educational Foundation, http://www.nraef.org

Partnership for Food Safety Education, http://www.fightbac.org

USDA Food Safety Information Center, http://foodsafety.nal.usda.gov

---

tested before entering their processing stream. This program is modeled after the program the beef industry successfully implemented.

Earthbound Farm reported that they will have heightened protocols fully implemented in all growing fields by spring 2007, such as certifying that seeds are free of pathogens prior to planting; certifying that soil amendments such as compost and fertilizers are free of contaminants before they are used; testing and monitoring water sources for harmful bacteria; regularly monitoring environmental conditions in the field; making frequent, unannounced inspections of growers' fields and equipment; training field harvesters on quality standards and sanitation; and refrigerating salad greens within the hour they're harvested and maintaining an unbroken cold chain.

Benbrook says, "I take my hat off to Natural Selection Foods. These are unprecedented preventative food safety measures."

Western Growers, an agriculture trade association whose members grow, pack, and ship 90% of the fresh fruits, nuts, and vegetables grown in California and 75% in Arizona (roughly one half of the nation's fresh produce), also announced that it would take action to initiate a California Marketing Agreement and a Marketing Order that would establish mandatory GAPs to strengthen spinach and leafy green food safety practices.

Education on the Farm-Food Safety Connection

The FDA and growers have pointed out that consumers need to be educated that fresh perishable produce and precut or peeled produce need to be stored in a clean refrigerator at temperatures of 40° F or below. The FDA, in conjunction with the Produce Marketing Association and the Partnership for Food Safety Education, has developed a national produce handling education campaign to help better educate consumers on handling produce.

"Dietitians need to know about food safety. We have to be spokespeople. We want people to have faith in the food supply," says Krakowski, who reports that something as simple as educating people to rinse fruits and vegetables and use vegetable brushes on produce before they are consumed is important. "Food safety is part of the dietary guidelines. It should be included when dietitians talk to their clients."

"I think some dietitians have a hard time seeing how agriculture relates, but it's all related to health," says Harmon, who notes that educating the public about food safety is an important part of the field. "The first message is to keep food safe in the kitchen, and then there's keeping it safe in the big picture, which involves a discussion about knowing how food is grown and how it is produced. We have a big job to do."

Sharon Palmer, RD, is a contributing editor at *Today's Dietitian* and a freelance food and nutrition writer in southern California.

For references, view article on our archive at www.TodaysDietitian.com.

Produce Safety: Back to Basics for Producers and Consumers

Feeling a little uneasy these days about the health-promoting properties of those fresh fruits and vegetables? Have we learned to love the invisible army of phytonutrients, vitamins, and minerals fighting the good fight for our long-term health, only to be reminded of the insidious presence of an equally invisible army of foodborne bacteria with the potential to make us sick?

According to the Centers for Disease Control and Prevention, there are approximately 76 million cases of foodborne illness reported in the United States each year. To reduce the incidence of foodborne illness, the actions taken to prevent produce contamination must be diligent and consistent, beginning on the farm and continuing through the entire food-handling process to consumer preparation.

Although proper cooking will kill most pathogens that may be present in or on a food, recent outbreaks in the United States have involved fresh produce that was not cooked before being consumed. Nevertheless, the consumption of raw fresh fruits and vegetables provides numerous valuable dietary nutrients. Therefore, it is important to consider ways to enhance the safety of these foods so that consumers can continue to enjoy fresh produce, whether it is cooked or uncooked.

Consumers want to reduce the risk in food; therefore, food producers and government regulators work tirelessly to do this as much as possible. There are also steps that consumers can take to reduce that risk. Still, an absolute absence of risk, even for food, simply is not possible.

Many factors can contribute to the risk of foodborne illness. Pathogens (any disease-producing agent) may be introduced by the exposure of foods to improperly processed manure used as fertilizer or to manure from animals on the farm. Exposure to foodborne pathogens may also occur because of the use of bad-quality water in irrigation or as a result of poor worker hygiene. Inferior storage and preparation practices, such as the storage of food at improper temperatures and cross-contamination among foods, can also further the growth of pathogens that are already present.

Food producers and suppliers, including farmers, processors, distributors, grocery stores, and restaurants that prepare and sell food to consumers, all play a significant role in reducing foodborne illness risk. Foods must be grown, harvested, packed, processed, and distributed in a manner that minimizes microbial contamination.

Produce growers and processors have recognized the importance of preventing contamination at each step from farm to fork, as the pathogens present on these foods are difficult to remove. For example, the natural curve and curling characteristics of lettuce and leafy greens provide a safe haven for microbial stowaways.

What Are Food Producers and Regulators Doing to Protect Consumers?

The actions that industry and government regulators have taken to protect consumers from foodborne illness can be broken down into four categories: (1) preventing contamination; (2) minimizing actual harm to the public if contamination has occurred; (3) improving communications among food producers, regulators, and the public; and (4) research into how and where foodborne illnesses arise in produce, and identify actions that can be taken to reduce these risks.

Numerous local actions have been ramped up as the result of the recent outbreaks. In January 2007, the produce industry—supported by industry representatives in the processing, distribution, and retail industries—called for the application of mandatory, strong, consistent, science-based, safety standards to both domestic and imported produce.

What Can Consumers Do to Protect Themselves?

It is important to remember that we do not live in a world free from risk. Thus, although consumers must understand that foodborne illness is a real risk, health care professionals can convey that prevention is possible and provide them with specific steps to prevent the consumption of foodborne pathogens. The Fight-BAC! campaign, managed by the Partnership for Food Safety Education is an excellent resource for consumer guidance for safe food handling procedures (www.fightbac.org). The four steps are simple and memorable:

- Clean: Wash hands and surfaces often
- Separate: Don't cross-contaminate
- Cook: Cook to proper temperature
- Chill: Refrigerate promptly

The FightBAC! Web site, as well as the International Food Information Council Foundation's brochure *A Consumer's Guide to Food Safety Risks* (http://ific.org/publications/other/consumersguideom.cfm), provide specific guidance for each step.

Fresh fruits and vegetables should be rinsed under running tap water. Fruits and vegetables with firm skins should be rubbed under running tap water or scrubbed with a clean cloth or paper towel. The use of detergent or bleach to wash produce is unnecessary and potentially hazardous, but even foods that will be peeled should be washed first. If pathogens are camped out on the rind of a cantaloupe, a perfectly clean knife could transfer the pathogen from the rind to the edible flesh with one slice.

Tips to Keep Your Kitchen Clean

Always wash all surfaces and utensils that come into contact with food with soap and hot water after each use. To kill bacteria, sanitize surfaces and utensil that come into contact with food with a solution of one to three tablespoons of household chlorine bleach per gallon of water, let stand two minutes; rinse, and allow the surface to air dry.

Creating and Sustaining Change

The incidence of foodborne illness can be reduced significantly, and consumers can play a leading role in making that happen. Together, the integrated actions of consumers, food suppliers, and regulators not only will reduce the incidence of foodborne illness, but also will sustain the wholesomeness of the food that we eat.

Reprinted from *Food Insight,* March/April 2007, published by the International Food Information Council Foundation.

UNIT 7

World Hunger, Nutrition, and Sustainability

Unit Selections

44. **In Search of Sustainability,** Karen Nachay
45. **A Question of Sustenance,** Gary Stix
46. **Pushing Beyond the Earth's Limits,** Lester R. Brown
47. **Draining Our Future: The Growing Shortage of Freshwater,** Lester R. Brown
48. **10 Reasons Why Organic Can Feed the World,** Ed Hamer and Mark Anslow

Key Points to Consider

- How extensive is global hunger and malnutrition? Give specific examples.

- What is the role of global food companies in world hunger and malnutrition?

- Offer several solutions to decreasing or eliminating food insecurity and malnutrition in the developing world.

- What are some steps you can take to reduce water consumption?

- How do your food choices affect the environment? Is it realistic for people to try buying organic foods, locally grown and in season?

Student Website
www.mhhe.com/cls

Internet References

Food and Agriculture Organization of the United Nations (FAO)
 www.fao.org/economic/ess/food-security-statistics/en/
Population Reference Bureau
 www.prb.org
World Health Organization (WHO)
 www.who.int/en

The cause of malnutrition worldwide is multifold, led by extreme poverty, inclement growing conditions, poor soil quality, and lack of access to clean water. Approximately 840 million people are malnourished in the developing world. Children under 5 years suffer long-term effects of malnutrition since adequate nutrition is essential for growth and brain development. Protein energy malnutrition weakens the immune system, leading to increased susceptibility to the biological contaminants in the unclean water supply of developing nations. Infectious disease kills approximately 10 million children each year due to impaired immunity secondary to malnutrition. Thus, the Director General of the Food and Agriculture Organization of the United Nations (FAO) launched, in 1994, a Special Program for Food Security (SPFS) for low-income, food-deficit countries (LIFDCs), which was endorsed by the World Food Summit held in Rome in 1996. They pledged to increase food production and access to food in LIFDCs so that the number of malnourished people would be reduced by half. They set goals to increase sustainable agricultural production within the cultural, political, and economic environment of each country to improve access to food, increase the role of trade, and to prepare for famine and food emergencies.

Malnutrition is the main culprit for lowered resistance to disease, infection, and death, especially in children. The malnutrition–infection combination results in stunted growth, lowered mental development in children, lowered productivity, and higher incidence of degenerative disease in adulthood. This directly affects the economies of developing countries. Over 1 billion people globally suffer from micronutrient malnutrition frequently called "hidden hunger." In addition, partnerships between the public and private sectors may prove valuable in combating malnutrition. Solutions to these problems such as building sustainability through indigenous knowledge and practices that are community based and environmentally friendly with emphasis on biofortification and dietary diversification may combat hunger and nutrient deficiencies in the future.

Nutrient deficiencies magnify the effect of disease, resulting in more severe symptoms and greater complications. For example, vitamin A deficiency leads to blindness in about 250,000–300,000 children annually and exacerbates the symptoms of measles. Iron deficiency, which is widespread among pregnant women and those in the child-bearing years in developing countries, increases the risk of death from hemorrhage in their offspring and reduces physical productivity and learning capacity. Finally, iodine deficiency causes brain damage and mental retardation. It is estimated that 1.5 billion people are at risk for iodine deficiency disorders.

Malnutrition does not only affect children and adults in developing countries, but is also prevalent in the United States. Thirty million Americans, of whom 11 million are children, experience food insecurity and hunger. In a country where one-fifth of the food is wasted and 130 pounds of food per person is disposed of, it is unacceptable that Americans go hungry. Gleaning is an initiative that is growing in popularity to make use of excess crops that lay unpicked in the fields. Gleaning programs locate excess produce from farms, harvest the produce, and distribute it to food insecure communities.

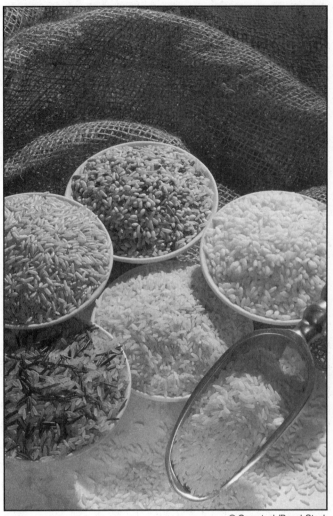

© Comstock/PunchStock

The primary nutrient deficiencies in this country, as in developing countries, are iron deficiency anemia, common in infants, young children, and teens, and lead poisoning. Undernourished pregnant women give birth to low-weight babies who suffer developmental delays and increases in mortality rate. Another group in the United States that experiences health problems due to hunger is the elderly.

One of the ways to feed the world is by organic farming. Organic crops use 25 percent less energy than chemically produced crops, produce higher yield, emit less greenhouse gases, and encourage biodiversity, which maintains soil fertility and supports natural pest control. These are just a few of the reasons we must begin to implement organic farming practices if we are going to feed the growing population.

Another alarming issue is that the earth's supply of fresh water is declining. Water tables all over the world are being depleted at a very fast rate. What many people don't realize though is that with a shortage of water also comes a shortage of food; water is necessary to raise livestock and grow crops. One of the articles in this unit raises awareness, reveals just how serious the world's water crisis is, and makes suggestions on how we can resolve the problem.

On the other hand, thanks to globalization, the Western diet is now being adopted all over the world. Developing countries that are dealing with problems of starvation usually in the rural areas are simultaneously dealing with problems of obesity in communities of stronger economic standing. This nutrition transition is becoming a challenge among scientists and policy makers as they try to offer solutions for two diametrically opposing problems.

Food security is now critical to consumers worldwide. The movement for purchasing local and seasonal foods with regard for the environment attempts to reconnect the consumer to the farmer, producer, or purveyor. In response to consumer demands, food companies are finding ways to improve the sustainability of their processing and packaging operations and be more environmentally conscious. From energy efficient processing plants to reducing or modifying packaging material, one article informs you on how these companies are trying to deal with the problems faced by our environment.

In Search of Sustainability

Seeking to reduce energy costs and to protect the environment, companies are exploring 'green' manufacturing practices and sustainable/renewable packaging applications.

KAREN NACHAY

Skyrocketing energy costs are hitting our pocketbooks, and a growing awareness of environmental issues is affecting our lifestyles. As a result, members of both the public and business communities are examining ways to reduce costs and promote their environmental consciousness by using renewable or sustainable sources of energy rather than nonrenewable sources like fossil fuels. As people reduce the number of miles they drive and switch from plastic to paper, or better yet, reusable cloth bags, they are also looking toward business to make sound changes. And many businesses are responding by installing technologies to help reduce energy usage and costs, redesigning packaging to use less material, or engineering innovative processing methods.

"It is no longer enough to create a quality product," said John Z. Blazevich, CEO of Contessa Premium Foods, Los Angeles, Calif., which opened the doors to a fully energy-efficient, eco-friendly frozen food plant earlier this year. "How you produce it is now the most important thing. Consumers are concerned about global warming and many blame big business for its role in it."

Companies are learning that this not only makes good sense for the environment, it makes good business sense, too. Information Resources Inc. recently conducted a survey that asked 22,000 U.S. consumers about their purchasing habits of products marketed as sustainable or green in four categories: eco-friendly products, eco-friendly packaging, organic, and fair treatment of employees and suppliers. The results revealed that about 30% of consumers look for eco-friendly products and packaging when choosing between brands. Consumers age 55 and older were much more likely to take these four categories into consideration when making a purchase. (See sidebar, "Green Products Gain Market Share," on page 192 for more information about the purchasing habits of consumers.)

"It's a new reality that manufacturers and retailers will need to address with new products and unique assortments to tap into emerging growth potential," said Andrew Salzman, Chief Marketing Officer, IRI. "Safeguarding the environment in whatever small way is becoming a consumer priority. And all successful consumer packaged goods industry mainstays live by one basic fact of life: The consumer's priorities are the industry's priorities."

Developing and implementing environmentally friendly initiatives and sourcing sustainable ingredients and raw materials are not always easy, as the process often requires a large investment, both financially and in the commitment from the company, its employees, and, quite often, the community. This article will provide information about what some food companies—both large and small—have done to improve the sustainable and eco-friendly nature of their processing and packaging operations.

Green Plants Save Energy

The food industry requires energy and water for processing, storage, and transport of food and beverage products, and the cost can be quite burdensome. Food processors, realizing the need to reduce their energy costs, as well as to lower greenhouse gas emissions, are harnessing the power of the wind and sun—sources of renewable energy—as well as recycling and reusing water from processing streams, installing energy-efficient equipment, and designing buildings with improved ventilation systems and more natural light. And even food by-products and organic food waste become sources of energy as part of companies' solid waste management and recycling efforts. For example, H.J. Heinz Co., Pittsburgh, Pa., in May announced plans to reduce greenhouse gas emissions through a series of initiatives, among them converting potato peels from its Ontario, Ore., facility into biofuel that will be sold to a local natural gas pipeline grid. And Miller Brewing Co., Milwaukee, Wis., operates a brewery in Irwindale, Calif., where brewery wastewater is recycled to generate bio-gas used to power electrical generators (Miller, 2008).

Frito-Lay, Plano, Texas, a division of PepsiCo, let the sun shine in earlier this year when it flipped the switch on a field of solar concentrators at its Modesto, Calif., *SunChips* manufacturing facility. Here, 54,000 sq ft of concave mirrors absorb sunlight while 192 solar collectors generate steam used to heat the cooking oil for the chips, thereby helping the company reduce its use of natural gas and the cost associated with it. The California Energy Commission provided a grant and the National Renewable Energy Laboratory, part of the U.S. Dept. of Energy, reviewed the design. Last year, the company installed a photovoltaic solar electric power system on

Fair Trade Helps More than the Environment

Check the packages of many different food products and you will see phrases such as "sustainably produced" and "fair trade" listed. These apply to a variety of products, including coffee, chocolate, tea, certain fruits, seafood, and wine. Both terms fall under the umbrella of sustainable agriculture, which refers to farming that does not irreversibly damage the land while at the same time improves or enhances the lives of farmers and members of their communities. Generally speaking, the farming methods employed minimize soil erosion and balance the amount of water used in irrigation with the amount that would be replenished naturally, all while reducing the amount of nonrenewable sources used to accomplish this. The 1990 Farm Bill describes sustainable agriculture as "an integrated system of plant and animal production practices having a site-specific application that will, over the long term, satisfy human food and fiber needs; enhance environmental quality and the natural resource base upon which the agricultural economy depends; make the most-efficient use of nonrenewable resources and on-farm resources and integrate, where appropriate, natural biological cycles and controls; sustain the economic viability of farm operations; and enhance the quality of life for farmers and society as a whole" (FACTA, 1990).

The goal of fair trade is to address global poverty by paying a fair price to farmers in Central and South America, Africa, and Asia for growing and harvesting such crops as coffee and cocoa. Food companies often work directly with farmers, suppliers, and exporters. According to the International Fair Trade Association (IFTA), a network of fair trade organizations from around the world, a fair price "covers not only the costs of production but enables production which is socially just and environmentally sound."

Paying farmers/producers a fair price is one of 10 standards that IFTA says fair trade organizations must follow. The others cited by the organization include creating economic opportunities for producers; improving transparency and accountability; helping producers to build their independence; promoting fair trade; promoting gender equity; ensuring safe and healthy working conditions; following child labor laws and regulations; respecting and protecting the environment; and maintaining trade relations. IFTA issues a certification mark to registered organizations that follow these fair trade standards.

A second organization, Fairtrade Labelling Organizations International (FLO), issues a certification mark for products that meet fair trade standards, as well as sets standards for 20 labeling initiatives such as Max Havelaar and TransFair USA used in 21 countries to label fair trade products.

Companies such as Starbucks, Cargill, Sara Lee, Hain Celestial Group, and many more that buy and sell coffee, cocoa, and other commodities participate in sustainable agriculture programs. Ingredients like vanilla can be certified as fair trade, and within the past several years, flavor manufacturers Virginia Dare and David Michael & Co. began offering it. At this year's IFT Annual Meeting and Food Expo in New Orleans, La., David Michael showcased its fair trade vanilla, which is certified by TransFair USA, in a *Double Bourbon and Cola* beverage made with vanilla ice cream.

Datamonitor predicts growth of 15.7% in the global sales of fair trade products for 2007–12. FLO reported that in the largest markets—the UK and the United States—sales of fair trade products grew by 72% and 46%, respectively, in 2007. The fastest-growing markets—Sweden and Norway—had sales increases of 166% and 110%, respectively.

the roof of its Arizona Service Center in Phoenix. The system produces no emissions and generates about 350,000 kWh of electricity to meet the daytime energy requirements for the facility, which is Frito-Lay's largest U.S. distribution center.

Other companies such as Decas Cranberry Products Inc., Carver, Mass., are investigating the use of wind as a way to generate energy. First used to grind grain and pump water, today's modern windmills—called wind turbines—are viewed as sustainable instruments in energy production. Decas in May began operating a wind turbine that should produce 3,279,000 kWh—or about half of the energy that the company uses per year. Ice cream manufacturer Mackie's, Aberdeenshire, Scotland, uses three wind turbines at its facility to meet about half of its total energy use of 3,000,000 kWh/year. A wind turbine icon and the phrase "made with 100% renewable energy" appear on the cartons of ice cream as a way, according to the company, to show its commitment to functioning as a carbon-neutral facility.

Certifying Green Buildings

Utilizing sustainable ways to generate energy recently earned Kettle Foods, Salem, Ore., a gold level certification for Leadership in Energy and Environmental Design (LEED) from the U.S.

Green Building Council (USGBC) for its new potato chip factory in Beloit, Wis. USGBC is a nonprofit organization with more than 15,000 members from across the building industry dedicated to sustainable construction. According to Jim Green, Kettle Foods spokesman, the company's goal was to be the first U.S. food manufacturing facility to earn the LEED gold certification, and it worked with engineers and architects who had experience with green building practices.

The company's 73,000-sq-ft building, which USGBC called "the greenest food manufacturing plant in the United States," contains energy-efficient equipment to reduce the use of natural gas and electricity and has the capacity to filter and reuse 1.65 million gallons of water used in the potato washers. The 18 wind turbines generate enough energy to produce 56,000 bags of potato chips per year and offset 100% of the building's electricity use. The company sourced more than 35% of building materials from within 500 miles of the facility's site. Even improving and protecting the indoor air quality was addressed by using zero-volatile organic compounds paints and increasing the ventilation for fresh air.

"The plant is green from the carpet, counters, and paint to the rooftop wind turbines and sophisticated water reclamation system that recycles potato wash water into gray water used to flush toilets," Green said.

Green Products Gain Market Share

Both manufacturers and consumers are embracing the green movement, according to data from market research company Mintel.

The percentage of consumers who purchased products made with recycled packaging and/or manufactured in an energy-efficient, environmentally friendly way jumped from 12% in August 2006 to 36% in December 2007 (Mintel, 2008b).

"We're seeing the green movement rapidly transition from niche to mainstream," said Colleen Ryan, Senior Analyst, Mintel, in a statement. "Major companies have jumped on board, promotional messages have changed, and the American public is increasingly looking at green products as a normal part of everyday life."

Mintel also reported that 328 products boasting an eco-friendly claim were launched in 2007. Compare that to only five of these product introductions in 2002 (Mintel, 2008a).

Mintel noted that while some of the food products labeled as eco-friendly were organic and natural, others focused on different environmental issues such as Green Energy Credits logos on packaging or support for health associations.

European consumers, too, are purchasing more products positioned as eco-friendly, including those that feature reduced packaging, are made with biodegradable packaging, and are labeled certified organic and/or fair trade. About 27% of European consumers bought these products in 2006, and in Europe, more than 60% of new product launches in 2007 were of these environmentally friendly products (Dodds, 2007).

USGBC also awarded LEED certification to Contessa for its "Green Cuisine Plant," the first LEED-certified frozen food facility in the world. The plant features a solar power system to generate electricity and a loading dock that prevents the loss of refrigerated air. But the biggest challenge the company faced was in trying to design an energy-efficient 4,000,000-cu-ft frozen food plant (almost entirely temperature-controlled). At that size, it is similar to running 200,000 refrigerators at the same time in the same place, said Blazevich, so it took plenty of creative thinking to design a plant that uses the least amount of energy possible. To accomplish this, the company installed a heat-redirection system that captures waste heat in the form of gas from refrigeration compressors and redirects the gas to a heat exchanger where it is condensed to a liquid that then heats water in a circulation system.

Plans are underway to maintain and improve the energy-efficient features of the plant. "We have an ongoing mission to fine tune the systems and features of our new Green Cuisine plant so that we can reduce water and energy consumption and even further reduce our greenhouse gas emissions," said Blazevich.

Although it cost the company an extra $6 million to improve the energy efficiency of the building, Blazevich said that it was the right thing to do for the sustainability of the planet.

"Two years ago, I converted my home to use geothermal energy, so I thought to myself, why not transfer this into the plant? I saw this as a great opportunity to address my business's output of greenhouse gases. If we don't do something about them, in 30 years we won't be living in the same place we have been."

Blazevich's efforts have not gone unrecognized. In addition to receiving the LEED certification, the company has fielded questions from and provided advice to companies seeking more information about energy-efficient building design. "From university engineers and major food manufacturers to major retailers, we have been approached to share our innovative patented technologies and processes," said Blazevich. "Food manufactures of all sizes will soon be expected to show that their back-end operations are as clean and responsible as the face they show the public."

Packing an Environmental Punch

Individuals trying to live a green lifestyle often urge companies to review the types of materials used to package products, develop ways to reduce packaging material, or adopt new material altogether. For example, after working closely with the Environmental Defense Fund (EDF) to address solid waste issues and develop ways to reduce and recycle, McDonald's discontinued the use of polystyrene foam "clamshell" boxes and switched to paper-based packaging for its sandwiches. EDF and McDonald's formed a task force in 1989, and EDF reported that in 1999, McDonald's eliminated 150,000 tons of packaging by redesigning or reducing the amount of material used to make a variety of items, including sandwich packaging, cups, napkins, and straws.

For the most part, processed food products need to be packaged in some type of package, be it paper, paperboard, plastic, or a combination of these. Even fresh produce, which is displayed unpackaged at the retail level, is transported from the point of origin to stores in crates, bags, and other containers. Packaging helps to keep food fresh, protect it from adulteration, and minimize damage and breakage due to shipping and handling. It also communicates important information about the product, how to prepare it, and what the nutrient content is.

Even though food manufacturers cannot eliminate packaging, they can redesign packages to reduce the amount of material used or to incorporate newly developed materials such as biodegradable plastic in their products' packaging. This is particularly important in the European Union where many countries are considering tougher legislation to encourage the use of less packaging material (Dodds, 2007). Reducing the weight of the package can also have a positive affect by reducing the amount of energy required to transport the products.

Other companies such as Nestlé and Tetra Pak support and encourage recycling efforts or use recyclable materials to produce their packages and products. In a number of countries around the world, Tetra Pak, Lausanne, Switzerland, has established plants to recycle its aseptic carton packages and campaigns to encourage recycling. Additionally, some packaging manufacturers are becoming more aware of depleting natural resources and opting to use materials from renewable sources.

According to Tetra Pak, about 75% of its raw material use in 2006 was for paperboard, which is used in the company's aseptic carton packaging material. To help ensure that the raw materials are sustainably sourced, the company collaborates with environmental organizations and nonprofit groups such as World Wildlife

Fund, Forest Stewardship Council, ProForest, Global Forest and Trade Network, and High Conservation Value Resource Network. Forest Stewardship Council (FSC) certifies forests and forest management around the world according to 10 principles and 57 criteria that address such issues as indigenous rights, labor rights, and environmental impact (FSC, 1996). The importance of the latter is to help maintain the integrity of the entire forest ecosystem: trees and other plant life, water, and soil.

"We have a corporate policy that more trees are planted than harvested in the process of making our packaging, and we conduct independent audits of our paper manufacturers to ensure this," said Laurens Van de Vijver, Vice President, Marketing and Product Placement, Tetra Pak U.S. & Canada.

These efforts, along with an initiative that encourages recycling, have allowed the company to position its packages as tools that, as Van de Vijver explained, help food and beverage companies meet their own sustainability goals and meet their own energy- and cost-savings goals. Also, since the packaging is lighter than plastic, glass, or steel, is non-breakable, and can be stacked closely during transport and storage, less fuel is required to transport the packages. All of this is increasingly important because rising costs of energy are quickly cutting into companies' bottom line.

"Industries across sectors are feeling the economic strain of rising fossil fuel and gas prices," said Van de Vijver. "This means that the availability of plastic packaging—made from petroleum—is less stable than the availability of feedstocks such as paper, which can be renewed through responsible harvesting and reforestation programs. Given this, it is important to look at beverage packaging options that minimize fossil fuel inputs by using fewer materials made from nonrenewable resources."

Bigger May Not Be Better

Choosing raw materials that are sourced or produced in ways that minimally affect the environment is a step that companies can take to become green. Designing packages to use more environmentally friendly material or use less material overall is another step. Unilever has made changes to product packaging, including *Knorr* vegetable mix and *Knorr Recipe Secrets* soup pouch (eliminated outer carton), *Lipton* soup (reduced the width of the outer box), and *Bertolli* frozen meal pouches (reduced the height of the package). According to the company, the changes have helped Unilever reduce the amount of corrugated material and other packaging matter as well as the number of pallets and trucks used to transport the products.

Two of the world's beverage industry giants recently announced environmental initiatives that include design changes to bottles.

PepsiCo Inc., Purchase, N.Y., reduced the plastic content of its new 500-mL bottles for noncarbonated beverages by 20%. Introduced in May, the bottle is used for *Lipton Iced Tea, Tropicana* juice drinks, *Aquafina FlavorSplash,* and *Aquafina Alive* products. Additionally, the company reduced by 10% the label size and by 5% the shrink wrap film used to wrap multipacks.

Taking on an effort like this is not as simple as one might think. According to Robert Lewis, Vice President of Worldwide Beverage Packaging and Equipment Development, PepsiCo, a team of employees from across the company took one year to complete the project, which included developing a bottle that was lighter and able to provide the same shelf life while withstanding the manufacturing and distribution process as well as the heavier bottle. The

It's Not Easy Being Green

Today's consumers are confronted with a barrage of advertising from companies touting their green products, celebrities exclaiming how they are reducing their carbon footprint, or officials telling us how we can reduce global warming by switching to compact fluorescent light bulbs. As more manufacturers promote their environmentally friendly products and sustainable business initiatives, some consumers are becoming confused and downright skeptical of what these companies are doing.

The Federal Trade Commission this year has held three public hearings and workshops in a series that will review its environmental marketing guidelines called the Green Guides. The guides, last updated in 1998, address eco-friendly marketing claims such as biodegradability, recyclability, and others and "help marketers avoid making environmental claims that are unfair or deceptive under Section 5 of the FTC Act, 15 U.S.C. 45" (CFR, 2007). The guides do not address new claims such as renewable energy certificates, carbon offsets, green packaging, green building claims, and sustainability. Since companies are using more and more ecofriendly marketing claims, especially these newer ones, on their products, FTC decided to move up the review process from 2009 to the beginning of this year.

"Consumers today have the option to purchase products and use them in ways that were unforeseen 15 years ago, when we first developed our guides, and consumer perceptions of old green claims may have evolved significantly over time," said Deborah Platt Majoras, FTC Chairman, at the hearing in January 2008. "Our robust review of these guides will allow us to explore emerging consumer protection issues and provide better direction to green marketers."

FTC will use the information gathered from these meetings to decide what modifications to the Green Guides are needed, particularly those that will benefit consumers and businesses, as well as deciding what steps should be taken to define the new green marketing claims.

"When such claims are used to sell products, consumer perception and substantiation issues may arise," reported FTC. "Also, in recent years, there has been an increase in the use of environmental seals and third-party certification programs purporting to verify the positive environmental impact of product packaging. Consumers may have varying interpretation of such seals and programs."

team submitted more than 30 bottle designs for consumer testing to determine the most aesthetically pleasing ones.

Coca-Cola Co., Atlanta, Ga., too, has redesigned some of its bottles for its carbonated and noncarbonated beverages. It introduced in 2007 a newly designed 20-oz polyethylene terephthalate (PET) contour bottle for its *Coca-Cola* brands. The bottle has 5%

less PET than the previous bottle. The company also reduced the plastic used in its *Dasani* bottles by 30%.

Earlier this year, the company announced a long-term plan to recycle or reuse 100% of the aluminum beverage cans it sells in the U.S. This followed an announcement last year that the company plans to invest more than $60 million to build the world's largest plastic bottle-to-bottle recycling plant to help meet its goal of recycling or reusing 100% of the company's PET plastic bottles in the U.S. The plant will be located in Spartanburg, S.C. When it is fully operational in 2009, it is expected that the plant will produce about 100 million lb of food-grade recycled PET plastic for reuse each year. Coca-Cola has invested in other recycling facilities in Austria, Switzerland, Mexico, and the Philippines.

One Word: Bioplastics

Environmentalists heavily criticize the use of plastic grocery bags and, more recently, plastic water bottles, so much so that natural and organic foods retailer Whole Foods Market—in conjunction with this year's Earth Day celebration on April 22—eliminated the use of plastic grocery bags in its 270 stores in the U.S., Canada, and the UK. Over the years, environmentalists and scientists studying environmental issues have said that plastic bags and bottles, particularly those that are petroleum-based, take up space in landfills and pollute the landscape. But developments in biodegradable ingredients now make it possible for more manufacturers to produce plastic bags, bottles, and packages made from bioplastics.

NatureWorks LLC, Minnetonka, Minn., a joint venture between Cargill Inc., and Teijin Ltd., produces the *NatureWorks* PLA (polyactide) line of polymers that are derived from the starch of standard field corn. The polymers are said to biodegrade when packages that are made from them are composted. Moisture and heat in the compost pile break the PLA polymer chains to smaller chains, and then ultimately to lactic acid. Microorganisms in the compost consume the lactic acid for nourishment.

Other biodegradable corn starch-based ingredients, these from Plantic Technologies Ltd., Melbourne, Australia, are used in plastic trays for some Marks & Spencer and Cadbury confectionery products. Last year, the company and DuPont Packaging and Industrial Polymers, Wilmington, Del., announced that they will collaborate to develop and sell renewably sourced polymers based on Plantic's technology.

While some bioplastics are made from crops like corn, wheat, and sugar cane, there are others that are made from petrochemical sources.

Bioplastics are both blessed and cursed, though. While producing the polymers uses less fuel and generates fewer greenhouse gases than petroleum-based polymers, they are still farmed industrially, which means that fuel is needed to operate the farming equipment and chemicals are used to fertilize the crops. Most bioplastics will degrade under the right conditions in composts to produce benign lactic acid, but will degrade very little, if at all, in tightly packed landfills in the absence of oxygen. If they do break down slightly in the landfill, they produce methane, a greenhouse gas. One additional drawback is the fact that bioplastics cannot be recycled with traditional plastics because of contamination issues.

Sustaining the Green Movement

So what does the future hold for eco-friendly practices, sustainably produced products, and the like? If companies continue to see value in these, i.e., consumers continue to purchase products that are promoted as eco-friendly or sustainable, they will produce more of these products as well as invest in corporate sustainable/environmental practices. Americans and Europeans lead the world as purchasers of eco-friendly products. Entering new markets may extend the reach of these products as well as educate consumers and those who work for government agencies and food companies on developing government policies and company initiatives that address environmental issues. Or will consumers who are dealing with the high costs for fuel, food, and other products decide that paying a premium for eco-friendly products is not worth it and retreat from purchasing these products?

Any single solution offered by the companies mentioned in this article will not immediately solve the problems faced by our environment; try as they might, the companies can only do so much, and there are still challenges that they must overcome. Remember, it's not easy being green. But perhaps these are the changes that need to take place to compel more people and companies to save precious resources and protect our environment.

References

CFR. 2007. Guides for the use of environmental marketing claims. Code of Federal Regulations 16CFRPart260. Nov. 27. 72: 66091-66093.

Dodds, A. 2007. The Future of Ethical Food and Drinks: Growth Opportunities in Organic and Sustainable Products and Packaging. Business Insights Ltd., London, UK.

FACTA. 1990. Food, Agriculture, Conservation, and Trade Act of 1990. Public Law 101-624, Title XVI, Subtitle A, Section 1603. NAL Call #KF1692.A31 1990.

FSC. 1996. FSC International Standard FSC Principles and Criteria for Forest Stewardship. FSC-STD-01-001 (version 4-0) EN. Forest Stewardship Council, Bonn, Germany.

Miller. 2008. Live Sustainably: The 2008 Sustainable Development Report. Miller Brewing Co., Milwaukee, Wis.

Mintel. 2008a. Mintel finds more new products boasting environmentally friendly claims. Press Release, Mintel, London, UK, April 9.

Mintel. 2008b. Americans go three shades greener in 16 months. Press Release, Mintel, London, UK, March.

Karen Nachay, a Member of IFT, is Assistant Editor of *Food Technology* magazine (knachay@ift.org).

A Question of Sustenance

Globalization ushered in a world in which more than a billion are overfed, yet hundreds of millions still suffer from hunger's persistent scourge.

GARY STIX

In 1963 some 200,000 Indians in West Bengal and Assam faced imminent starvation. A few years later drought caused severe food shortages in the nearby state of Bihar. Against a backdrop of such reports, biologist Paul Ehrlich speculated in his 1968 book *The Population Bomb* that, within just a few years, hundreds of millions would starve to death, as inexorable population growth outstripped limited resources.

This neo-Malthusian scenario never came to pass. For India, the green revolution in agriculture averted a "ship to mouth" existence in which foreign food aid would be needed indefinitely to stave off Ehrlich's worst-case prognostications. In the ensuing 40 years, India has undergone a radical makeover and now graces magazine covers as an emerging economic giant. The turn-of-the-century developing world now often confronts more of a problem with fat than it does with famine—a sociological spin-off of globalization known as the nutrition transition. The millennium marked the first time that the overweight equaled the number of the undernourished worldwide, and, as a demographic, the overnourished 1.3 billion now surpass the hungry by several hundred million.

Rich and poor now fret about many of the same things at the dinner table. Coca-Colonization—a term that even crops up in academic papers—has built a global infrastructure for *comida chatarra,* the Mexican label for junk food. Coca-Cola distributors ink exclusive agreements down to the level of neighborhood *tiendas,* supplying shopkeepers with refrigerators and point-of-sale materials. Mexicans now take in more calories from sugared drinks than Americans do. In tandem, the rise of the U.S.-style supermarket has promoted widespread adoption of corn, soy and other vegetable oils.

The green revolution forestalled mass starvation, but comparable technological ingenuity has largely failed to stem global expansion in waist sizes. An understanding of the endocrinology, neurology and genetics of obesity has slowly emerged. Scientists have even discovered a gene for fidgeting that promotes the burning of calories. But these insights have yet to produce a good diet pill. The weight-loss drug combination known as Fen-Phen was yanked from the market in 1997 after reports of heart problems. And orlistat (alli) is now sold without

a prescription—a consequence, according to some doctors, of its mixed record of effectiveness as a prescription medicine. If it really worked well, physician prescriptions would have brought in blockbuster billions in yearly revenues to GlaxoSmithKline.

Drugmakers have not given up. They are investigating molecules that block brain and gut chemicals that stimulate appetite, along with others that increase the rate of energy expenditure. But a drug will not address the psychological foibles that threaten to undermine the best of treatments. Recent behavioral research shows that gulping diet pills encourages consumers to yield to temptations for double bacon cheeseburgers and weekends of sitting on the couch watching *Sopranos* reruns. Side effects, too, are a constant preoccupation when tweaking pathways that regulate something as primal as eating. In June, Sanofi Aventis withdrew an application for a proposed weight-loss drug, rimonabant (Acomplia), that may provoke suicidal thoughts. An FDA advisory panel had recommended against its approval.

Following a regimen of eating less and exercising more seems like the simplest bet. Yet even a puritanical way of life comes loaded with controversy. A 2005 study revealed that the moderately overweight have a lower overall death rate than those with bathroom-scale readings in the healthy range. Ever since, the academic nutrition community, steeped in the rhetoric of obesity epidemics, has lobbed broadsides at those blasphemous results.

If most diets do not work in the long run—as much evidence does suggest—what are the overweight to do without a pill or a plan? The fit-but-fat movement advocates staying active combined with diminished worries about one's body mass index. Embracing cultural norms, rather than epidemiology, a few take this argument further. Rural women from Niger shun thinness, and some urban, male hip-hoppers (Heavy D and the Boo-Yaa T.R.I.B.E. among them) embrace excess adiposity, giving new meaning to the word "phat."

The nutrition transition is by no means monolithic. A visitor to a modest home in Indonesia might find a corpulent child sitting on a living room couch alongside an undernourished sibling, a testament to the paradoxical effects of diets loaded with sugar and vegetable oils. The world produces enough food to feed everyone from West Palm Beach to Pyongyang. But getting rice from paddy to bowl often still poses challenges. Although the number of the world's hungry has fallen, undernourishment persists: hundreds of millions do not receive enough calories every day.

The green revolution, meanwhile, may be pushing its own limits of growth. Whereas cereal production has climbed steadily since the 1960s, when farmers in the developing world first started planting hybrid grains and deploying fertilizers, irrigation and pesticides, the amount of land available for farming remains the same. Heavy pesticide usage may also limit further gains because of pollution of drinking water.

Will Gene Follow Green?

In theory, a "gene revolution" based on genetically modified crops could make up for the inadequacies of the green revolution. The adoption of new practices in the 1960s, fueled by subsidies from governments and transnational groups, took place almost overnight and boosted yields immediately, but biotech crops for the developing world have yet to prove themselves. The private sector purveys genetically modified organisms (GMOs), sometimes charging prohibitive rates that put seed stocks beyond the budgets of small- and medium-size Third World farms. Although a few developing countries have tried GMO corn or soybeans with some success, the promise of the technology as an aid to a specific region's development—gene-altered crops that can survive drought or grow in saline soil—has yet to be realized on a commercial scale.

Fat and famine coexist in developing countries, but the industrial world wrestles with its own peculiar dietary confusion. Carefully constructed dietary food plans prescribe an exact number of daily servings for meat, dairy, fruits and vegetables. Despite its revision in recent years, the U.S. Department of Agriculture's food pyramid still receives a heaping portion of disdain from many nutritionists.

The scientific basis for precision national meal planning is decidedly scant. Most food research relies on tracking a single nutrient and fails to identify other contributors, whether genetic or behavioral, that can lead to such killers as coronary artery disease or diabetes. The necessity of oversimplification helps to explain the constant overturning of the prevailing wisdom with studies claiming that eating more fiber does not prevent cancer and that low-fat diets do nothing to prevent heart disease and colorectal cancer. Marion Nestle, author of "Eating Made Simple," . . . tries to sort things out for the perplexed supermarket patron by coining a mantra: eat less, move more, consume plenty of fruits, vegetables and whole grains, and eschew junk food.

Entreaties to keep it simple do not stray far from what might be called the "Mark Twain diet." Twain reduced the complexities of dietary energy balances to a single sentence: "Part of the secret of success in life is to eat what you like and let the food fight it out inside." Other neo-Twainians—Michael Pollan, author of the much heralded *The Omnivore's Dilemma* (Penguin, 2006), among them—argue for the pleasures of food, while forgoing nutritionism, the quest for nutrients as medicine, a pursuit that may, paradoxically, fail to enhance health. Pollan urges the consumer to "pay more, eat less" by buying organics or other quality foodstuffs that conserve taste along with nutritional value. If one follows his reasoning, the culinary arts and nutritional sciences need not remain at loggerheads. Both should roundly reject the vitamin-fortified meal-replacement bar.

Pushing Beyond the Earth's Limits

The future will see not just more mouths to feed, but a growing demand for higher-quality, more resource-intensive food. The world's farmers may not be up to the many challenges of meeting those demands.

LESTER R. BROWN

During the last half of the twentieth century, the world economy expanded sevenfold. In 2000 alone, its growth exceeded that of the entire nineteenth century. Economic growth, now the goal of governments everywhere, has become the status quo. Stability is considered a departure from the norm.

As the economy grows, its demands are outgrowing the earth, exceeding many of the planet's natural capacities. While the world economy multiplied sevenfold in just 50 years, the earth's natural life-support systems remained essentially the same. Water use tripled, but the capacity of the hydrological system to produce fresh water through evaporation changed little. The demand for seafood increased fivefold, but the sustainable yield of oceanic fisheries was unchanged. Fossil-fuel burning raised carbon dioxide (CO_2) emissions fourfold, but the capacity of nature to absorb it changed little, leading to a buildup of CO_2 in the atmosphere and a rise in the earth's temperature. As human demands surpass the earth's natural capacities, expanding food production becomes more difficult.

Losing Agricultural Momentum

Environmentalists have been saying for years that, if the environmental trends of recent decades continued, the world would one day be in trouble. What was not clear was what form the trouble would take and when it would occur. Now it has become increasingly clear that tightening food supplies will be our greatest trouble and that it will emerge within the next few years. In early 2004, China's forays into the world market to buy 8 million tons of wheat marked what could be the beginning of the global shift from an era of grain surpluses to one of grain scarcity.

World grain production is a basic indicator of dietary adequacy at the individual level and of overall food security at the global level. After nearly tripling from 1950 to 1996, the grain harvest stayed flat for seven years in a row, through 2003, showing no increase at all. And production fell short of consumption in each of the last four of those years. The shortfalls of nearly 100 million tons in 2002 and again in 2003 were the largest on record.

Consumption exceeded production for four years, leading world grain stocks to drop to the lowest level in 30 years. The last time stocks were this low, in 1972–1974, wheat and rice prices doubled. Importing countries competed vigorously for inadequate supplies. A politics of scarcity emerged, and some countries, such as the United States, restricted exports.

In 2004, a combination of stronger grain prices at planting time and the best weather in a decade yielded a substantially larger harvest for the first time in eight years. Yet even with a harvest that was up 124 million tons from that in 2003, the world still consumed all the grain it produced, leaving none to rebuild stocks. If stocks cannot be rebuilt in a year of exceptional weather, when can they?

From 1950 to 1984, world grain production expanded faster than population, raising the grain produced per person per year from 250 kilograms to the historic peak of 339 kilograms—an increase of 34%. This positive development initially reflected recovery from the disruption of World War II, and then later solid technological advances. The rising tide of food production lifted all ships, largely eradicating hunger in some countries and substantially reducing it in many others.

But since 1984, growth in grain harvests has fallen behind growth in population. The amount of grain produced per person fell to 308 kilograms in 2004.

Africa is suffering the most, with a decline in grain produced per person that is unusually steep and taking a heavy human toll. Soils are depleted of nutrients, and the amount of grainland per person has been shrinking steadily due to population growth in recent decades. But in addition, Africa must now contend with the loss of adults to AIDS, which is depleting the rural workforce and undermining agriculture. In two of the last three years, grain production per person in sub-Saharan Africa has been below 120 kilograms—dropping to a level that leaves millions of Africans on the edge of starvation.

Several long-standing environmental trends are contributing to the global loss of agricultural momentum. Among these are the cumulative effects of soil erosion on land productivity, the loss of cropland to desertification, and the accelerating conversion of cropland to nonfarm uses. All are taking a toll, although their relative roles vary among countries.

In addition, farmers are seeing fewer new technologies to dramatically boost production. The high-yielding varieties of wheat, rice, and corn that were developed a generation or so ago doubled and tripled yields, but there have not been any dramatic advances in the genetic yield potential of grains since then.

Similarly, the use of fertilizer has now plateaued or even declined slightly in key food-producing countries. The rapid growth in irrigation that characterized much of the last half century has also slowed. Indeed, in some countries the irrigated area is shrinking.

And now, two newer environmental trends are slowing the growth in world food production: falling water tables and rising temperatures. The bottom line is that it is now more difficult for farmers to keep up with the growing demand for grain. The rise in world grainland productivity, which averaged over 2% a year from 1950 to 1990, fell to scarcely 1% a year in the last decade of the twentieth century. This will likely drop further in the years immediately ahead.

If the rise in land productivity continues to slow and if population continues to grow by 70 million or more per year, governments may begin to define national security in terms of food shortages, rising food prices, and the emerging politics of scarcity. Food insecurity may soon eclipse terrorism as the overriding concern of national governments.

Food Challenges Go from Local to Global

The world economy is making excessive demands on the earth. Evidence of this can be seen in collapsing fisheries, shrinking forests, expanding deserts, rising CO_2 levels, eroding soils, rising temperatures, falling water tables, melting glaciers, deteriorating grasslands, rising seas, rivers that are running dry, and disappearing species.

Nearly all of these environmentally destructive trends contribute to global food insecurity. For example, even a modest rise of 1°F in temperature in mountainous regions can substantially increase rainfall and decrease snowfall. The result is more flooding during the rainy season and less snowmelt to feed rivers during the dry season, when farmers need irrigation water.

Or consider the collapse of fisheries and the associated leveling off of the oceanic fish catch. During the last half century, the fivefold growth in the world fish catch that satisfied much of

the growing demand for animal protein pushed oceanic fisheries to their limits and beyond. Now, in this new century, we cannot expect any growth at all in the catch. The Food and Agriculture Organization warns that all future growth in animal protein supplies can only come from that produced on land, not the sea, putting even more pressure on the earth's land and water resources.

Until recently, the economic effects of environmental trends, such as overfishing, overpumping, and overplowing, were largely local. Among the many examples are the collapse of the cod fishery off Newfoundland from overfishing that cost Canada 40,000 jobs, the halving of Saudi Arabia's wheat harvest as a result of aquifer depletion, and the shrinking grain harvest of Kazakhstan as wind erosion claimed half of its cropland.

Now, if world food supplies tighten, we may see the first global economic effect of environmentally destructive trends. Rising food prices could be the first economic indicator to signal serious trouble in the deteriorating relationship between the global economy and the earth's ecosystem. The short-lived 20% rise in world grain prices in early 2004 may turn out to be a warning tremor before the quake.

Two New Challenges

As world demand for food has tripled, so too has the use of water for irrigation. As a result, the world is incurring a vast water deficit. But the trend is largely invisible because the deficit takes the form of aquifer overpumping and falling water tables. Falling water levels are often not discovered until wells go dry.

The world water deficit is a relatively recent phenomenon. Only within the last half century have powerful diesel and electrically driven pumps given us the pumping capacity to deplete aquifers. The worldwide spread of these pumps since the late 1960s and the drilling of millions of wells have in many cases pushed water withdrawal beyond the aquifers' recharge from rainfall. As a result, water tables are now falling in countries that are home to more than half of the world's people, including China, India, and the United States—the three largest grain producers.

Groundwater levels are falling throughout the northern half of China. Under the North China Plain, they are dropping 1–3 meters (3–10 feet) a year. In India, they are falling in most states, including the Punjab, the country's breadbasket. And in the United States, water levels are falling throughout the southern Great Plains and the Southwest. Overpumping creates a false sense of food security: It enables us to satisfy growing food needs today, but it almost guarantees a decline in food production tomorrow when the aquifer is depleted.

It takes a thousand tons of water to produce a single ton of grain, so food security is closely tied to water security. Seventy percent of world water use is for irrigation, 20% is used by industry, and 10% is for residential purposes. As urban water use rises while aquifers are being depleted, farmers are faced with a shrinking share of a shrinking water supply.

Meanwhile, temperatures are rising and concern about climate change is intensifying. Scientists have begun to focus on the precise relationship between temperature and crop yields. Crop ecologists at the International Rice Research Institute in the Philippines and at the U.S. Department of Agriculture (USDA) have jointly concluded that each 1°C rise in temperature during the growing season cuts 10% off the yields of wheat, rice, and corn.

Over the last three decades, the earth's average temperature has climbed by nearly 0.7°C; the four warmest years on record came during the last six years. In 2002, record-high temperatures and drought shrank grain harvests in both India and the United States. In 2003, Europe bore the brunt of the intense heat. The record-breaking August heat wave claimed 35,000 lives in eight nations and withered grain harvests in virtually every country from France to Ukraine.

In a business-as-usual scenario, the earth's average temperature will rise by 1.4°–5.8°C (2°–10°F) during this century, according to the Intergovernmental Panel on Climate Change. These projections are for the earth's average temperature, but the rise is expected to be much greater over land than over the oceans, in the higher latitudes than in the equatorial regions, and in the interior of continents than in the coastal regions. This suggests that increases far in excess of the projected average are likely for regions such as the North American breadbasket—the region defined by the Great Plains of the United States and Canada and the U.S. corn belt. Today's farmers face the prospect of temperatures higher than any generation of farmers since agriculture began.

The Japan Syndrome

When studying the USDA world grain database more than a decade ago, I noted that, if countries are already densely populated when they begin to industrialize rapidly, three things happen in quick succession to make them heavily dependent on grain imports: Grain consumption climbs as incomes rise, grainland area shrinks, and grain production falls. The rapid industrialization that drives up demand simultaneously shrinks the cropland area. The inevitable result is that grain imports soar. Within a few decades, countries can go from being essentially self-sufficient to importing 70% or more of their grain. I call this the "Japan syndrome" because I first recognized this sequence of events in Japan, a country that today imports 70% of its grain.

In a fast-industrializing country, grain consumption rises rapidly. Initially, rising incomes permit more direct consumption of grain, but before long the growth shifts to the greater indirect consumption of grain in the form of grain-intensive livestock products, such as pork, poultry, and eggs.

Once rapid industrialization is under way, the grainland area begins to shrink within a few years. As a country industrializes and modernizes, cropland gets taken over by industrial and residential developments and by roads, highways, and parking lots to accommodate more cars and drivers. When farmers are left with fragments of land that are too small to be cultivated

economically, they often simply abandon their plots, seeking employment elsewhere.

As rapid industrialization pulls labor out of the countryside, it often leads to less double cropping, a practice that depends on quickly harvesting one grain crop once it is ripe and immediately preparing the seedbed for the next crop. With the loss of workers as young people migrate to cities, the capacity to do this diminishes. As incomes rise, diets diversify, generating demand for more fruits and vegetables. This in turn leads farmers to shift land from grain to these more profitable, high-value crops.

Japan was essentially self-sufficient in grain when its grain harvested area peaked in 1955. Since then the grainland area has shrunk by more than half. The multiple-cropping index has dropped from nearly 1.4 crops per hectare per year in 1960 to scarcely one crop today. Some six years after Japan's grain area began to shrink, the shrinkage overrode the rise in land productivity and overall production began to decline. With grain consumption climbing and production falling, grain imports soared. By 1983, imports accounted for 70% of Japan's grain consumption, a level they remain at today.

South Korea and Taiwan are tracing Japan's pattern. In both cases, the decline in grain area was followed roughly a decade later by a decline in production. Perhaps this should not be surprising, since the forces at work in the two countries are exactly the same as in Japan. And, like Japan, both South Korea and Taiwan now import some 70% of their total grain supply.

Based on the sequence of events in these three countries that affected grain production, consumption, and imports—the Japan syndrome—it was easy to anticipate the precipitous decline in China's grain production that began in 1998. The obvious question now is which other countries will enter a period of declining grain production because of the same combination of forces. Among those that come to mind are India, Indonesia, Bangladesh, Pakistan, Egypt, and Mexico.

Of particular concern is India, with a population of nearly 1.1 billion now and growing by 18 million a year. In recent years, India's economic growth has accelerated, averaging 6%–7% a year. This growth, only slightly slower than that of China, is also beginning to consume cropland. In addition to the grainland shrinkage associated with the Japan syndrome, the extensive overpumping of aquifers in India—which will one day deprive farmers of irrigation water—will also reduce grain production.

Exactly when rapid industrialization in a country that is densely populated will translate into a decline in grain production is difficult to anticipate. Once crop production begins to decline, countries often try to reverse the trend. But the difficulty of achieving this can be seen in Japan, where a rice support price that is four times the world market price has failed to expand production.

The China Factor

China—the most-populous country in the world—is now beginning to experience the Japan syndrome. The precipitous fall in China's grain production since 1998 is perhaps the most

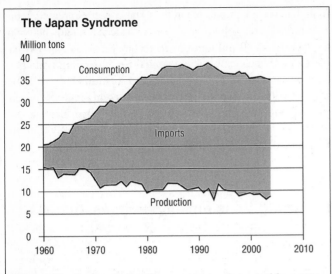

The Japan Syndrome

Figure 1   Grain production, consumption, and imports in Japan, 1960–2004. As consumption of grain increased with an improving economy, Japan reached out to the world's supermarkets to compensate for falling production. Now there is fear that a bigger, hungrier consumer, China, will sink the global economy as it experiences its own "Japan syndrome."

Source: USDA, cited in *Outgrowing the Earth* by Lester R. Brown.

alarming recent world agricultural event. After an impressive climb from 90 million tons in 1950 to a peak of 392 million tons in 1998, China's grain harvest fell in four of the next five years, dropping to 322 million tons in 2003. For perspective, this decline of 70 million tons exceeds the entire grain harvest of Canada.

The decline resulted when China's farmers began converting cropland to nonfarm uses and shifting grainland to higher-value fruits and vegetables. And, as happened in Japan, better jobs in some of the more prosperous regions lured away the rural labor needed for multiple cropping, thus reducing productivity.

China is also losing grainland to the expansion of deserts and the loss of irrigation water, due to both aquifer depletion and diversion of water to cities. Unfortunately for China, none of the forces that are shrinking the grainland area are easily countered.

Between 1998 and 2003, five consecutive harvest shortfalls dropped China's once massive stocks of grain to their lowest level in 30 years. With stocks now largely depleted, China's leaders—all of them survivors of the great famine of 1959–1961, when 30 million people starved to death—are worried. For them, food security is not a trivial issue.

China desperately wants to reverse the recent fall in grain production and has tried to encourage farmers to grow more grain. In March 2004, Beijing expanded the agricultural budget by one-fifth ($3.6 billion) and raised the support price for the early rice crop by 21%. These two emergency measures did reverse the grain harvest decline temporarily,

but whether they can reverse the trend over the longer term is doubtful.

When China turns to the outside world for commodities, it can overwhelm world markets. When wheat prices within China started climbing in the fall of 2003, the government dispatched wheat-buying delegations to Australia, Canada, and the United States. They purchased 8 million tons, and overnight China became the world's largest wheat importer. China has been the world's fastest-growing economy since 1980, and the economic effects of this massive expansion can be seen in the rest of the world.

But China is also putting enormous pressure on its own natural resource base. The northern half of the country is literally drying out. Water tables are falling, rivers are going dry, and lakes are disappearing. The World Bank warns of "catastrophic consequences for future generations" if China's water use and supply cannot quickly be brought back into balance. More immediately, if China cannot quickly restore a balance between the consumption of water and the sustainable yield of its aquifers and rivers, its grain imports will likely soar in the years ahead.

For people not living in China, it is difficult to visualize how quickly deserts are expanding. Like invading armies, expanding deserts are claiming ever more territory. Old deserts are advancing and new ones are forming, like guerrilla forces striking unexpectedly, forcing Beijing to fight on several fronts. Throughout northern and western China, some 24,000 villages have either been abandoned or partly depopulated as drifting sand has made farming untenable.

China's food problems now are not hunger and starvation, as the nation now has a substantial cushion between consumption levels and minimal nutrition needs. Rather, the concern is rising food prices and the effect that this could have on political stability. China's leaders are striving for a delicate balance between food prices that will encourage production in the countryside but maintain stability in the cities.

If smaller countries like Japan, South Korea, and Taiwan import 70% or more of their grain, the impacts on the global economy are not so dramatic. But if China turns to the outside world to meet even 20% of its grain needs—which would be close to 80 million tons—it will create a huge challenge for grain exporters. The resulting rise in world grain prices could destabilize governments in low-income, grain-importing countries. The entire world thus has a stake in China's efforts to stabilize its agricultural resource base.

The Challenge Ahead

We must not underestimate the challenges that the world faces over the next half century. There will be a projected 3 billion more people to feed, and 5 billion who will want to improve their diets by eating more meat, which requires more grain (as livestock feed) to produce. Meanwhile, the world's farmers will still be fighting soil erosion and the loss of cropland to nonfarm uses, as well as newer challenges, such as falling water tables, the diversion of irrigation water to cities, and rising temperatures.

The World Food Summit of 1996 in Rome set a goal of halving the number of hungry people by 2015. That would require reducing the ranks of the hungry by 20 million a year. While some progress was made in the 1990s, it has not been enough. And things have gotten even worse: By the end of the century, the number of hungry people in the world began to increase, rising to 798 million in 2001. This increase in hunger is not too surprising, given the lack of growth in the world grain harvest during this period.

Looming over this darkening horizon is the prospect that other countries will soon fall victim to the Japan syndrome of accelerating economic growth and shrinking grain harvests. Will India's grain production peak and start declining in the next few years, much as China's did after 1998? Or will India be able to hold off the loss of cropland to nonfarm uses and the depletion of aquifers long enough to eradicate most of its hunger? There are signs that the shrinkage in India's grain area—a precursor to the shrinkage of overall production—may have begun.

Because aquifer depletion is recent, it is taking agricultural analysts into uncharted territory. Water tables are falling simultaneously in many countries and at an accelerating rate, but we cannot be certain exactly when aquifers will be depleted and precisely how much this will reduce food production. And in a world of rising temperatures, there is added reason to be concerned about world food security.

On another front, in Africa the spread of HIV/AIDS is threatening the food security of the entire continent as the loss of able-bodied field workers shrinks harvests. In sub-Saharan Africa, disease begets hunger and hunger begets disease. In some villages, high HIV-infection rates have claimed an entire generation of young adults, leaving only the elderly and children. Without a major intervention from the outside world, the continuing spread of the virus—combined with the hunger that is cutting life expectancy in half in some countries—could take Africa back to the Dark Ages.

In a world where the food economy has been shaped by an abundance of cheap oil, tightening world oil supplies will further complicate efforts to eradicate hunger. Modern mechanized agriculture requires large amounts of fuel for tractors, irrigation pumps, and grain drying. Rising oil prices may soon translate into rising food prices.

Feeding the World

If grain imports continue to grow in Asia, where half the world's people live, and if harvests continue to shrink in Africa, the second-most populous continent, we have to ask where tomorrow's grain will come from. The countries that dominated world grain exports for the last half century—the United States, Canada, Australia, and Argentina—may not be able to export much beyond current levels.

The United States has produced as much as 350 million tons of grain a year several times over the last two decades,

though never much more than this. The country exported about 100 million tons of grain a year two decades ago, but only an average of 80 million tons in recent years, as demand has increased domestically. The potential for expanding grain production and export in both Canada and Australia is constrained by relatively low rainfall in their grain-growing regions. Argentina's grain production has actually declined over the last several years as land has shifted to soybeans, principally used for feeding livestock rather than people.

In a world of rising temperatures, there is added reason to be concerned about world food security.

By contrast, Russia and Ukraine should be able to expand their grain exports, at least modestly, as population has stabilized or is declining. There is also some unrealized agricultural production potential in these countries. But northern countries heavily dependent on spring wheat typically have lower yields, so Russia is unlikely to become a major grain exporter. Ukraine has a somewhat more promising potential if it can provide farmers with the economic incentives they need to expand production. So, too, do Poland and Romania.

Yet, the likely increases in exports from these countries are small compared with the prospective import needs of China and, potentially, India. It is worth noting that the drop in China's grain harvest of 70 million tons over five years is equal to the grain exports of Canada, Australia, and Argentina combined.

Argentina can expand its already large volume of soybean exports, but its growth potential for grain exports is limited by the availability of arable land. The only country that has the potential to substantially expand the world's grainland area is Brazil, with its vast cerrado—a savannah-like region on the southern edge of the Amazon basin. Because its soils require the heavy use of fertilizer and because transporting grain from Brazil's remote interior to distant world markets is costly, it would likely take substantially higher world grain prices for Brazil to emerge as a major exporter. Beyond this, would a vast expansion of cropland in Brazil's interior be sustainable? Or is its vulnerability to soil erosion likely to prevent it from making a long-term contribution? And what will be the price paid in the irretrievable loss of ecosystems and plant and animal species?

In sum, ensuring future food security is a formidable, multifaceted problem. To solve it, the world will need to:

- Check the HIV epidemic before it so depletes Africa's adult population that starvation stalks the land.
- Arrest the steady shrinkage in grainland area per person.
- Eliminate the overgrazing that is converting grasslands to desert.

- Reduce soil erosion losses to below the natural rate of new soil formation.
- Halt the advancing deserts that are engulfing cropland.
- Check the rising temperature that threatens to shrink harvests.
- Arrest the fall in water tables.
- Protect cropland from careless conversion to nonfarm uses.

LESTER R. BROWN is president of the Earth Policy Institute, 1350 Connecticut Avenue, N.W., Suite 403, Washington, D.C. 20036.

This article draws from his most recent book, *Outgrowing the Earth: The Food Security Challenge in an Age of Falling Water Tables and Rising Temperatures* (W.W. Norton, 2005), which is available from the Futurist Bookshelf, www.wfs.org/bkshelf.htm. For additional information, visit www.earth-policy.org/Books/Out/index.htm.

Draining Our Future

The Growing Shortage of Freshwater

Global demand for freshwater has tripled in the last half century and will continue to grow along with population increases and economic development. Shrinking water supplies endanger not only the natural environment, but also food and energy supplies and even statehood and international stability.

LESTER R. BROWN

The world is incurring a vast water deficit—one that is largely invisible, historically recent, and growing fast. Globally, demand for water has tripled over the last half century, and millions of irrigation wells have been drilled, pushing water withdrawals beyond recharge rates. In other words, we're now mining groundwater.

Governments have failed to limit pumping to the sustainable yield of aquifers. The result: Water tables are now falling in countries that contain more than half the world's people, including the big three grain producers—China, India, and the United States.

The link between water and food is strong: We each drink on average nearly four liters of water per day in one form or another, while 500 times as much water is required to produce our daily food totals. Seventy percent of all water use is for irrigation, compared with 20% used by industry and 10% used for residential purposes. With the demand for water growing in all three categories, competition among sectors is intensifying—and agriculture almost always loses. While most people recognize that the world is facing a future of water shortages, not everyone has connected the dots to see that this also means a future of food shortages.

World's Water Tables Are Dropping

Scores of countries are overpumping aquifers as they struggle to satisfy their growing water needs. Most aquifers are replenishable, but when they are depleted—as may happen in India, for instance—the maximum rate of pumping will be automatically reduced to the rate of recharge.

Fossil aquifers, however, are not replenishable. If the vast U.S. Ogallala aquifer or the Saudi aquifer, for example, become depleted, pumping comes to an end. Farmers who lose their irrigation water have the option of returning to lower-yield dryland farming if rainfall permits. But in more arid regions, such as in the southwestern United States or the Middle East, the loss of irrigation water means the end of agriculture.

Falling water tables are already adversely affecting harvests in some countries, including China, which rivals the United States as the world's largest grain producer. A 2001 groundwater survey revealed that the water table is falling fast under the North China Plain—an area that produces more than half of the country's wheat and a third of its corn. Overpumping has largely depleted the shallow aquifer, forcing well drillers to turn to the region's deep aquifer, which is not replenishable.

The World Bank warns, "Anecdotal evidence suggests that deep wells [drilled] around Beijing now have to reach 1,000 meters [more than half a mile] to tap fresh water, adding dramatically to the cost of supply." In unusually strong language for a Bank report, it foresees "catastrophic consequences for future generations" unless water use and supply can quickly be brought back into balance.

Falling water tables, the conversion of cropland to nonfarm uses, and the loss of farm labor in provinces that are rapidly industrializing are combining to shrink China's grain harvest. The wheat crop, grown mostly in semiarid northern China, is particularly vulnerable to water shortages. After peaking at 123 million tons in 1997, the harvest has fallen, coming in at 105 million tons in 2007, a drop of 15%.

According to the World Bank, China is mining underground water in three adjacent river basins in the north—those of the Hai, the Yellow, and the Huai. Since it takes 1,000 tons of water to produce one ton of grain, the Hai basin's shortfall of nearly 40 billion tons of water per year means that, when the aquifer is depleted, the grain harvest will drop by 40 million tons— enough to have fed 120 million Chinese.

As serious as water shortages are in China, they are even more serious in India, where the margin between food consumption and survival is so precarious. India's grain harvest, squeezed both by water scarcity and the loss of cropland to nonfarm uses, has plateaued since 2000. This helps explain why India reemerged as a leading wheat importer in 2006. Some 15% of India's food supply is produced by mining groundwater, the World Bank reports. In other words, 175 million Indians are fed with grain produced with water from irrigation wells that will soon go dry.

As water tables fall, the energy required for pumping rises. In both India and China, the rising electricity demand from irrigation is satisfied largely by building coal-fired power plants.

In the United States, according to the Department of Agriculture, the underground water table has dropped by more than 30 meters (100 feet) in parts of Texas, Oklahoma, and Kansas—three leading grain-producing states. As a result, wells have gone dry on thousands of farms in the southern Great Plains, forcing farmers to return to lower-yielding dryland farming. Although this mining of underground water is taking a toll on U.S. grain production, irrigated land accounts for only one-fifth of the U.S. grain harvest, compared with close to three-fifths of the harvest in India and four-fifths in China.

Other countries affected by falling water tables include:

- **Pakistan,** where future irrigation water cutbacks as a result of aquifer depletion will undoubtedly reduce grain harvest.
- **Iran,** which is overpumping its aquifers by an average of 5 billion tons of water per year, the water equivalent of one-third of its annual grain harvest. Villages in eastern Iran are being abandoned as wells go dry, generating a flow of "water refugees."
- **Saudi Arabia,** which is as water-poor as it is oil-rich. With plunging fossil water reservoirs, irrigated agriculture in Saudi Arabia could last for another decade or so and then will largely vanish.
- **Yemen,** with a water table falling by roughly 2 meters a year as water use outstrips the sustainable yield of aquifers. With its population growing at 3% a year and water tables falling everywhere, Yemen is fast becoming a hydrological basket case. Its grain production has fallen by two-thirds over the last 20 years, and it now imports four-fifths of its grain supply.
- **Israel,** which is depleting both of its principal aquifers, despite being a pioneer in raising irrigation water productivity. Because of severe water shortages, Israel has banned the irrigation of wheat. Conflicts between Israelis and Palestinians over the allocation of water are ongoing.
- **Mexico,** where population is projected to reach 132 million by 2050 and where demand for water is outstripping supply. More than half of all the water extracted from underground is from aquifers that are being overpumped.

Since the overpumping of aquifers is occurring in many countries more or less simultaneously, the depletion of aquifers and the resulting harvest cutbacks could come at roughly the same time. And the accelerating depletion of aquifers means this day may come soon, creating potentially unmanageable food scarcity.

Rivers Running Dry and Lakes Shrinking

Falling water tables are largely hidden, but we can see rivers that are drained dry or reduced to a trickle before they reach the sea. The Colorado—the major river in the southwestern United States—and the Yellow—the largest river in northern China—are two rivers where this phenomenon can be seen. Others include the Nile, the lifeline of Egypt; the Indus, which supplies most of Pakistan's irrigation water; and the Ganges in India's densely populated Gangetic basin. Many smaller rivers have disappeared entirely.

Compounding the growing demand for water is the demand for hydroelectric power, which has grown even faster. Dams and diversions of river water have drained many rivers dry. As water tables have fallen, the springs that feed rivers have gone dry, reducing river flows.

Since 1950, the number of large dams (more than 15 meters high) has increased from 5,000 to 45,000. Each dam deprives a river of some of its flow. Engineers like to say that dams built to generate electricity take only a river's energy, not its water, but this is not entirely true. Reservoirs increase evaporation. The annual loss of water from a reservoir in arid or semiarid regions, where evaporation rates are high, is typically equal to 10% of its storage capacity.

The Colorado River now rarely makes it to the sea. With the states of Colorado, Utah, Arizona, Nevada, and California depending heavily on the Colorado's water, there is little, if any, water left when it reaches the Gulf of California. This excessive demand for water is destroying the river's ecosystem, including its fisheries.

Pakistan, like Egypt, is essentially a river-based civilization, heavily dependent on the Indus. This river, originating in the Himalayas and flowing southwestward to the Indian Ocean, not only provides surface water, but it also recharges aquifers that supply the irrigation wells dotting the Pakistani countryside. In the face of Pakistan's growing population and water demand, the Indus, too, is starting to run dry in its lower reaches.

The same problem exists with the overused Tigris and Euphrates rivers, which originate in Turkey and flow through Syria and Iraq en route to the Persian Gulf. Large dams erected in Turkey and Iraq have reduced water flow to the once "fertile crescent," helping to destroy 80% of the vast wetlands that formerly enriched the delta region.

In river systems such as the Colorado, the Yellow, the Nile, and many others around the world, virtually all the water in the basin is being used. Inevitably, if people upstream get more water, those downstream will get less. Allocating water among competing interests, within and among societies, is part of an emerging politics of resource scarcity.

Lakes, too, are shrinking or even disappearing, including some of the world's best known: Lake Chad in Central Africa, the Aral Sea in Central Asia, and the Sea of Galilee (also known as Lake Tiberias).

With the Jordan's flow further diminished as it passes through Israel, the Dead Sea is shrinking even faster than the Sea of Galilee. Over the past 40 years, its water level has dropped by some 25 meters (nearly 80 feet). It could disappear entirely by 2050.

Of all the shrinking lakes and inland seas, none has gotten as much attention as the Aral Sea. Its ports, once centers of commerce, are now abandoned, looking like the ghost mining towns of the American West. Once one of the world's largest freshwater bodies, the Aral has lost four-fifths of its volume since 1960, as Soviet planners diverted water from its feeding rivers to an expanding cotton and textile industry. By 1990, an aerial view of the dry, salt-covered seabed resembled the surface of the Moon.

As the sea shrank, the salt concentrations climbed until the fish died. The thriving fishery that once yielded 50,000 tons of seafood per year disappeared, as did the jobs on the fishing boats and in the fish processing factories.

Lakes are disappearing on every continent and for the same reasons: excessive diversion of water from rivers and over-pumping of aquifers. No one knows exactly how many lakes have disappeared over the last half century, but we do know that thousands of them now exist only on old maps.

Farmers Losing to Cities

Water tensions among countries are more likely to make the headlines, but it is the jousting for water between cities and farms within countries that preoccupies local political leaders. The economics of water use do not favor farmers in this competition, simply because it takes so much water to produce food. For example, while it takes only 14 tons of water to make a ton of steel worth $560, it takes 1,000 tons of water to grow a ton of wheat worth $200. In countries preoccupied with expanding the economy and creating jobs, agriculture becomes the residual claimant.

Many of the world's largest cities are located in watersheds where all available water is being used. Cities in such watersheds—Mexico City, Cairo, and Beijing, for example—can increase their water consumption only by importing water from other basins or taking it from agriculture. Increasingly, the world's cities are meeting their growing needs by taking irrigation water from farmers. Among the U.S. cities doing so are San Diego, Los Angeles, Las Vegas, Denver, and El Paso.

The competition between farmers and cities for underground water resources is intensifying throughout India. Nowhere is this more evident than in Chennai (formerly Madras), a city of 7 million on the east coast of south India. The government has failed to supply water for some of the city's residents, so a thriving tank-truck industry has emerged to bring in water that it buys from farmers.

For farmers surrounding the city, the price of water far exceeds the value of the crops they can produce with it. Unfortunately, the 13,000 tankers hauling the water to Chennai are mining the underground water resources. Water tables are falling and shallow wells have gone dry. Eventually even the deeper wells will go dry, depriving these communities of both their food supply and their livelihood.

Chinese farmers along the Juma River downstream from Beijing discovered in 2004 that the river had suddenly stopped flowing. A diversion dam had been built near the capital to take river water for Yanshan Petrochemical, a state-owned industry. The farmers protested bitterly, but it was a losing battle. For the 120,000 villagers downstream from the diversion dam, the loss of water could cripple their ability to make a living from farming.

Literally hundreds of cities in other countries are meeting their growing water needs by taking the water that farmers count on. In western Turkey, for example, the historic city of Izmir now relies heavily on well fields (a network of wells connected by pipe) from the neighboring agricultural district of Manisa.

In the U.S. southern Great Plains and Southwest, where virtually all water is now spoken for, the growing water needs of cities and thousands of small towns can be satisfied only by taking water from agriculture.

Colorado has one of the world's most active water markets. Fast-growing cities and towns in a state with high immigration are buying irrigation water rights from farmers and ranchers. And in 2003, San Diego made a 75-year deal to buy annual rights to 247 million tons of water from farmers in the nearby Imperial Valley—the largest farm-to-city water transfer in U.S. history. Without irrigation water, the highly productive land owned by these farmers is wasteland. The farmers who are selling their water rights would like to continue farming, but city officials are offering far more for the water than the farmers could possibly earn by irrigating crops.

Whether it is outright government expropriation, farmers being outbid by cities, or cities simply drilling deeper wells than farmers can afford, the world's farmers are losing the water war. They are faced with not only a shrinking water supply in many situations, but also a shrinking share of that shrinking supply. Slowly but surely, fast-growing cities are siphoning water from the world's farmers even as they try to feed some 70 million more people each year.

Scarcity Crosses National Borders

Water scarcity has historically been a local issue. It was up to national governments to balance water supply and demand. Now, scarcity crosses national boundaries via the international grain trade. It takes a thousand tons of water to produce one ton of grain, so importing grain is the most efficient way to import water. In effect, countries are using grain to balance their water books. Similarly, trading in grain futures is in a sense trading in water futures.

After China and India, there is a second tier of smaller countries with large water deficits. Algeria, Egypt, and Mexico already import much of their grain. Pakistan, too, may soon turn to world markets for grain, with a population outgrowing its water supply.

From Morocco to Iran, the Middle East and North Africa region has become the world's fastest-growing grain import market. The demand for grain is driven both by rapid population growth and by rising affluence, thanks largely to oil exports. Virtually every country in the region is pressing against its water limits, so the growing urban demand for water can be satisfied only by taking irrigation water from agriculture.

Egypt has become a major importer of wheat in recent years, vying with Japan for the top spot as the world's leading wheat importer. Egypt now imports close to 40% of its total grain supply, a dependence that reflects a population that is outgrowing the grain harvest produced with the Nile's water. And Algeria imports well over half of its grain.

The water now required to produce a year's worth of grain and other farm products imported into the Middle East and North Africa nearly equals the annual flow of the Nile River at Aswan. In effect, the region's water deficit can be thought of as another Nile flowing into the region in the form of imported food.

It is often said that future wars in the Middle East will more likely be fought over water than oil, but in reality the competition for water is taking place in world grain markets. The countries that are financially the strongest, not necessarily those that are militarily the strongest, will fare best in this competition.

Knowing where grain deficits will be concentrated tomorrow requires looking at where water deficits are developing today. Thus far, the countries importing much of their grain have been smaller ones. Now we are looking at fast-growing water deficits in both China and India, each with more than a billion people.

As noted earlier, overpumping is a way of satisfying growing food demand that virtually guarantees a future drop in food production when aquifers are depleted. Many countries are essentially creating a "food bubble economy"—one in which food production is artificially inflated by the unsustainable mining of groundwater. At what point does water scarcity translate into food scarcity?

David Seckler and his colleagues at the International Water Management Institute, the world's premier water research group, summarized this issue well: "Many of the most populous countries of the world—China, India, Pakistan, Mexico, and nearly all the countries of the Middle East and North Africa—have literally been having a free ride over the past two or three decades by depleting their groundwater resources. The penalty for mismanagement of this valuable resource is now coming due and it is no exaggeration to say that the results could be catastrophic for these countries and, given their importance, for the world as a whole."

Water Scarcity Yields Political Stresses

We typically measure well-being in economic terms—in income per person—but water well-being is measured in cubic meters or tons of water per person. A country with an annual supply of 1,700 cubic meters of water per person is well supplied with water, able to comfortably meet agricultural, industrial, and residential needs. Below this level, stresses begin to appear. When water supply drops below 1,000 cubic meters per person, people face scarcity. Below 500 cubic meters, acute scarcity, they suffer from hydrological poverty—living without enough water to produce food or, in some cases, even for basic hygiene.

The world's most severe water stresses are found in North Africa and the Middle East. While Morocco and Egypt have fewer than 1,000 cubic meters per person per year, Algeria, Tunisia, and Libya have fewer than 500. Some countries, including Saudi Arabia, Yemen, Kuwait, and Israel, have less than 300 cubic meters per person per year. A number of sub-Saharan countries are also facing water stress, including Kenya and Rwanda.

While national averages indicate an adequate water supply in each of the world's three most populous countries—China, India, and the United States—regions within these countries also suffer from acute water shortages. Water is scarce throughout the northern half of China. In India, the northwestern region suffers extreme water scarcity. For the United States, the southwestern states from Texas to California are experiencing acute water shortages.

Although the risk of international conflict over water is real, so far there have been remarkably few water wars. Water tensions tend to build more within societies, particularly where water is already scarce and population growth is rapid. Recent years have witnessed conflicts over water in scores of countries, such as the competition between cities and farmers in countries like China, India, and Yemen. In other countries, the conflicts are between tribes, as in Kenya, or between villages, as in India and China, or between upstream and downstream water users, as in Pakistan or China. In some countries, local water conflicts have led to violence and death, as in Kenya, Pakistan, and China.

In Pakistan's arid southwest province of Balochistan, water tables are falling everywhere as a fast-growing local population swelled by Afghan refugees is pumping water far faster than aquifers can recharge. The provincial capital of Quetta is facing a particularly dire situation. And Iraq is concerned that dam building on the Euphrates River in Turkey and Syria will leave it without enough water to meet its basic needs. The flow into Iraq of the Euphrates River has shrunk by half over the last few decades.

Many of the countries high on the list of failing states are those where populations are outrunning their water supplies.

At the global level, most of the projected population growth of nearly 3 billion by 2050 will come in countries where water tables are already falling. The states most stressed by the scarcity of water tend to be those in arid and semiarid regions, with fast-growing populations and a resistance to family planning. Many of the countries high on the list of failing states are those where populations are outrunning their water supplies: Sudan, Iraq, Somalia, Chad, Afghanistan, Pakistan, and Yemen, for instance. Unless population can be stabilized in these countries, the continually shrinking supply of water per person will put still more stress on already overstressed governments.

Although spreading water shortages is a daunting problem, we have the technologies needed to raise water use efficiency, thus buying time to stabilize population size. Prominent among these technologies are those for more water-efficient irrigation, industrial water recycling, and urban water recycling.

Raising Water Productivity

Raising irrigation efficiency is central to raising water productivity overall. Using more water-efficient irrigation technologies and shifting to crops that use less water permit the expansion of irrigated area even with a fixed water supply. Eliminating water and energy subsidies that encourage wasteful water use allows water prices to rise to market levels. Higher water prices encourage all water users to use water more efficiently. In many countries, local rural water users associations that directly involve users in water management have raised water productivity.

Evaporation, percolation, and runoff also reduce irrigation's efficiency. In surface water projects—that is, dams that deliver water to farmers through a network of canals—crop usage of irrigation water never reaches 100%. Water policy analysts Sandra Postel and Amy Vickers found that "surface water irrigation efficiency ranges between 25% and 40% in India, Mexico, Pakistan, the Philippines, and Thailand; between 40% and 45% in Malaysia and Morocco; and between 50% and 60% in Israel, Japan, and Taiwan." In hot arid regions, the evaporation of irrigation water is far higher than in cooler humid regions.

In 2004, China's Minister of Water Resources Wang Shucheng shared details of China's plans to raise irrigation efficiency from 43% in 2000 to 55% in 2030. The steps included raising the price of water, providing incentives for adopting more irrigation-efficient technologies, and developing the local institutions to manage this process. Reaching these goals, he felt, would assure China's future food security.

Raising irrigation water efficiency typically means shifting from the less-efficient flood or furrow system to overhead sprinklers or drip irrigation, the gold standard of irrigation efficiency. Switching from flood or furrow to low-pressure sprinkler systems reduces water use by an estimated 30%, while switching to drip irrigation typically cuts water use in half.

A few small countries—Cyprus, Israel, and Jordan—rely heavily on drip irrigation. Among the big three agricultural producers, this more efficient technology is used on 1%–3% of irrigated land in India and China and on roughly 4% in the United States.

In recent years, small-scale drip-irrigation systems—virtually a bucket with flexible plastic tubing to distribute the water—have been developed to irrigate small vegetable gardens with roughly 100 plants (covering 25 square meters). Somewhat larger drum systems irrigate 125 square meters. In both cases,

the containers are elevated slightly, so that gravity distributes the water. Large-scale drip systems using plastic lines that can be moved easily are also becoming popular. These simple systems can pay for themselves in one year. By simultaneously reducing water costs and raising yields, they can dramatically raise incomes of smallholders.

In the Punjab, with its extensive double cropping of wheat and rice, fast-falling water tables led the state farmers' commission in 2007 to recommend a delay in transplanting rice from May to late June or early July. This would reduce irrigation water use by roughly one-third, since transplanting would coincide with the arrival of the monsoon. This reduction in groundwater use would help stabilize the water table, which has fallen from 5 meters below the surface to 30 meters in parts of the state.

Institutional shifts—specifically, moving the responsibility for managing irrigation systems from government agencies to local water users associations—can facilitate the more efficient use of water. In many countries, farmers are organizing locally so they can assume this responsibility. Since they have an economic stake in good water management, they tend to do a better job than a distant government agency.

Mexico is a leader in developing water users associations. As of 2002, farmers associations managed more than 80% of Mexico's publicly irrigated land. One advantage of this shift for the government is that the cost of maintaining the irrigation system is assumed locally, reducing the drain on the treasury. This means that associations often need to charge more for irrigation water, but for farmers the production gains from managing their water supply themselves more than outweigh this additional outlay.

Low water productivity is often the result of low water prices. In many countries, subsidies lead to irrationally low water prices, creating the impression that water is abundant when in fact it is scarce. As water becomes scarce, it needs to be priced accordingly.

What is needed now is a new mind-set, a new way of thinking about water use. For example, shifting to more water-efficient crops wherever possible boosts water productivity. Rice production is being phased out around Beijing because rice is such a thirsty crop. Similarly, Egypt restricts rice production in favor of wheat.

Any measures that raise crop yields on irrigated land also raise the productivity of irrigation water. Similarly, any measures that convert grain into animal protein more efficiently in effect increase water productivity.

For people consuming unhealthy amounts of livestock products, moving down the food chain reduces water use. In the United States, where annual consumption of grain as food and feed averages some 800 kilograms (four-fifths of a ton) per person, a modest reduction in the consumption of meat, milk, and eggs could easily cut grain use per person by 100 kilograms. For 300 million Americans, such a reduction would cut grain use by 30 million tons and irrigation water use by 30 billion tons.

Reducing water use to the sustainable yield of aquifers and rivers worldwide involves a wide range of measures not only in agriculture but throughout the economy. The more obvious steps, in addition to more water-efficient irrigation practices and more water-efficient crops, include adopting more water-efficient industrial processes and using more water-efficient household appliances. Recycling urban water supplies is another obvious step to consider in countries facing acute water shortages.

Unless we commit to a plan for restoring water security, our water planet's future will be thirstier, hungrier, and more precarious. The good news is that momentum is building to reverse the damaging environmental and resource trends that we ourselves have set in motion.

LESTER R. BROWN is president of the Earth Policy Institute, 1350 Connecticut Avenue, N.W., Suite 403, Washington, D.C. 20036. Web site www.earthpolicy.org.

Originally published in the May/June 2008 issue of *The Futurist*. Copyright © 2008 by World Future Society, 7910 Woodmont Avenue, Suite 450, Bethesda, MD 20814. Telephone: 301/656-8274; Fax: 301/951-0394; http://www.wfs.org. Used with permission from the World Future Society.

10 Reasons Why Organic Can Feed the World

Can organic farming feed the world? Ed Hamer and Mark Anslow say yes, but we must farm and eat differently.

ED HAMER AND MARK ANSLOW

1. Yield

Switching to organic farming would have different effects according to where in the world you live and how you currently farm.

Studies show that the less-industrialised world stands to benefit the most. In southern Brazil, maize and wheat yields doubled on farms that changed to green manures and nitrogen-fixing leguminous vegetables instead of chemical fertilisers. In Mexico, coffee-growers who chose to move to fully organic production methods saw increases of 50 percent in the weight of beans they harvested. In fact, in an analysis of more than 286 organic conversions in 57 countries, the average yield increase was found to be an impressive 64 percent.

The situation is more complex in the industrialised world, where farms are large, intensive facilities, and opinions are divided on how organic yields would compare.

Research by the University of Essex in 1999 found that, although yields on US farms that converted to organic initially dropped by between 10 and 15 percent, they soon recovered, and the farms became more productive than their all-chemical counterparts. In the UK, however, a study by the Elm Farm Research Centre predicted that a national transition to all-organic farming would see cereal, rapeseed and sugar beet yields fall by between 30 and 60 percent. Even the Soil Association admits that, on average in the UK, organic yields are 30 percent lower than non-organic.

So can we hope to feed ourselves organically in the British Isles and Northern Europe? An analysis by former *Ecologist* editor Simon Fairlie in *The Land journal* suggests that we can, but only if we are prepared to rethink our diet and farming practices. In Fairlie's scenario, each of the UK's 60 million citizens could have organic cereals, potatoes, sugar, vegetables and fruit, fish, pork, chicken and beef, as well as wool and flax for clothes and biomass crops for heating. To achieve this we'd each have to cut down to around 230 g of beef (½ lb), compared to an average of 630 g (1½ lb) today, 252 g of pork/bacon, 210 g of chicken and just under 4 kg (9 lb) of dairy produce each week—considerably more than the country enjoyed in 1945. We would probably need to supplement our diet with homegrown vegetables, save our food scraps as livestock feed and reform the sewage system to use our waste as an organic fertiliser.

2. Energy

Currently, we use around 10 calories of fossil energy to produce one calorie of food energy. In a fuel-scarce future, which experts think could arrive as early as 2012, such numbers simply won't stack up.

Studies by the Department for Environment, Food and Rural affairs over the past three years have shown that, on average, organically grown crops use 25 percent less energy than their chemical cousins. Certain crops achieve even better reductions, including organic leeks (58 percent less energy) and broccoli (49 percent less energy).

When these savings are combined with stringent energy conservation and local distribution and consumption (such as organic box schemes), energy-use dwindles to a fraction of that needed for an intensive, centralised food system. A study by the University of Surrey shows that food from Tolhurst Organic Produce, a smallholding in Berkshire, which supplies 400 households with vegetable boxes, uses 90 percent less energy than if non-organic produce had been delivered and bought in a supermarket.

Organic farms even have the potential to become energy exporters.

Far from being simply 'energy-lite', however, organic farms have the potential to become self-sufficient in energy—or even to become energy exporters. The 'Dream Farm' model, first proposed by Mauritius-born agro-scientist George Chan, sees farms feeding manure and waste from livestock and crops into biodigesters, which convert it into a methane-rich gas to be used for creating heat and electricity. The residue from these bio-digesters is a crumbly, nutrient-rich fertiliser, which can be spread on soil to increase crop yields or further digested by algae and used as a fish or animal feed.

3. Greenhouse Gas Emissions and Climate Change

Despite organic farming's low-energy methods, it is not in reducing demand for power that the techniques stand to make the biggest savings in greenhouse gas emissions.

The production of ammonium nitrate fertiliser, which is indispensable to conventional farming, produces vast quantities of nitrous oxide—a greenhouse gas with a global warming potential some 320 times greater than that of CO_2. In fact, the production of one tonne of ammonium nitrate creates 6.7 tonnes of greenhouse gases (CO_2e), and was responsible for around 10 percent of all industrial greenhouse gas emissions in Europe in 2003.

The techniques used in organic agriculture to enhance soil fertility in turn encourage crops to develop deeper roots, which increase the amount of organic matter in the soil, locking up carbon underground and keeping it out of the atmosphere. The opposite happens in conventional farming: high quantities of artificially supplied nutrients encourage quick growth and shallow roots. A study published in 1995 in the journal *Ecological Applications* found that levels of carbon in the soils of organic farms in California were as much as 28 percent higher as a result. And research by the Rodale Institute shows that if the US were to convert all its corn and soybean fields to organic methods, the amount of carbon that could be stored in the soil would equal 73 percent of the country's Kyoto targets for CO_2 reduction.

Organic farming might also go some way towards salvaging the reputation of the cow, demonised in 2007 as a major source of methane at both ends of its digestive tract. There's no doubt that this is a problem: estimates put global methane emissions from ruminant livestock at around 80 million tonnes a year, equivalent to around two billion tonnes of CO_2, or close to the annual CO_2 output of Russia and the UK combined. But by changing the pasturage on which animals graze to legumes such as clover or birdsfoot trefoil (often grown anyway by organic farmers to improve soil nitrogen content), scientists at the Institute of Grassland and Environmental Research believe that methane emissions could be cut dramatically. Because the leguminous foliage is more digestible, bacteria in the cow's gut are less able to turn the fodder into methane. Cows also seem naturally to prefer eating birdsfoot trefoil to ordinary grass.

4. Water Use

Agriculture is officially the most thirsty industry on the planet, consuming a staggering 72 percent of all global freshwater at a time when the UN says 80 percent of our water supplies are being overexploited.

This hasn't always been the case. Traditionally, agricultural crops were restricted to those areas best suited to their physiology, with drought-tolerant species grown in the tropics and water-demanding crops in temperate regions. Global trade throughout the second half of the last century led to a worldwide production of grains dominated by a handful of high-yielding cereal crops, notably wheat, maize and rice. These thirsty cereals—the 'big three'—now account for more than half of the world's plant-based calories and 85 percent of total grain production.

Organic agriculture is different. Due to its emphasis on healthy soil structure, organic farming avoids many of the problems associated with compaction, erosion, salinisation and soil degradation, which are prevalent in intensive systems. Organic manures and green mulches are applied even before the crop is sown, leading to a process known as 'mineralisation'—literally the fixing of minerals in the soil. Mineralised organic matter, conspicuously absent from synthetic fertilisers, is one of the essential ingredients required physically and chemically to hold water on the land.

Organic management also uses crop rotations, undersowing and mixed cropping to provide the soil with near-continuous cover. By contrast, conventional farm soils may be left uncovered for extended periods prior to sowing, and again following the harvest, leaving essential organic matter fully exposed to erosion by rain, wind and sunlight.

In the US, a 25-year Rodale Institute experiment on climatic extremes found that, due to improved soil structure, organic systems consistently achieve higher yields during periods both of drought and flooding.

5. Localisation

The globalisation of our food supply, which gives us Peruvian apples in June and Spanish lettuces in February, has seen our food reduced to a commodity in an increasingly volatile global marketplace. Although year-round availability makes for good marketing in the eyes of the biggest retailers, the costs to the environment are immense.

Friends of the Earth estimates that the average meal in the UK travels 1,000 miles from plot to plate. In 2005, Defra released a comprehensive report on food miles in the UK, which valued the direct environmental, social and economic costs of food transport in Britain at £9 billion each year. In addition, food transport accounted for more than 30 billion vehicle kilometres, 25 percent of all HGV journeys and 19 million tonnes of carbon dioxide emissions in 2002 alone.

The organic movement was born out of a commitment to provide local food for local people, and so it is logical that organic marketing encourages localisation through veg boxes, farm shops and stalls. Between 2005 and 2006, organic sales made through direct marketing outlets such as these increased by 53 percent, from £95 to £146 million, more than double the sales growth experienced by the major supermarkets. As we enter an age of unprecedented food insecurity, it is essential that our consumption reflects not only what is desirable, but also what is ultimately sustainable. While the 'organic' label itself may inevitably be hijacked, 'organic and local' represents a solution with which the global players can simply never compete.

6. Pesticides

It is a shocking testimony to the power of the agrochemical industry that in the 45 years since Rachel Carson published her pesticide warning *Silent Spring*, the number of commercially available synthetic pesticides has risen from 22 to more than 450.

According to the World Health Organization there are an estimated 20,000 accidental deaths worldwide each year from pesticide exposure and poisoning. More than 31 million kilograms of pesticide were applied to UK crops alone in 2005, 0.5 kilograms for every person in the country. A spiralling dependence on pesticides throughout recent decades has resulted in a catalogue of repercussions, including pest resistance, disease susceptibility, loss of natural biological controls and reduced nutrient-cycling.

Organic farmers, on the other hand, believe that a healthy plant grown in a healthy soil will ultimately be more resistant to pest damage. Organic systems encourage a variety of natural methods to enhance soil and plant health, in turn reducing incidences of pests, weeds and disease.

First and foremost, because organic plants grow comparatively slower than conventional varieties they have thicker cell walls, which provide a tougher natural barrier to pests. Rotations or 'break-crops', which are central to organic production, also provide a physical obstacle to pest and disease lifecycles by removing crops from a given plot for extended periods. Organic systems also rely heavily on a rich agro-ecosystem in which many agricultural pests can be controlled by their natural predators.

Inevitably, however, there are times when pestilence attacks are especially prolonged or virulent, and here permitted pesticides may be used. The use of organic pesticides is heavily regulated and the International Federation of Organic Agriculture Movements (IFOAM) requires specific criteria to be met before pesticide applications can be justified.

There are in fact only four active ingredients permitted for use on organic crops: copper fungicides, restricted largely to potatoes and occasionally orchards; sulphur, used to control additional elements of fungal diseases; Retenone, a naturally occurring plant extract, and soft soap, derived from potassium soap and used to control aphids. Herbicides are entirely prohibited.

7. Ecosystem Impact

Farmland accounts for 70 percent of UK land mass, making it the single most influential enterprise affecting our wildlife. Incentives offered for intensification under the Common Agricultural Policy are largely responsible for negative ecosystem impacts over recent years. Since 1962, farmland bird numbers have declined by an average of 30 percent. During the same period more than 192,000 kilometres of hedgerows have been removed, while 45 percent of our ancient woodland has been converted to cropland.

By contrast, organic farms actively encourage biodiversity in order to maintain soil fertility and aid natural pest control. Mixed farming systems ensure that a diversity of food and nesting sites are available throughout the year, compared with conventional farms where autumn sow crops leave little winter vegetation available.

Organic production systems are designed to respect the balance observed in our natural ecosystems. It is widely accepted that controlling or suppressing one element of wildlife, even if it is a pest, will have unpredictable impacts on the rest of the food chain. Instead, organic producers regard a healthy ecosystem as essential to a healthy farm, rather than a barrier to production.

In 2005, a report by English Nature and the RSPB on the impacts of organic farming on biodiversity reviewed more than 70 independent studies of flora, invertebrates, birds and mammals within organic and conventional farming systems. It concluded that biodiversity is enhanced at every level of the food chain under organic management practices, from soil microbiota right through to farmland birds and the largest mammals.

8. Nutritional Benefits

While an all-organic farming system might mean we'd have to make do with slightly less food than we're used to, research shows that we can rest assured it would be better for us.

In 2001, a study in the *Journal of Complementary Medicine* found that organic crops contained higher levels of 21 essential nutrients than their conventionally grown counterparts, including iron, magnesium, phosphorus and vitamin C. The organic crops also contained lower levels of nitrates, which can be toxic to the body.

Other studies have found significantly higher levels of vitamins—as well as polyphenols and antioxidants—in organic fruit and veg, all of which are thought to play a role in cancer-prevention within the body.

Scientists have also been able to work out why organic farming produces more nutritious food. Avoiding chemical fertiliser reduces nitrates levels in the food; better-quality soil increases the availability of trace minerals, and reduced levels of pesticides mean that the plants' own immune systems grow stronger, producing higher levels of antioxidants. Slower rates of growth also mean that organic food frequently contains higher levels of dry mass, meaning that fruit and vegetables are less pumped up with water and so contain more nutrients by weight than intensively grown crops do.

Milk from organically fed cows has been found to contain higher levels of nutrients in six separate studies, including omega-3 fatty acids, vitamin E, and beta-carotene, all of which can help prevent cancer. One experiment discovered that levels of omega-3 in organic milk were on average 68 percent higher than in non-organic alternatives.

But as well as giving us more of what we do need, organic food can help to give us less of what we don't. In 2000, the UN Food and Agriculture Organization (FAO) found that organically produced food had 'lower levels of pesticide and veterinary drug residues' than non-organic did. Although organic farmers are allowed to use antibiotics when absolutely necessary to treat disease, the routine use of the drugs in animal feed—common on intensive livestock farms—is forbidden. This means a shift to organic livestock farming could help tackle problems such as the emergence of antibiotic-resistant bacteria.

9. Seed-Saving

Seeds are not simply a source of food; they are living testimony to more than 10,000 years of agricultural domestication. Tragically, however, they are a resource that has suffered unprecedented neglect. The UN FAO estimates that 75 percent of the genetic diversity of agricultural crops has been lost over the past 100 years.

Traditionally, farming communities have saved seeds year-on-year, both in order to save costs and to trade with their neighbours. As a result, seed varieties evolved in response to local climatic and seasonal conditions, leading to a wide variety of fruiting times, seed size, appearance and flavour. More importantly, this meant a constant updating process for the seed's genetic resistance to changing climatic conditions, new pests and diseases.

By contrast, modern intensive agriculture depends on relatively few crops—only about 150 species are cultivated on any significant scale worldwide. This is the inheritance of the Green Revolution, which in the late 1950s perfected varieties Filial 1, or F1 seed technology, which produced hybrid seeds with specifically desirable genetic qualities. These new high-yield seeds were widely adopted, but because the genetic makeup of hybrid F1 seeds becomes diluted following the first harvest, the manufacturers ensured that farmers return for more seed year-on-year.

With its emphasis on diversity, organic farming is somewhat cushioned from exploitation on this scale, but even Syngenta, the world's third-largest biotech company, now offers organic seed lines. Although seed-saving is not a prerequisite for organic production, the holistic nature of organics lends itself well to conserving seed.

In support of this, the Heritage Seed Library, in Warwickshire, is a collection of more than 800 open-pollinated organic varieties, which have been carefully preserved by gardeners across the country. Although their seeds are not yet commercially available, the Library is at the forefront of addressing the alarming erosion of our agricultural diversity.

Seed-saving and the development of local varieties must become a key component of organic farming, giving crops the potential to evolve in response to what could be rapidly changing climatic conditions. This will help agriculture keeps pace with climate change in the field, rather than in the laboratory.

10. Job Creation

There is no doubt British farming is currently in crisis. With an average of 37 farmers leaving the land every day, there are now more prisoners behind bars in the UK than there are farmers in the fields.

Although it has been slow, the decline in the rural labour force is a predictable consequence of the industrialisation of agriculture. A mere one percent of the UK workforce is now employed in land-related enterprises, compared with 35 percent at the turn of the last century.

The implications of this decline are serious. A skilled agricultural workforce will be essential in order to maintain food security in the coming transition towards a new model of post-fossil fuel farming. Many of these skills have already been eroded through mechanisation and a move towards more specialised and intensive production systems.

Organic farming is an exception to these trends. By its nature, organic production relies on labour-intensive management practices. Smaller, more diverse farming systems require a level of husbandry that is simply uneconomical at any other scale. Organic crops and livestock also demand specialist knowledge and regular monitoring in the absence of agrochemical controls.

93,000 new jobs would be created if all farming in the UK converted to organic.

According to a 2006 report by the University of Essex, organic farming in the UK provides 32 percent more jobs per farm than comparable non-organic farms. Interestingly, the report also concluded that the higher employment observed could not be replicated in non-organic farming through initiatives such as local marketing. Instead, the majority (81 percent) of total employment on organic farms was created by the organic production system itself. The report estimates that 93,000 new jobs would be created if all farming in the UK were to convert to organic.

Organic farming also accounts for more younger employees than any other sector in the industry. The average age of conventional UK farmers is now 56, yet organic farms increasingly attract a younger more enthusiastic workforce, people who view organics as the future of food production. It is for this next generation of farmers that Organic Futures, a campaign group set up by the Soil Association in 2007, is striving to provide a platform.

ED HAMER is a freelance journalist. **MARK ANSLOW** is the *Ecologist*'s senior reporter.

Test-Your-Knowledge Form

We encourage you to photocopy and use this page as a tool to assess how the articles in *Annual Editions* expand on the information in your textbook. By reflecting on the articles you will gain enhanced text information. You can also access this useful form on a product's book support website at www.mhhe.com/cls.

NAME: DATE:

_____

TITLE AND NUMBER OF ARTICLE:

_____

BRIEFLY STATE THE MAIN IDEA OF THIS ARTICLE:

_____

LIST THREE IMPORTANT FACTS THAT THE AUTHOR USES TO SUPPORT THE MAIN IDEA:

_____

WHAT INFORMATION OR IDEAS DISCUSSED IN THIS ARTICLE ARE ALSO DISCUSSED IN YOUR TEXTBOOK OR OTHER READINGS THAT YOU HAVE DONE? LIST THE TEXTBOOK CHAPTERS AND PAGE NUMBERS:

_____

LIST ANY EXAMPLES OF BIAS OR FAULTY REASONING THAT YOU FOUND IN THE ARTICLE:

_____

LIST ANY NEW TERMS/CONCEPTS THAT WERE DISCUSSED IN THE ARTICLE, AND WRITE A SHORT DEFINITION:

We Want Your Advice

ANNUAL EDITIONS revisions depend on two major opinion sources: one is our Advisory Board, listed in the front of this volume, which works with us in scanning the thousands of articles published in the public press each year; the other is you—the person actually using the book. Please help us and the users of the next edition by completing the prepaid article rating form on this page and returning it to us. Thank you for your help!

ANNUAL EDITIONS: Nutrition 10/11

ARTICLE RATING FORM

Here is an opportunity for you to have direct input into the next revision of this volume.
We would like you to rate each of the articles listed below, using the following scale:

1. **Excellent: should definitely be retained**
2. **Above average: should probably be retained**
3. **Below average: should probably be deleted**
4. **Poor: should definitely be deleted**

Your ratings will play a vital part in the next revision.
Please mail this prepaid form to us as soon as possible.
Thanks for your help!

RATING	ARTICLE	RATING	ARTICLE
	1. Mission Organic 2010: Healthy People, Healthy Planet		24. Why We Overeat
	2. A Burger and Fries (Hold the Trans Fats)		25. Still Hungry?
	3. Fast Food: Would You Like 1000 Calories with That?		26. The Health Diet Face-Off
	4. Smarter—and Healthier—Supermarket Shopping Made Simple		27. Will Your Child Be Fat?: How to Prevent Obesity—for Babies on Up
	5. Eat Like a Greek		28. Are We Setting the Stage for Obesity and Poor Oral Health?
	6. The Slow Food Movement Picks up Speed		29. Cancer: How Extra Pounds Boost Your Risk
	7. Schools Can Taste Good		30. The World Is Fat
	8. The Potential of Farm-to-College Programs		31. Miscommunicating Science
	9. Produce to the People		32. Shaping up the Dietary Supplement Industry
	10. Color Me Healthy: Eating for a Rainbow of Benefits		33. Why People Use Vitamin and Mineral Supplements
	11. Antioxidants: Fruitful Research and Recommendations		34. "Fountain of Youth" Fact and Fantasy
	12. Confusion at the Vitamin Counter: Too Little or Too Much?		35. Brain Food
	13. Minerals Matter: The Wrong Amounts Can Harm You		36. Phytosterols: Mother Nature's Cholesterol Fighters
	14. Fiber Free-for-All		37. The Benefits of Flax
	15. The Fairest Fats of Them All (and Those to Avoid)		38. Is Your Food Contaminated?
	16. Omega-3 Madness		39. Dirty Birds: Even 'Premium' Chickens Harbor Dangerous Bacteria
	17. Food for Thought: Exploring the Potential of Mindful Eating		40. Fear of Fresh: How to Avoid Food-Borne Illness from Fruits & Vegetables
	18. Eating Disorders in Childhood: Prevention and Treatment Supports		41. Irradiation of Fresh Fruits and Vegetables
	19. The Diet-Inflammation Connection		42. The E. Coli Outbreak: Lettuce Learn a Lesson
	20. The Best Diabetes Diet for Optimal Outcomes		43. Produce Safety: Back to Basics for Producers and Consumers
	21. Diet Does Matter: Nutrition's Role in Cancer Prevention and Treatment		44. In Search of Sustainability
	22. Alzheimer's—The Case for Prevention		45. A Question of Sustenance
	23. Living Longer: Diet		46. Pushing Beyond the Earth's Limits
			47. Draining Our Future: The Growing Shortage of Freshwater
			48. 10 Reasons Why Organic Can Feed the World

ABOUT YOU

Name

Date

Are you a teacher? ☐ A student? ☐
Your school's name

Department

Address

City

State

Zip

School telephone #

YOUR COMMENTS ARE IMPORTANT TO US!

Please fill in the following information:
For which course did you use this book?

Did you use a text with this ANNUAL EDITION? ☐ yes ☐ no
What was the title of the text?

What are your general reactions to the Annual Editions concept?

Have you read any pertinent articles recently that you think should be included in the next edition? Explain.

Are there any articles that you feel should be replaced in the next edition? Why?

Are there any World Wide Websites that you feel should be included in the next edition? Please annotate.

May we contact you for editorial input? ☐ yes ☐ no
May we quote your comments? ☐ yes ☐ no

NOTES

NOTES

NOTES

NOTES

NOTES

NOTES